Health Assessment

made Incredibly Easy!

Fourth Edition

Laura M. Willis, DNP, APRN-CNP
Family Nurse Practitioner/Lead APC
Bon Secours Mercy Health
Wittenberg University Health Center
Springfield, Ohio

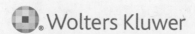
. Wolters Kluwer

Philadelphia · Baltimore · New York · London
Buenos Aires · Hong Kong · Sydney · Tokyo

Vice President and Publisher: Julie K. Stegman
Manager, Nursing Education and Practice Content: Jamie Blum
Acquisitions Editor: Joyce Berendes
Development Editor: Phoebe Jordan-Reilly
Editorial Coordinator: Varshaanaa SM
Marketing Manager: Amy Whitaker
Production Project Manager: Frances Gunning
Manager, Graphic Arts & Design: Stephen Druding
Art Director, Illustration: Jennifer Clements
Manufacturing Coordinator: Bernard Tomboc
Prepress Vendor: TNQ Tech

Fourth edition

9 8 7 6 5 4 3 2 1

Printed in Mexico

Library of Congress Cataloging-in-Publication Data

ISBN-13: 978-1-975222-22-2

Cataloging in Publication data available on request from publisher.

shop.lww.com

QUADM0624

Dedication

To my sons and my husband—my reasons.

Contributors and consultants

Diego Acero, MSN, BSN
Nurse Practitioner
Transplant Surgery
Northshore University Hospital
Astoria, New York

Leigh Ann Trujillo, DNP, MSN
Manager of Quality and Risk
Community Stroke and Rehabilitation
  Center
Crown Point, Indiana

Cheryl Brown, DNP, MEd, ENP, FNP-BC
Family Nurse Practitioner
Urgent Care and Village Medicine
Maniilaq Association & Alaska Native
  Tribal Health Consortium
Midway, Arkansas

Alan Eddison, DNP, APRN, NP-C
11471 SW Halton St
Port St Lucie, Florida

Mary K. Jones, DNP, CNM, ENP-BC, FNP-BC,
  PMHNP-BC
Assistant Professor
Psychiatric Nursing
Frontier Nursing University
Byesville, Ohio

Rachel Koransky-Matson, DNP, MSN, FNP-C
Diabetes Nurse Practitioner
Nutrition
Northern Light Mayo
Exeter, Maine

Katrin Moskowitz, DNP, FNP, PMHNP
APRN
New England Mind Matters
Torrington, Connecticut

Luke Pohlman, AGACNP-BC
Certified Nurse Practitioner
ICU
Premier Health
Xenia, Ohio

Lauren Pohlman, BSN, RN
Emergency Department
Bon Secours Mercy Health
Xenia, Ohio

Estella J. Wetzel, DNP, APRN, FNP-C
Regional Clinical Faculty, Instructor
Family Nurse Practitioner
Frontier Nursing University
Ohio, Beavercreek

Laura M. Willis, DNP, APRN-CNP
Family Nurse Practitioner/Lead APC
Bon Secours Mercy Health
Wittenberg University Health Center
Springfield, Ohio

Victoria Wilson, BSN, RN, CHPN
Travel Float Nurse
Education Department
Ohio's Hospice
Liberty Township, Ohio

Not another boring foreword

If you're like me, you're too busy to wade through a foreword that uses pretentious terms and umpteen dull paragraphs to get to the point. So let's cut right to the chase! Here's why this book is so terrific:

1. It will teach you all the important things you need to know about assessment. (And it will leave out all the fluff that wastes your time.)
2. It will help you remember what you've learned.
3. It will make you smile as it enhances your knowledge and skills.

Don't believe me? Try these recurring logos on for size:

Peak technique illustrates and describes the best ways to perform specific physical examination techniques.

Bridging the gap explains cultural variables that may influence the health assessment.

Handle with care pinpoints age-related variations in assessment findings.

Interpretation station provides sure-fire guidelines for interpreting assessment findings quickly and easily.

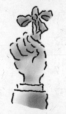

Memory jogger helps the reader remember important points.

Just for fun—provides quick-study information in a gamelike format.

See? I told you! And that's not all. Look for key points in the margins throughout this book. They will be there to explain key concepts, provide important care reminders, and offer reassurance.

I hope you find this book helpful. Best of luck throughout your career!

Dr. Laura M. Willis, DNP, APRN-CNP

Contents

Dedication   iii
Contributors and consultants   iv
Not another boring foreword   v

PART I Beginning the assessment

1	Health history	3
2	Fundamental physical assessment techniques	23
3	Nutritional assessment	41
4	Mental health assessment	57

PART II Assessing body systems

5	Skin, hair, and nails	75
6	Neurologic system	103
7	Eyes	137
8	Ears, nose, and throat	163
9	Cardiovascular system	193
10	Respiratory system	231
11	Breasts and axillae	269
12	Gastrointestinal system	287
13	Female genitourinary system	315
14	Male genitourinary system	367
15	Musculoskeletal system	389

Appendices and index

Practice makes perfect	422
Glossary	445
Selected references	448
Index	451

Part I

Beginning the assessment

1 **Health history** 3

2 **Fundamental physical assessment techniques** 23

3 **Nutritional assessment** 41

4 **Mental health assessment** 57

Chapter 1

Health history

Just the facts

In this chapter, you'll learn:

♦ reasons for performing a health history
♦ techniques for communicating effectively during a health history assessment
♦ essential steps in a complete health history
♦ questions specific to each step of a health history.

A look at the health history

Knowing how to complete an accurate and thorough assessment—from taking the health history to performing the physical examination—can help you uncover significant problems and develop an appropriate care plan.

Any assessment involves collecting two kinds of data: objective and subjective. *Objective data* are obtained through observation and are verifiable. For instance, a red, swollen arm in a patient who's complaining of arm pain is an example of data that can be seen and verified by someone other than the patient. *Subjective data* can't be verified by anyone other than the patient; they're gathered solely from the patient's own account—for example, "My head hurts" or "I have trouble sleeping at night."

Exploring past and present

You'll use a health history to gather subjective data about the patient and explore past and current problems. To begin, ask the patient about their general physical and emotional health; then ask them about specific body systems and structures.

Skills for getting the scoop

Keep in mind that the accuracy and completeness of your patient's answers largely depend on your skill as an

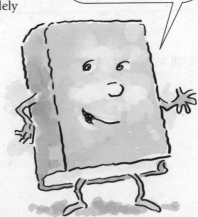

Here's a way to remember the two types of data: you "observe" objective data, whereas only the "subject" provides subjective data.

interviewer. Therefore, before you start asking questions, review the following communication guidelines.

Beginning the interview

To get the most out of your patient interview, before you begin, you'll need to create an environment in which the patient feels comfortable. During the interview, you'll want to use various communication strategies to make sure you communicate effectively.

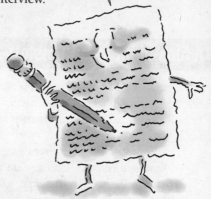

Take a moment to set the stage. A supportive, encouraging approach will make your patient much more forthcoming and will enable you to provide optimal care.

Create the proper environment

Before asking your first question, try to establish a rapport with the patient and explain what you'll cover during the interview. Consider the following guidelines when selecting a location for the interview.

Settling in

- Choose a quiet, private, well-lit interview setting. Such a setting makes it easier for you and your patient to interact and helps the patient feel more at ease.
- Make sure that the patient is comfortable. Sit facing them, 3′ to 4′ (1 to 1.5 m) away.
- Introduce yourself and explain that the purpose of the health history and assessment is to identify key problems and gather information to aid in planning care.
- Reassure the patient that everything they say will be kept confidential.
- Tell the patient how long the interview will last and ask them what they expect from the interview.
- Use touch sparingly. Many people aren't comfortable with strangers hugging, patting, or touching them.

Watch what you say

- Assess the patient to see if language barriers exist. For example, does the patient speak and understand English? Can the patient hear you? (See *Overcoming interview obstacles*.)
- Speak slowly and clearly, using easy-to-understand language. Avoid using medical terms and jargon.
- Ask the patient how they would like you to address them. Don't call them by their first name unless they ask you to. Avoid using terms of endearment, such as "honey" or "sweetie." Treating the patient with respect encourages them to trust you and provide more accurate and complete information.

Overcoming interview obstacles

With a little creativity, you can overcome barriers to interviewing. For example, if a patient doesn't speak English, your facility may have a list of interpreters you can call on for help. A trained medical interpreter—one who's familiar with medical terminology, knows interpreting techniques, and understands the patient's rights—would be ideal. Be sure to tell the interpreter to translate the patient's speech verbatim.

Avoid using one of the patient's family members or friends as an interpreter. Doing so violates the patient's right to confidentiality.

Breaking the sound barrier
Does your patient have a condition that affects their hearing? You can overcome this barrier, too. First, make sure the light is bright enough for the patient to see your lips move. Then face them and speak slowly and clearly but not loudly. If necessary, have the patient use an assistive device, such as a hearing aid or an amplifier. You can also write your questions on paper and have the patient answer by either speaking or writing back. If the patient uses sign language, see if your facility has a sign-language interpreter.

Communicate effectively

Realize that you and the patient communicate nonverbally as well as verbally. Being aware of these forms of communication will aid you in the interview process.

Nonverbal communication strategies

To make the most of nonverbal communication, follow these guidelines:

- Listen attentively and make eye contact frequently. (See *Overcoming cultural barriers*.)
- Use reassuring gestures, such as nodding your head, to encourage the patient to keep talking.
- Watch for nonverbal clues that indicate the patient is uncomfortable or unsure about how to answer a question. For example, they might lower their voice or glance around uneasily.
- Be aware of your own nonverbal behaviors that might cause the patient to stop talking or become defensive. For example, if you cross your arms, you might appear closed off from the patient. If you stand while they're sitting, you might appear superior. If you glance at your watch, you might appear to be bored or rushed, which could keep the patient from answering questions completely.

Overcoming cultural barriers

To maintain a good relationship with your patient, remember that their behaviors and beliefs may differ from your own because of their cultural background. For example, many people in the United States make eye contact when talking with others. However, people from some cultures or backgrounds may find eye contact disrespectful or aggressive. Be aware of these differences and respond appropriately.

- Observe the patient closely to see if they understand each question. If they don't appear to understand, repeat the question using different words or familiar examples. For instance, instead of asking, "Do you have respiratory difficulty after exercising?" ask, "Do you have to sit down after walking around the block?"

Verbal communication strategies

Verbal communication strategies range from alternating between open-ended and closed questions to employing such techniques as silence, facilitation, confirmation, reflection, clarification, summarization, and conclusion.

An open...

Asking open-ended questions such as "How did you fall?" lets the patient respond more freely. The patient's response may provide answers to many other questions. For instance, from the patient's answer, you might learn that they have previously fallen, that they were unsteady on their feet before they fell, and that they fell just before eating dinner. Armed with this information, you might deduce that the patient had a syncopal episode caused by hypoglycemia.

...and shut case

You may also choose to ask closed questions. Although these questions are unlikely to provide extra information, they may encourage the patient to give clear, concise feedback. (See *Two ways to ask*.)

Peak technique

Two ways to ask

You can ask your patient two types of questions: open-ended and closed.

Open-ended questions

Open-ended questions prompt the patient to express feelings, opinions, and ideas. They also help you gather more information than closed questions do. Open-ended questions facilitate nurse-patient rapport because they show that you're interested in what the patient has to say. Examples of such questions include:
- What caused you to come to the hospital tonight?
- How would you describe the problems you're having with your breathing?
- What lung problems, if any, do other members of your family have?

Closed questions

Closed questions elicit yes-or-no answers or one- to two-word responses. They limit the development of nurse-patient rapport. Closed questions can help you "zoom in" on specific points, but they don't provide the patient the opportunity to elaborate. Examples of closed questions include:
- Do you ever get short of breath?
- Are you the only one in your family with lung problems?

Silence is golden

Another communication technique is to allow moments of *silence* during the interview. Besides encouraging the patient to continue talking, silence gives you a chance to assess their ability to organize thoughts. You may find this technique difficult (most people are uncomfortable with silence), but the more often you use it, the more comfortable you'll become.

Give 'em a boost

Using such phrases as "please continue," "go on," and even "uh-huh" encourages the patient to continue with their story. Known as *facilitation*, this communication technique shows the patient that you're interested in what they are saying.

Confirmation conversation

Confirmation helps ensure that you and the patient are on the same track. For example, you might say, "If I understand you correctly, you said…" and then repeat the information the patient gave. This communication technique helps to clear misconceptions that you or the patient might have.

Check and reflect

Try using *reflection* (repeating something the patient has just said) to help you obtain more-specific information. For example, a patient with a stomachache might say, "I know I have an ulcer." If so, you can repeat the statement as a question, "You know you have an ulcer?" Then the patient might say, "Yes. I had one before and the pain is the same."

Clear skies

When information is vague or confusing, use the communication technique of *clarification*. For example, if your patient says, "I can't stand this," you might respond, "What can't you stand?" or "What do you mean by 'I can't stand this'?" Doing so gives the patient an opportunity to explain the statement.

Put the landing gear down…

Get in the habit of summarizing the information the patient gave you. Known as *summarization*, this communication technique ensures that the data you've collected are accurate and complete. Summarization also signals that the interview is about to end.

...and come in for a safe landing

Signal the patient when you're ready to end the interview. Known as *conclusion*, this signal gives the patient the opportunity to gather their thoughts and make any pertinent final statements. You can do this by saying, "I think I have all the information I need now. Is there anything you would like to add?"

Reviewing general health

You've just learned how to ask questions. Now it's time to learn the right questions to ask when reviewing the patient's general physical and emotional health. Also, remember to maintain a professional attitude throughout this process.

Asking the right questions

A complete health history requires information from each of the following categories, optimally obtained in this order:
1. biographic data
2. presenting problem
3. medical history (past and current)
4. family history
5. psychosocial history
6. activities of daily living.
    Many facilities have a health history form or computer program that prompts the interviewer to gather specific required information. (See *Components of a complete health history*.)

Biographic data

Start the health history by obtaining biographic information from the patient. Do this first so you don't forget to gather this information after you become involved in details of the patient's health. Ask the patient for their name, address, telephone number, birth date, age, marital status, religion, and nationality. Find out with whom they live and get the name and telephone number of a person to contact in case of an emergency.

Also, ask the patient about their health care, including who their primary doctor is and how the patient gets to the doctor's office. Ask if they have ever been treated for their current problem and, if so, when they received treatment. Finally, ask if they have an advance directive in place. If they do, request a copy to place in their chart. (See *Advance directives*, page 10.)

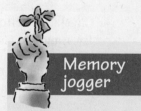

Memory jogger

To remember the categories, you should cover in your health history, think: Being Prepared Makes For Proper Assessment:

Biographic data

Presenting problem

Medical history

Family history

Psychosocial history

Activities of daily living.

Components of a complete health history

You can use this health history form as a guide when gathering a patient's health history information.

BIOGRAPHICAL DATA

Name _____

Address _____

Date of birth _____

Advance directive explained: ☐ Yes ☐ No

Living will on chart: ☐ Yes ☐ No

Name and phone of two people to call if necessary:

NAME   RELATIONSHIP   PHONE #

_____

_____

CHIEF COMPLAINT

History of present illness

_____

_____

CURRENT MEDICATIONS

DRUG AND DOSE   FREQUENCY   LAST DOSE

_____

MEDICAL HISTORY

Allergies

☐ Tape   ☐ Iodine   ☐ Latex   ☐ No known allergies

☐ M Drug: _____

☐ Food: _____

☐ Environmental: ___

☐ Blood reaction: ___

☐ Other: _____

Be sure to include prescription drugs, over-the-counter drugs, herbal preparations, and vitamins and supplements.

Childhood illnesses

DATE

_____

_____

Previous hospitalizations

(Illness, accident or injury, surgery, blood transfusion)   DATE

_____

_____

Health problems

	Yes	No		Yes	No
Arthritis	☐	☐	Hypertension	☐	☐
Blood problem (anemia, sickle cell, clotting, bleeding)	☐	☐	Kidney problem	☐	☐
			Liver problem	☐	☐
Cancer	☐	☐	Lung problem (asthma, bronchitis, emphysema, pneumonia, TB, shortness of breath)	☐	☐
Diabetes mellitus	☐	☐			
Eye problem (cataracts, glaucoma)	☐	☐	Stroke	☐	☐
Heart disease (heart failure, MI, valve disease)	☐	☐	Thyroid problem	☐	☐
			Ulcers (duodenal, peptic)	☐	☐
Hiatal hernia	☐	☐	Psychological disorder	☐	☐
HIV/AIDS	☐	☐			

Obstetric history (females)

Last menstrual period _____

Gravida _____   Para _____

Menopause ☐ Yes ☐ No

Psychosocial history

Coping strategies

Feelings of safety

Ask about the patient's feelings of safety to help identify physical, psychological, emotional, and sexual abuse issues.

Social history

Smoker ☐ No ☐ Yes (# packs/day_____ # years_____)

Alcohol ☐ No ☐ Yes (type _____ amount/day_____)

Illicit drug use ☐ No ☐ Yes (type _____)

Religious and cultural observations

_____

Activities of daily living

Diet and exercise regimen_____

Elimination patterns_____

Sleep patterns _____

Work and leisure activities _____

Use of safety measures (seat belt, bike helmet, sunscreen)_____

Ask about the patient's family medical history, including history of diabetes or heart disease.

Health maintenance history   DATE

Colonoscopy _____

Dental examination _____

Eye examination _____

Immunizations _____

Mammography _____

FAMILY MEDICAL HISTORY

	Yes	No	Who (parent, grandparent, sibling)
Arthritis	☐	☐	
Cancer	☐	☐	
Diabetes mellitus	☐	☐	
Heart disease (heart failure, MI, valve disease)	☐	☐	
Hypertension	☐	☐	
Stroke	☐	☐	

Handle with care

Advance directives

The Patient Self-Determination Act allows patients to prepare advance directives—written documents that state their wishes regarding health care in the event they become incapacitated or unable to make decisions. Older patients in particular may have interest in advance directives because they tend to be concerned with end-of-life issues.

Direction for directives

If a patient doesn't have an advance directive in place, the health care facility must provide them with information about it, including how to establish one.

An advance directive may include:
• power of attorney for health care that authorizes a specific person to make medical decisions if the patient can no longer do so
• specific medical treatment the patient wants or doesn't want
• instructions regarding pain medication and comfort—specifically, whether the patient wishes to receive certain treatment even if the treatment may hasten their death
• information the patient wants to relay to their loved ones
• name of the patient's primary health care provider
• any other wishes.

Take a hint

Your patient's answers to basic questions can provide important clues about their personality, medical problems, and reliability. If they can't furnish accurate information, ask them for the name of a friend or relative who can. Document the source of the information and whether an interpreter was used to obtain the information.

Presenting problem

Try to pinpoint why the patient is seeking health care, or their *presenting problem*. Document this information in the patient's exact words to avoid misinterpretation. Ask how and when the symptoms developed, what led the patient to seek medical attention, and how the problem has affected their life and ability to function.

Alphabet soup

To ensure that you don't omit pertinent data, use the PQRSTU mnemonic device, which provides a systematic approach to obtaining information. (See *PQRSTU: What's the story?*)

Medical history

Ask the patient about past and current medical problems, such as hypertension, diabetes, and back pain. Typical questions include:
• Have you ever been hospitalized? If so, when and why?
• What childhood illnesses did you have?

Peak technique

PQRSTU: What's the story?

Use the PQRSTU mnemonic device to fully explore your patient's presenting problem. When you ask the questions below, you'll encourage them to describe their symptoms in greater detail.

Precipitating or palliative	**Quality or quantity**	**Region or radiation**	**Severity**	**Timing or temporal**	**Understanding**
Ask the patient:	Ask the patient:	Ask the patient:	Ask the patient:	Ask the patient:	Ask the patient:
• What precipitates the symptom?	• What does the symptom feel like, look like, or sound like?	• Where in the body does the symptom occur?	• How severe is the symptom? How would you rate it on a scale of 1 to 10, with 10 being the most severe?	• When did the symptom begin?	• What do you think caused the symptom?
• Do stress, anger, certain physical positions, or other factors trigger the symptom or make it worse?	• Are you having the symptom right now? If so, is it more or less severe than usual?	• Does the symptom appear in other regions? If so, where?	• Does the symptom seem to be diminishing, intensifying, or staying the same?	• Was the onset sudden or gradual?	• How do you feel about the symptom? Do you have fears associated with it?
• What makes the symptom lessen or subside?	• To what degree does the symptom affect your normal activities?			• How often does the symptom occur?	• How is the symptom affecting your life?
				• How long does the symptom last?	• What are your expectations of the health care team?

- Are you being treated for any problem? If so, for what reason and who's your doctor?
- Have you ever had surgery? If so, when and why?
- Are you allergic to anything in the environment or to any medications or foods? If so, what kind of allergic reaction do you have?
- Are you taking medications, including over-the-counter preparations, such as aspirin, vitamins, or cough syrup? If so, what are you taking them for? How much do you take and how often do you take them? Do you use home remedies such as homemade ointments? Do you use herbal preparations or take dietary supplements? Do you use other alternative or complementary therapies,

such as acupuncture, therapeutic massage, or chiropractic? Do you use any illegal substances? If so, how much and how often?

Family history

Questioning the patient about their family's health is a good way to uncover their risk of having certain illnesses. Typical questions include:

- Are your parent or parents and siblings living? If not, how old were they when they died? What were the causes of their deaths?
- If they're alive, do they have diabetes, high blood pressure, heart disease, asthma, cancer (if so, what kind?), sickle cell anemia, hemophilia, cataracts, glaucoma, or other illnesses?

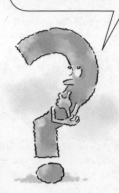

Want to know if a patient is at risk for certain illnesses? Ask about their family's health history.

Psychosocial history

Find out how the patient feels about themselves, their place in society, and their relationships with others. Ask about their occupation (past and current), education, economic status, and responsibilities. Typical questions include:

- How have you coped with medical or emotional crises in the past? (See *Asking about abuse*.)
- Has your life changed recently? If yes, in what ways? What changes in your personality or behavior have you noticed?

The ties that bind

- How adequate is the emotional support you receive from family and friends?

Peak technique

Asking about abuse

Abuse is a tricky subject. Anyone can be a victim of abuse: a significant other, a spouse, an older adult patient, a child, or a parent. Also, abuse can come in many forms: physical, psychological, emotional, and sexual. So, when taking a health history, ask two open-ended questions to explore abuse: When do you feel safe at home? When don't you feel safe?

Watch the reaction

Even if you don't immediately suspect an abusive situation, be aware of how your patient reacts to open-ended questions. Is the patient defensive, hostile, confused, or frightened? Assess how they interact with you and others. Do they seem withdrawn or frightened or show other inappropriate behavior? Keep their reactions in mind when you perform your physical assessment.

Remember, if the patient tells you about any type of abuse, you're obligated to report it. Inform the patient that you must report the incident to local authorities.

- How close do you live to health care facilities? Can you get to them easily?
- Do you have health insurance?
- Do you have any financial concerns?

Activities of daily living

Find out what's normal for the patient by asking them to describe a typical day. Make sure you ask about the following areas in your assessment.

Diet and elimination

Ask the patient about appetite, special diets, and food allergies. Ask them to describe what they have eaten in the past 48 hours. Find out the amount and type of fluids they drink in a typical day. Who cooks and shops at their house? Ask about the frequency of bowel movements and laxative use. Do they have any problems or concerns related to elimination?

Exercise and sleep

Ask the patient about daily exercise. Find out if they have a special exercise program and, if so, why. Ask them to describe it. Ask how many hours they sleep at night, what their sleep pattern is like, and whether they feel rested after sleep. Ask them if they have any difficulties with sleep.

Work and leisure

Ask the patient what they do for a living and what they do during their leisure time. Do they have hobbies?

Use of tobacco, alcohol, and other drugs

Ask the patient if they smoke cigarettes or use tobacco. Determine how many packs per year they use if the patient does smoke. If they don't currently smoke, ask if they've ever smoked. If they answer "yes," when did they quit? Do they drink alcohol? If so, what type of alcohol do they drink and how much each day? Ask if they use illicit drugs, such as marijuana and cocaine. If so, what type and how often?

Fudging the facts

Patients may understate the amount they drink because of embarrassment. If you're having trouble getting what you believe are honest answers to such questions, you might try overestimating the amount. For example, you might say, "You told me you drink beer. Do you drink about a six-pack per day?" The patient's response might be, "No, I drink about half that."

Religious observances

Ask the patient if they have religious beliefs that affect diet, dress, or health practices. Patients will feel reassured when you make it clear that you understand these points.

Maintaining a professional attitude

Don't let your personal opinions interfere with this part of the assessment. Maintain a professional, neutral approach and don't offer advice. For example, don't suggest that the patient enter a drug rehabilitation program. That type of response puts them on the defensive and they might not answer subsequent questions honestly.

Also, avoid making patronizing statements, such as "The doctor knows what's best for you." Such statements make the patient feel inferior and break down communication. Finally, don't use leading questions such as, "You don't do drugs, do you?" to get the answer you're hoping for. This type of question, based on your own value system, can make the patient feel defensive and might prevent them from responding honestly.

Reviewing structures and systems

The last part of the health history is a systematic assessment of the patient's body structures and systems. A thorough assessment requires that you follow a process while asking specific questions.

Follow a process

Always start at the top of the head and work your way down the body. This helps keep you from skipping any areas. When questioning an older patient, remember that they may have difficulty hearing or communicating. (See *Overcoming communication problems in older patients*.)

Ask specific questions

Information gained from a health history forms the basis for your care plan and enables you to distinguish physical changes and devise a holistic approach to treatment. As with other nursing skills, the only way you can improve your interviewing technique is with practice, practice, and more practice. (See *Evaluating a symptom*.)

Here are some key questions to ask your patient about each body structure and system.

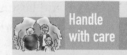

Handle with care

Overcoming communication problems in older patients

An older patient might have sensory or memory impairment or a decreased attention span. If your patient is confused or has trouble communicating, you may need to rely on a family member for some or all of the health history.

Evaluating a symptom

Your patient is vague in describing their presenting problem. Using your interviewing skills, you discover their problem is related to abdominal distention. Now what? This flowchart will help you decide what to do next, using abdominal distention as the patient's presenting problem.

Ask the patient to identify the symptom that's bothering them.

Form a first impression. Does the patient's condition alert you to an emergency? For example, do they say the bloating developed suddenly? Do they mention that other signs or symptoms occur with it, such as sweating and light-headedness? (Both indicate hypovolemia.)

Yes

Take a brief history.

Perform a focused physical examination to quickly determine the severity of the patient's condition.

No

Take a thorough history. Note GI disorders that can lead to abdominal distention.

Thoroughly examine the patient. Observe for abdominal asymmetry. Inspect the skin, auscultate for bowel sounds, percuss and palpate the abdomen, and measure abdominal girth.

Evaluate your findings. Are emergency signs or symptoms present, such as abdominal rigidity and abnormal bowel sounds?

Yes

Intervene appropriately to stabilize the patient, and notify the doctor immediately.

After the patient's condition stabilizes, review your findings to consider possible causes, such as trauma, large-bowel obstruction, mesenteric artery occlusion, and peritonitis.

No

Review your findings to consider possible causes, such as cancer, bladder distention, cirrhosis, heart failure, and gastric dilation.

Devise an appropriate care plan. Position the patient comfortably, administer analgesics, and prepare the patient for diagnostic tests.

Head first

Do you get headaches? If so, where are they and how painful are they? How often do they occur, and how long do they last? Does anything trigger them, and how do you relieve them? Have you ever had a head injury? Do you have lumps or bumps on your head?

Vision quest

When was your last eye examination? Do you wear glasses or contacts? Do you have glaucoma, cataracts, or color blindness? Does light bother your eyes? Do you have excessive tearing or drainage; blurred vision; double vision; or dry, itchy, burning, inflamed, or swollen eyes? Have you ever had eye surgery? If yes, what type and when?

An earful

Do you have loss of balance, ringing in your ears, deafness, or poor hearing? If so, when did it start? Have you ever had ear surgery? If so, why and when? Do you wear a hearing aid? Are you having pain, swelling, or discharge from your ears? If so, has this problem occurred before and how frequently?

Nose knows

Have you ever had nasal surgery? If so, why and when? Have you ever had sinusitis or nosebleeds? If so, when did it happen and how was it treated? Do you have nasal problems that impair your ability to smell or that cause breathing difficulties, frequent sneezing, or discharge?

Past the lips and over the gums

Do you have mouth sores, a dry mouth, loss of taste, a toothache, or bleeding gums? If so, when did it start? Do you wear dentures and, if so, do they fit properly? Do you have a sore throat, fever, or chills? How often do you get a sore throat, and have you seen a doctor for this?

Do you have difficulty swallowing? If so, is the problem with solids or liquids? Is it a constant problem or does it accompany a sore throat or another problem? What, if anything, makes it go away? How long have you had this problem?

Neck check

Do you have swelling, soreness, lack of movement, stiffness, or pain in your neck? If so, did something specific cause it to happen such as too much exercise? How long have you had this symptom? Does anything relieve it or make it worse?

Respiratory research

Do you ever have trouble breathing? When? What makes it better or worse? How many pillows do you use at night? Does breathing cause pain or wheezing? Do you have a cough? If so, do you cough up sputum? What color is it? How much sputum do you produce? Do you have night sweats?

Have you ever been treated for pneumonia, asthma, emphysema, or frequent respiratory tract infections? If so, when and what was the treatment? Have you ever had a chest x-ray or tuberculin skin test? If so, when and what were the results?

Do you use oxygen? How much and how often? Have you ever had surgery for a lung problem? If so, what was the reason for the surgery? What type of surgery did you have and when? Do you ever use an inhaler? When and for what reason?

Heart health hunt

Do you have chest pain, palpitations, irregular heartbeat, fast or slow heartbeat, shortness of breath, or a persistent cough? If so, when did it start? Does anything make it better or worse? Have you ever had an electrocardiogram? If so, when and what were the results? Do you have a pacemaker or an internal defibrillator? If so, when did you receive it and why? Have you ever had any other type of heart surgery? If so, when and why? What type of surgery was it?

Do you have high blood pressure, peripheral vascular disease, swelling of the ankles and hands, varicose veins, cold extremities, or intermittent pain in your legs? If so, when did it start? How is it treated?

Breast test

Ask patients with female breasts these questions: Do you perform monthly breast self-examinations? Have you noticed a lump, a change in breast or nipple contour, breast pain, or discharge from your nipples? Have you ever had breast cancer? If yes, when and how was it treated? If not, has anyone else in your family had it? Have you ever had a mammogram? When and what were the results?

Ask patients with male breasts these questions: Do you have pain in your breast tissue? Have you noticed lumps or a change in contour?

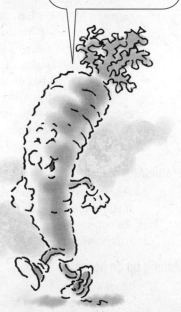

Asking these questions will help you get to the root of the patient's problem.

Stomach symptom search

Do you have nausea, vomiting, loss of appetite, heartburn, abdominal pain, frequent belching, or passing of gas? If yes, how often and when does it occur and what makes it better or worse? Have you lost or gained weight recently? How much and over what period of time? How often do you have a bowel movement, and what color, odor, and consistency are your stools? Have you noticed a change in your regular elimination pattern? Do you use laxatives frequently?

Have you had hemorrhoids, rectal bleeding, hernias, gallbladder disease, or liver disease? If yes, when and how was it treated? Have you ever had surgery on your stomach? If yes, when, for what reason, and what type of surgery?

Renal rundown

Do you have urinary problems, such as burning during urination, incontinence, urgency, retention, reduced urinary flow, and dribbling? If yes, when did it start? What makes it better or worse? Do you get up during the night to urinate? If so, how many times? What color is your urine? Have you ever noticed blood in it? Have you ever been treated for kidney stones? If yes, when and how were you treated?

Reproduction review

Some of the following questions depend on the reproductive body parts your patient has.

How old were you when you started menstruating? How often do you get your period, and how long does it usually last? Do you have pain or pass clots? If you're postmenopausal, at what age did you stop menstruating? If you're in the transitional stage, what perimenopausal symptoms are you experiencing? Have you ever been pregnant? If so, how many times? What was the method of delivery? How many pregnancies resulted in live births? How many resulted in miscarriages? Have you had an abortion?

What's your method of birth control? Do you have multiple sex partners? Do you have anal sex? Have you ever had a vaginal infection or a sexually transmitted infection (STI)? When was your last gynecologic examination and Papanicolaou test? What were the results? Have you ever had surgery for a gynecologic problem? If so, when and for what reason?

Do you perform monthly testicular self-examinations? Have you ever had a prostate examination and, if so, when? Have you noticed penile pain, discharge, or lesions or testicular lumps? Have you had a vasectomy?

Monitoring muscle

Do you have difficulty walking, sitting, or standing? If yes, when did it start? What makes it better or worse? Are you steady on your feet, or do you lose your balance easily? Do you have arthritis, gout, a back injury, muscle weakness, or paralysis?

Boning up on bones

Have you ever fractured a bone? When and how was it treated? Do you have joint pain? If yes, which joints? When did it start? What makes it better or worse?

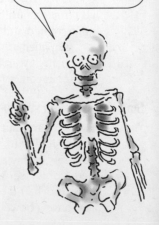

I know I'm muscling in here, and I don't mean to put your nose out of joint, but don't forget to ask about your patient's bones!

CNS scrutiny

Have you ever had a seizure? If yes, when? Do you know what type of seizure you had? Did anything in particular trigger it? Do you ever experience tremors, twitching, numbness, tingling, or loss of sensation in a part of your body? Have you noticed any problem with your memory? If so, when did it start? (See *Tips for assessing a patient with a severe illness*.)

Endocrine inquiry

Have you been unusually tired lately? When did it start? Does anything make it better or worse? Do you feel hungry or thirsty more often than usual? Have you lost weight for unexplained reasons? How well can you tolerate heat or cold? Have you noticed changes in your hair texture or color? Have you been losing hair?

Circulatory study

Have you ever been diagnosed with anemia or blood abnormalities? If yes, when and what was the diagnosis? How was it treated? Do you bruise or bleed easily or become fatigued quickly? Have you ever had a blood transfusion? If so, what was the reason, and did you have any type of adverse reaction?

Psychological survey

Do you ever experience mood swings? Do you ever feel anxious, depressed, or unable to concentrate? How often does this happen? Are you feeling unusually stressed? Do you ever feel unable to cope? When? What makes these feelings better or worse?

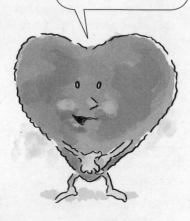

Throughout your initial assessment, be aware of the patient's emotional status. Keep in mind that stress levels and emotional well-being can affect every body system.

Peak technique

Tips for assessing a patient with a severe illness

When the patient's condition doesn't allow a full assessment—for instance, if the patient is in severe pain—get as much information as possible from other sources. With a patient with a severe illness, keep these key points in mind:
- Identify yourself to the patient and their family.
- Stay calm to gain their confidence and allay anxiety.

- Stay on the lookout for important information. For example, if a patient seeks help for ringing in their ears, don't overlook their casual mention of a periodic "racing heartbeat."
- Avoid jumping to conclusions. Don't assume that the patient's symptom is related to their admitting diagnosis. Use a systematic approach and collect the appropriate information; then draw conclusions.

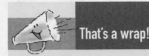
That's a wrap!

Health history review

Obtaining assessment data
- Collect objective data (data that are obtained through observation and are verifiable).
- Collect subjective data (data that can be verified only by the patient).

Patient interview
- Select a quiet, private setting.
- Choose terms carefully and avoid using medical jargon.
- Use appropriate body language.
- Confirm patient statements to avoid misunderstanding.
- Use open-ended questions when possible.

Effective communication
- Use silence effectively.
- Encourage responses.
- Use repetition and reflection to help clarify meaning.
- Use clarification to eliminate misunderstandings.
- Summarize and conclude with "Is there anything else?"

Components of a complete health history
- Biographic data, such as the patient's name, address, birth date, and emergency contact information
- Presenting problem
- Past and current medical history
- Family history
- Psychosocial history (feelings about self, place in society, and relationships with others)
- Activities of daily living

Review of structures and systems
Head
- Headaches
- Past or current head injury

Eyes
- Vision
- Use of glasses or contact lenses
- History of glaucoma, cataracts, color blindness
- Tearing or drainage; blurred vision; double vision; dry, itchy, burning, or inflamed eyes
- History of eye surgery

Ears
- Hearing and balance
- History of ear surgery
- Use of hearing aids
- Ear pain or swelling
- Discharge from ears

Nose
- History of nasal surgery
- Breathing or smelling difficulties
- History of sinusitis or nosebleeds

Mouth and throat
- Dentures
- Mouth sores or dryness
- Loss of taste
- Toothache or bleeding gums
- Throat soreness or difficulty swallowing

Neck
- Swelling
- Soreness
- Lack of movement, stiffness, or pain

Respiratory
- Shortness of breath
- Pain or wheezing with breathing
- Cough (productive or nonproductive) and sputum description
- History of pneumonia, asthma, emphysema, or frequent respiratory tract infections
- Tuberculin skin test or chest x-ray results
- History of lung surgery

Cardiovascular
- Chest pain, palpitations, irregular or fast heartbeat, shortness of breath, persistent cough
- Results of electrocardiogram
- History of high blood pressure, peripheral vascular disease, swelling of the extremities, varicose veins, or intermittent pain in the legs
- History of pacemaker or internal defibrillator
- History of cardiac surgery

Breasts
- Monthly breast self-examination
- Lumps, changes in breast or nipple contour, pain, discharge from nipples
- History of breast cancer (personal and family)
- Results of mammograms

GI
- Recent weight changes
- Frequency and characteristics of bowel movements
- Laxative use

(Continued)

Health history review *(continued)*

- Nausea, vomiting, loss of appetite, heartburn, abdominal pain, frequent belching, passing of gas
- Hemorrhoids, rectal bleeding, hernias, gallbladder disease, liver disease
- History of abdominal surgery

Kidney
- Color of urine
- Nighttime urination
- Burning, incontinence, urgency, retention, reduced urinary flow, or dribbling
- History of kidney stones

Reproductive
- Menstruation and menopause
- Pregnancies
- Birth control
- Papanicolaou test results
- Vaginal infections

- STIs
- History of gynecologic surgery
- Monthly testicular self-examinations
- Results of prostate examinations
- Birth control or vasectomy
- Penile pain, discharge, or lesions
- Testicular lumps

Musculoskeletal
- Balance
- Difficulty walking, sitting, or standing
- History of arthritis, gout, back injury, muscle weakness, paralysis, or joint pain
- History of fractures

Neurologic
- Tremors, twitching, numbness, tingling, or loss of sensation

- History of seizures
- History of memory loss

Endocrine
- Unusual fatigue or tiredness
- Hunger and thirst
- Unexplained weight loss or gain
- Tolerance of heat and cold
- Hair loss or changes in color or texture

Hematologic
- History of anemia, blood abnormalities, or blood transfusions
- Fatigue, bruising, or bleeding

Psychological
- Mood swings
- Anxiety, depression, or difficulty concentrating
- Stress and coping mechanisms

Quick quiz

1. Leading questions may initiate untrue or inaccurate responses because such questions:
    A. encourage short or vague answers.
    B. require an educational level the patient may not possess.
    C. prompt the patient to try to give a particular answer.
    D. confuse the patient.

Answer: C. Because of how they're phrased, leading questions may prompt the patient to give the answer you're looking for.

2. When obtaining a health history from a patient, ask first about:
    A. family history.
    B. presenting problem.
    C. health insurance coverage.
    D. biographic data.

Answer: D. Take care of the biographic data first; otherwise, you might get involved in the patient history and forget to ask basic questions.

3. Silence is a communication technique used during an interview to:
   A. show respect.
   B. change the topic.
   C. encourage the patient to continue talking.
   D. clarify information.

Answer: C. Silence allows the patient to collect their thoughts and continue to answer your questions.

4. Data are considered subjective if you obtain them from:
   A. the patient's verbal account.
   B. your observations of the patient's actions.
   C. the patient's records.
   D. x-ray reports.

Answer: A. Data from the patient's own words are subjective.

5. "If I understand you correctly, you said…" is an example of the interviewing technique:
   A. clarification.
   B. confirmation.
   C. reflection.
   D. facilitation.

Answer: B. The phrase is an example of confirmation, a technique that can help confirm information the patient has provided.

6. Which of the following questions is considered open-ended?
   A. Does your pain last through the night?
   B. Have you ever had heart surgery?
   C. Do you frequently get headaches?
   D. How would you describe your pain?

Answer: D. Open-ended questions require the patient to express feelings, opinions, or ideas. They elicit more than just a simple yes-or-no response.

Scoring

☆☆☆ If you answered all six questions correctly, bravo! You're an intrepid interviewer.

☆☆ If you answered four or five questions correctly, that's cool! You're a hip historian.

☆ If you answered fewer than four questions correctly, that's okay! This is only the first chapter. You'll have many more opportunities to answer questions.

Chapter 2

Fundamental physical assessment techniques

Just the facts

In this chapter, you'll learn:

◆ types of equipment used in a physical assessment and the proper ways to use them

◆ skills for performing an initial observation of the patient

◆ ways to prepare your patient for an assessment

◆ techniques for performing inspection, palpation, percussion, and auscultation.

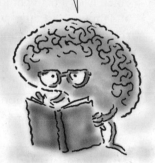

Performing a physical assessment calls for the use of critical thinking. What clues do your findings give you about the larger picture?

A look at physical assessment

During the physical assessment, you'll use all of your senses and a systematic approach to collect information about your patient's health. As you proceed through the physical examination, you can also teach your patient about their body. For instance, you can explain how to evaluate for swollen lymph nodes or why the patient should monitor the appearance of a mole. More than anything else, successful assessment requires critical thinking. How does one finding fit in the big picture? An initial assessment guides your care plan, allowing you to give your patient the individualized care they deserve.

Collecting the tools

Before starting a physical assessment, you will need a variety of tools; these may include cotton balls, gloves, an ophthalmoscope, an otoscope, a penlight, a percussion hammer, safety pins, and a stethoscope. (For a more complete list, see *Assessment tools*, page 24.)

Assessment tools

Tools used for assessment include:
- blood pressure cuff
- cotton balls
- gloves
- metric ruler (clear)
- near-vision and visual acuity charts
- ophthalmoscope
- otoscope
- penlight
- percussion hammer
- safety pins
- scale with height measurement
- skin calipers
- specula (nasal and vaginal)
- stethoscope
- tape measure (cloth or paper)
- thermometer
- tuning fork
- wooden tongue blade.

Two heads are better than one

Use a stethoscope with a diaphragm and a bell. The diaphragm has a flat, thin, plastic surface that picks up high-pitched sounds such as breath sounds. The bell has a smaller, open end that picks up low-pitched sounds, such as third and fourth heart sounds.

All the better to see you with...

You'll need a penlight to illuminate the inside of the patient's nose and mouth, cast tangential light on lesions, and evaluate pupillary reactions. An ophthalmoscope enables you to examine the internal structures of the eye; an otoscope enables you to examine the external auditory canal and tympanic membrane.

Other tools include cotton balls and safety pins to test sensation and pain differentiation, a percussion hammer to evaluate deep tendon reflexes, and gloves to protect the patient and you.

Performing a general survey

After assembling the necessary tools, move on to the first part of the physical assessment: forming your initial impressions. Does the patient seem comfortable or do they seem like they are in distress? After your initial impression, obtain their baseline data, including height, weight, and vital signs. This information will direct the rest of your assessment.

Observing the patient

A patient's behavior and appearance can offer subtle clues about their health. Carefully observe them for unusual behavior or signs of stress or illness.

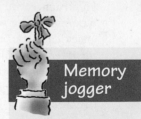

Memory jogger

Remembering that the bell of a stethoscope is used to hear low-pitched sounds and the diaphragm is used to hear high-pitched sounds is easy: *Bell* and *low* both contain the letter l.

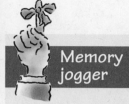

Memory jogger

Use the mnemonic **SOME TEAMS** as a checklist to help you remember what to look for when observing a patient:

Symmetry—Are the face and body symmetrical?

Old—Do they appear their stated age?

Mental acuity—Are they alert, confused, agitated, or inattentive?

Expression—Do they appear ill, in pain, or anxious?

Trunk—Are they lean, stocky, overweight, or barrel chested?

Extremities—Are their fingers clubbed? Do they have joint abnormalities or edema?

Appearance—Are they clean and appropriately dressed?

Movement—How are their posture, gait, and coordination?

Speech—Is their speech relaxed, clear, strong, understandable, and appropriate? Does it sound stressed?

Preparing the patient

If possible, introduce yourself to the patient before the assessment, preferably when they're dressed. Meeting you under less-threatening circumstances might decrease their anxiety when you perform the assessment. Creating a good rapport with your patient is vital for making a patient feel comfortable. (See *Tips for assessment success*.)

Keep in mind that the patient may be worried that you'll find a problem. They may also consider the assessment an invasion of their privacy because you're observing and touching sensitive, private, and perhaps painful body areas.

No surprises

Before you start, briefly explain what you're planning to do, why you're doing it, how long it will take, what position changes it will require, and what equipment you'll use. As you perform the assessment, explain each step in detail. A well-prepared patient won't be surprised or feel unexpected discomfort, so they'll trust you more and cooperate better.

Put your patient at ease but know where to draw the line. Maintain professionalism during the examination. Humor can help put the patient at ease, but avoid sarcasm and keep jokes in good taste.

Peak technique

Tips for assessment success

Before starting the physical assessment, follow these guidelines:
• Eliminate as many distractions and disruptions as possible.
• Ask your patient to void before beginning the physical assessment.
• Have your patient change into a gown to ensure the patient is covered, but body systems can be readily accessible.
• Wash your hands before and after the assessment—preferably in the patient's presence.
• Have all the necessary equipment on hand and in working order.
• Make sure the examination room is well lit and warm.
• Warm your hands and equipment before touching the patient.
• Be aware of your nonverbal communication and possible negative reactions from the patient.
• Communicate with your patient so they understand what you are doing and why you're doing it.

Get it down on paper

Document your findings up to this point in a concise paragraph. Include only essential information that communicates your overall impression of the patient. For example, if your patient has a lesion, simply note it now. You'll describe the lesion in detail when you complete the physical assessment.

Recording vital signs and statistics

Accurate measurements of your patient's height, weight, vital signs (which include the patient's temperature, heart rate, blood pressure, respiration rate, and oxygen saturation) along with the patient's current pain level provide critical information about body functions. The first time you assess a patient, record their baseline vital signs and statistics. Afterward, take measurements at regular intervals, depending on the patient's condition and your facility's policy. A series of readings usually provides more valuable information than a single set. (See *Tips for interpreting vital signs*.)

Height and weight

Height and weight are important parameters for evaluating nutritional status, calculating medication dosages, and assessing fluid loss or gain. Take the patient's baseline height and weight so you can gauge future weight changes or calculate medication dosages in an emergency. (See *Measuring height and weight*.) Keep this information handy so you can refer to it quickly, if needed. Note that these measurements differ for pediatric patients. (See *Obtaining pediatric measurements*, page 28.)

Body temperature

Body temperature is measured in degrees Fahrenheit (F) or degrees Celsius (C). Normal body temperature ranges from 96.7° to

Tips for interpreting vital signs

Always analyze vital signs at the same time because two or more abnormal values provide important clues to your patient's problem. For example, a rapid, thready pulse along with low blood pressure may signal shock, or a low respiratory rate with a low oxygen saturation may indicate hypoxia.

Accuracy

If you obtain an abnormal value, take the vital sign again to make sure it's accurate. Remember that normal readings vary with the patient's age. For example, temperature decreases with age, and respiratory rate may increase with age or with an underlying disease.

Individuality

Also remember that an abnormal value for one patient may be a normal value for another. Each patient has their own baseline values, which is what makes recording vital signs during the initial assessment so important.

Peak technique

Measuring height and weight

Ask the patient to remove their shoes and to dress in a hospital gown. Then use these techniques to measure their height and weight.

Balancing the scale
Slide both weight bars on the scale to zero. The balancing arrow should stop in the center of the open box. If the scale has wheels, lock them before the patient gets on.

Measuring height
Ask the patient to step on the scale and turn their back to it. Move the height bar over their head and lift the horizontal arm. Then lower the bar until the horizontal arm touches the top of their head. Now read the height measurement from the height bar.

Measuring weight
Slide the lower weight into the groove representing the largest increment below the patient's estimated weight. For example, if you think the patient weighs 145 lb (65.8 kg), slide the weight into the groove for 100 lb (45.4 kg).

Slide the upper weight across until the arrow on the right stops in the middle of the open box. If the arrow hits the bottom, slide the weight to a lower number. If the arrow hits the top, slide the weight to a higher number.

The patient's weight is the sum of these numbers. For example, if the lower weight is on 150 lb (68 kg) and the upper weight is on 12 lb (5.4 kg), the patient weighs 162 lb (73.5 kg).

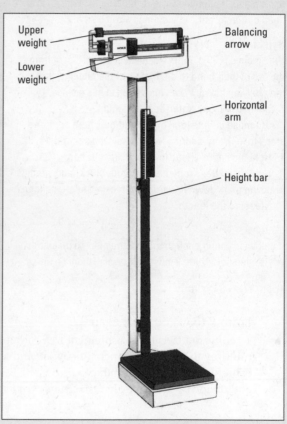

100.5° F (35.9° to 38.1° C), depending on the route used for measurement. A fever is an elevation in oral body temperature over 98.6° F (37° C) but is generally not considered significant until it rises above 100.4° F (38° C). Hyperthermia describes an oral temperature above 106° F (41.1° C); hypothermia, a rectal temperature below 95° F (35° C). Older adults tend to be 0.5° C cooler when compared to children and young adults due to the decreased muscle mass and lower immunity response (Geneva II et al., 2019).

Handle with care

Obtaining pediatric measurements

The height and weight of an infant or a young child are measured differently from those of an adult. In addition to obtaining height and weight, you'll include the child's head circumference in your measurements.

Height

Until a child is 36 months old, measure their height from the top of their head to the bottom of their heel while they're lying down. When measured in this fashion, height is commonly referred to as length.

Because infants tend to flex and curl, here are three steps to make measuring length easy and accurate:
1. Hold the infant's head in the midline position.
2. Hold their knees together with your other hand, gently pressing them down toward the table until fully extended.
3. Measure the length.

Weight

If a child is young enough to have their length measured while lying down, you'll most likely weigh them on an infant scale. Infant scales may be digital or use a balancing arrow. To obtain the weight, the infant or child either sits or lies down in a "bucket" or other enclosed area.

To prevent injury, never turn away from a child on a scale or leave them unattended. You can usually use an adult scale to weigh children older than age 2 or 3.

Head circumference

You should measure a child's head circumference until they're 36 months old. This measurement reflects the growth of the cranium and its contents. It is important to note that children assigned male at birth have head circumference 1 cm larger compared to children assigned female at birth (CDC, 2001).

To measure a child's head circumference, place a flexible measuring tape around the child's head at the widest point, from the frontal bone of the forehead and around the occipital prominence at the back of the head.

From F to C and back again

To convert a Celsius measurement to a Fahrenheit measurement, multiply the Celsius temperature by 1.8 and add 32. To convert Fahrenheit to Celsius, subtract 32 from the Fahrenheit temperature and divide by 1.8. (See *How temperature readings compare*, page 29.)

Pulse

The patient's pulse reflects the amount of blood ejected with each heartbeat. To assess the pulse, palpate one of the patient's arterial pulse points and note the rate, rhythm, and amplitude of the pulse. A normal pulse for an adult is between 60 and 100 beats/minute.

The radial pulse is commonly the most accessible. However, in cardiovascular emergencies, you should palpate for the femoral or carotid pulse. These vessels are larger and closer to the heart and more accurately reflect the heart's activity. (See *Pinpointing pulse sites*.)

Feeling the beat

To palpate for a pulse, use the pads of your index and middle fingers. Press the area over the artery until you feel pulsations. If the rhythm

How temperature readings compare

You can take your patient's temperature in four ways. The chart below describes each method.

Method	Normal temperature	Used with
Oral	97.7° to 99.5° F (36.5° to 37.5° C)	Adults and older children who are awake, alert, oriented, and cooperative
Axillary (armpit)	96.7° to 98.5° F (35.9° to 36.9° C)	Infants, young children, and patients with impaired immune systems when infection is a concern
Rectal	98.7° to 100.5° F (37.1° to 38.1° C)	Infants, young children, and confused or unconscious patients
Tympanic (ear)	98.2° to 100° F (36.8° to 37.8° C)	Adults, children, conscious and cooperative patients, and confused or unconscious patients

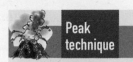

Peak technique

Pinpointing pulse sites

You can assess your patient's pulse rate at several sites, including those shown in the illustration below.

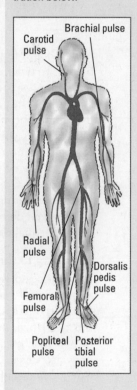

is regular, count the beats for 30 seconds and then multiply by 2 to get the number of beats per minute. If the rhythm is irregular or your patient has a pacemaker, count the beats for 1 minute.

When taking the patient's pulse for the first time (or when obtaining baseline data), count the beats for 1 minute.

Palpation pointers

Avoid using your thumb to count a patient's pulse because the thumb has a strong pulse of its own. If you need to palpate the carotid arteries, avoid exerting a lot of pressure, which can stimulate the vagus nerve and cause reflex bradycardia. Also, never palpate both carotid pulses at the same time. Putting pressure on both sides of the patient's neck can impair cerebral blood flow and function.

Off beat

When you note an irregular pulse:

- Evaluate whether the irregularity follows a pattern—for example, whether it follows a "regular" irregular pattern, such as a pause every third beat.
- Auscultate the apical pulse while palpating the radial pulse. You should feel the pulse every time you hear a heartbeat.
- Measure the difference between the apical pulse rate and radial pulse rate, a measurement called the *pulse deficit*. Measuring the pulse deficit allows you to evaluate indirectly the ability of each cardiac contraction to eject sufficient blood into the peripheral circulation.

Leaps and bounds

You also need to assess the pulse amplitude. To do this, use a numerical scale or descriptive term to rate or characterize the strength. Numerical scales differ slightly among facilities, but the following scale is commonly used:

- *absent pulse*—not palpable, measured as 0
- *weak or thready pulse*—hard to feel, easily obliterated by slight finger pressure, measured as +1
- *normal pulse*—easily palpable, obliterated by strong finger pressure, measured as +2
- *bounding pulse*—readily palpable, forceful, not easily obliterated by pressure from the fingers, measured as +3.

Respirations

As you count respirations, be aware of the depth and rhythm of each breath. To determine the respiratory rate, count the number of respirations for 60 seconds. A rate of 12 to 20 breaths/minute is normal for an adult. If the patient knows you're counting how often they breathe, they may subconsciously alter the rate. To avoid this, count their respirations while you take their pulse.

Pay attention as well to the depth of the patient's respirations by watching their chest rise and fall. Is their breathing shallow, moderate, or deep? Observe the rhythm and symmetry of their chest wall as it expands during inspiration and relaxes during expiration. Be aware that skeletal deformity, fractured ribs, and collapsed lung tissue can cause unequal chest expansion.

Accessory to the act...of breathing

Use of accessory muscles can enhance lung expansion when oxygenation drops. Patients with chronic obstructive pulmonary disease (COPD) or respiratory distress may use accessory muscles, like neck muscles (including sternocleidomastoid muscles) and abdominal muscles, for breathing. Patient position during normal breathing may also suggest problems such as COPD, because patients with COPD are usually noted to be sitting and leaning forward with their hands on their knees or another hard, sturdy surface. Normal respirations are quiet and easy, so note any abnormal sounds, such as crackles, wheezing, or stridor.

Blood pressure

Blood pressure measurements are helpful in evaluating cardiac output, fluid and circulatory status, and arterial resistance. Blood pressure measurements consist of systolic and diastolic readings. The systolic reading reflects the maximum pressure exerted on the arterial wall at the peak of left ventricular contraction. Normal systolic pressure ranges from 100 to 119 mm Hg.

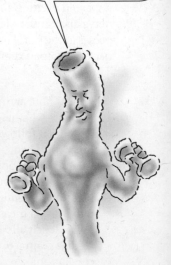

The systolic reading is the maximum pressure exerted on the arterial wall at the peak of left ventricular contraction. But don't worry, that kind of pressure doesn't bother a healthy artery like me!

The diastolic reading reflects the minimum pressure exerted on the arterial wall during left ventricular relaxation. This reading is generally more significant than the systolic reading because it evaluates arterial pressure when the heart is at rest. Normal diastolic pressure ranges from 60 to 79 mm Hg. (See *Blood pressure variations*.)

Unpronounceable and indispensable

The sphygmomanometer, a device used to measure blood pressure, consists of an inflatable cuff, a pressure manometer, and a bulb with a valve. To record a blood pressure, the cuff is centered over an artery, inflated, and deflated. (See *Using a sphygmomanometer*.)

As the cuff deflates, listen with a stethoscope for Korotkoff sounds, which indicate the systolic and diastolic pressures. Blood pressure can be measured from most extremity pulse points. The brachial artery is used for most patients because of its accessibility. (See *Tips for hearing Korotkoff sounds*.)

Bridging the gap

Blood pressure variations

Blood pressure may vary depending on the patient's race or sex. For example, Black women tend to have higher systolic blood pressure than White women, regardless of age. While the exact cause of this difference is not known, it is believe to be related to genetics, environmental, and lifestyle factors.

With this in mind, carefully monitor the blood pressure of your Black female patients, being alert for signs of hypertension. Early detection and treatment—combined with lifestyle changes—can help prevent such complications as stroke and kidney disease.

Peak technique

Using a sphygmomanometer

Here's how to use a sphygmomanometer properly:
• For accuracy and consistency, position your patient with their upper arm at heart level and their palm turned up.
• Have your patients sit straight back against a chair with legs planted firmly on the floor.
• Apply the cuff snugly, 1" (2.5 cm) above the brachial pulse.
• The bladder inside the cuff should encircle 80% of the arm circumference in an adult and 100% of the arm circumference in a child younger than age 13. A cuff that's too small may give a false abnormally high reading.
• Position the manometer in line with your eye level.
• Palpate the brachial or radial pulse with your fingertips while inflating the cuff.
• Inflate the cuff to 30 mm Hg above the point where the pulse disappears.

• Place the bell of your stethoscope over the point where you felt the pulse, as shown in the photo. Using the bell helps you better hear Korotkoff sounds, which indicate pulse.
• Release the valve slowly and note the point at which Korotkoff sounds reappear. The start of the pulse sound indicates the systolic pressure.
• The sounds will become muffled and then disappear. The last Korotkoff sound you hear is the diastolic pressure.

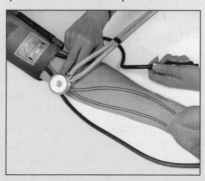

Tips for hearing Korotkoff sounds

If you have difficulty hearing Korotkoff sounds, try to intensify them by increasing vascular pressure below the cuff. Here are two techniques.

Have the patient raise their arm

Palpate the brachial pulse and mark its location with a pen to avoid losing the pulse spot. Apply the cuff and have the patient raise their arm above their head. Then inflate the cuff about 30 mm Hg above the patient's systolic

pressure. Have them lower their arm until the cuff reaches heart level, deflate the cuff, and take a reading.

Have the patient make a fist

Position the patient's arm at heart level. Inflate the cuff to 30 mm Hg above the patient's systolic pressure and ask them to make a fist. Have them rapidly open and close their hand approximately 10 times; then deflate the cuff and take the reading.

Performing a physical assessment

During the physical assessment, use drapes so only the area being examined is exposed. Develop a pattern for your assessments, starting with the same body system and proceeding in the same sequence. Organize your steps to minimize the number of times the patient needs to change position. By using a systematic approach, you'll also be less likely to forget an area.

A tetrad of techniques

No matter where you start your physical assessment, you'll use four techniques: inspection, palpation, percussion, and auscultation. Use these techniques in sequence except when you perform an abdominal assessment. Because palpation and percussion can alter bowel sounds, the sequence for assessing the abdomen is inspection, auscultation, percussion, and palpation. Let's look at each step in the sequence, one at a time.

Inspection

Inspect the patient using vision, smell, and hearing to observe normal conditions and deviations. Performed correctly, inspection can reveal more than other techniques. Touch is not part of the inspection process and is utilized in the palpation/percussion part of the physical assessment.

Inspection begins when you first meet the patient and continues throughout the health history and physical examination. As you assess each body system, observe for color, size, location, movement, texture, symmetry, body posture, gait, behavior, odors, and sounds.

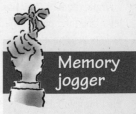

Memory jogger

To remember the order in which you should perform assessment of most systems, just think, "I'll Properly Perform Assessment":

Inspection

Palpation

Percussion

Auscultation.

Palpation

Palpation requires you to touch the patient with different parts of your hands, using varying degrees of pressure. In palpation, your hands are your tools, so ensure that your fingernails are short and your hands are warm. Avoid quick, short taps, as these can be difficult for the patient to anticipate. Always palpate tender areas last. Tell your patient the purpose of your touch and what you're feeling with your hands. (See *Types of palpation.*)

Check out these features

As you palpate each body system, evaluate the following features:
- texture—rough or smooth?
- temperature—warm, hot, or cold?
- thickness—thick or thin?

Peak technique

Types of palpation

The two types of palpation, light and deep, provide different types of assessment information.

Light palpation
Perform light palpation to feel for surface abnormalities. Depress the skin ½" to ¾" (1 to 2 cm) with your finger pads, using the lightest touch possible. Assess for texture, tenderness, temperature, moisture, elasticity, pulsations, superficial organs, swelling, crepitus, pain, and masses.

Deep palpation
Deep palpation is used to feel internal organs and masses for size, shape, tenderness, symmetry, and mobility. Depress the skin 1½" to 2" (4 to 5 cm) with firm, deep pressure. If necessary, use one hand on top of the other to exert firmer pressure.

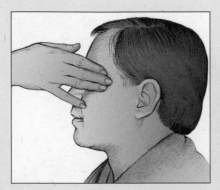

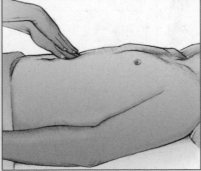

- moisture—dry, wet, or moist?
- firmness—soft or hard?
- motion—still or vibrating?
- consistency of structures—solid or fluid filled?
- patient response—any pain or tenderness?

Percussion

Percussion involves tapping your fingers or hands quickly and sharply against parts of the patient's body, usually the chest or abdomen. The technique helps you locate organ borders, identify organ shape and position, and determine if an organ is solid or filled with fluid or gas. (See *Types of percussion*.)

Peak technique

Types of percussion

You can perform percussion using the direct or indirect method.

Direct percussion

Direct percussion reveals pain/tenderness. Using one or two fingers, tap directly on the body part. Ask the patient to tell you which areas are painful and watch their face for signs of discomfort. This technique is commonly used to assess an adult patient's sinuses for tenderness or assessing newborn/infant lungs.

Indirect percussion

Indirect percussion, the most used type of percussion, elicits sounds that give clues to the makeup of the underlying tissue. Press the distal part of the middle finger of your nondominant hand firmly on the body part. Keep the rest of your hand off the body surface. Flex the wrist of your dominant hand. Using the middle finger of your dominant hand, tap quickly and directly over the point where your other middle finger touches the patient's skin. Listen to the sounds produced.

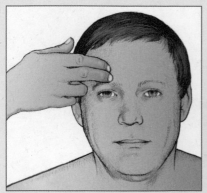

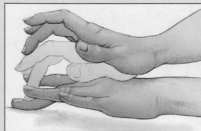

Sounds and their sources

As you practice percussion, you'll recognize different sounds. Each sound is related to the structure underneath. This chart offers a quick guide to percussion sounds and their sources.

Sound	Quality of sound	Where it's heard	Source
Tympany	Drumlike/high pitched	Over enclosed air	Air in bowel/bladder
Resonance	Hollow/low pitched	Over areas of part air and part solid	Normal lung
Hyperresonance	Booming/low pitched	Over air	Lung with emphysema
Dullness	Thudlike	Over solid tissue	Liver, spleen, heart
Flatness	Flat/more quiet than dullness	Over dense tissue	Muscle, bone

Subtle sounds

Percussion requires a skilled touch and an ear trained to detect slight variations in sound. Organs and tissues, depending on their density, produce sounds of varying loudness, pitch, and duration. For instance, air-filled cavities such as the lungs produce markedly different sounds than solid or dense tissue. (See *Sounds and their sources*.)

As you percuss, move gradually from areas of resonance to those of dullness and then compare sounds. Also, compare sounds on one side of the body with those on the other side.

Auscultation

Auscultation, usually the last step, involves listening for various breath, heart, and bowel sounds with a stethoscope. As you identify different sounds while assessing a body system, make sure you note the intensity and location of each sound. To prevent the spread of infection among patients, clean the heads and end pieces of the stethoscope with alcohol or a disinfectant before each use. (See *Using a stethoscope*, page 36.)

Peak technique

Using a stethoscope

Even if using a stethoscope is second nature to you, it might still be a good idea to brush up on your technique. First, your stethoscope should have these features:
• snug-fitting ear plugs, which you'll position toward your nose
• tubing no longer than 15″ (38.1 cm) with an internal diameter no greater than ⅛″ (0.3 cm)
• diaphragm
• bell.

How to auscultate

Hold the *diaphragm* firmly against the patient's skin, enough to leave a slight ring afterward. Hold the *bell* lightly against the patient's skin, just enough to form a seal. Holding the bell too firmly causes the skin to act as a diaphragm, obliterating low-pitched sounds.

Hair on the patient's chest may cause friction on the end piece, which can mimic abnormal breath sounds such as crackles. You can minimize this problem by lightly wetting the hair before auscultating.

A few more tips

Also keep these points in mind:
• Provide a quiet environment.
• Make sure the area to be auscultated is exposed. Don't try to auscultate over a gown or bed linens because they can interfere with sounds.
• Warm the stethoscope head in your hand before placing it on the patient.
• Close your eyes to help focus your attention.
• Listen to and try to identify the characteristics of one sound at a time.

Recording your findings

Begin your documentation with general information, including the patient's age, race, sex, general appearance, height, weight, body mass, vital signs, communication skills, behavior, awareness, orientation, and level of cooperation. Next, precisely record all information you obtained using the four physical assessment techniques. (See *Documenting your findings*.)

Just as you should follow an organized sequence in your examination, you should also follow an organized pattern for recording your findings. Document all information about one body system, for example, before proceeding to another.

Documenting your findings

Whether documenting an initial assessment of a patient admitted to your unit or writing a routine assessment note after a home visit, you'll need to use the appropriate form. The illustration below is an example of part of an initial assessment form similar to one you might use.

GENERAL INFORMATION

Name _Joe Smith_   Date _6/28/24_

Age _55_   Sex _M_   Height _163 cm_   Weight _57 kg_

T _98.6° F_ P _76_ R _14_ B/P(R) _150/90 sitting_ (L) _____

Room _328_   Patient's stated reason   Allergies _penicillin,_

Admission time _0800_   for hospitalization _____   _codeine_

Admission date _6/28/24_   _Trouble breathing and_

Doctor _Manzel_   _coughing a lot._   Current medications _None_

Admitting diagnosis

Pneumonia

Name	Dosage	Last taken

GENERAL SURVEY

Pt. is in no acute distress, is slender, and appears younger than stated
age. Is alert and well-groomed. Communicates well. Makes eye contact
and expresses appropriate concern throughout exam.—C. Smith, RN

Locate landmarks

Use anatomic landmarks in your descriptions so other people caring for the patient can compare their findings with yours. Using specific terminology like medial, lateral, proximal, distal, superior, and inferior is a great way to help explain landmarks of abnormal findings. For instance, you might describe a wound as "1½" × 2½" located 2½" inferior to the umbilicus at the midclavicular line."

With some structures, such as the tympanic membrane and breast, you can pinpoint a finding by its position on a clock. For instance, you might write "breast mass at 3 o'clock." If you use this method, however, make sure others recognize the same landmark for the 12 o'clock reference point.

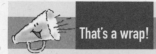
That's a wrap!

Physical assessment review

Performing a physical assessment
• Introduce yourself and help alleviate the patient's anxiety.
• Explain the entire procedure, including expected duration.
• Briefly document essential information.

Body temperature
• Remember that normal body temperature ranges from 96.7° to 100.5° F (35.9° to 38.1° C).
• To convert from Celsius to Fahrenheit, multiply the Celsius temperature by 1.8 and add 32.
• To convert from Fahrenheit to Celsius, subtract 32 from the Fahrenheit temperature and divide by 1.8.

Pulse
• Remember that a normal pulse is between 60 and 100 beats/minute.
• To palpate a pulse, press the area over the artery using the pads of your index and middle fingers until you feel pulsations.
• Avoid using your thumb to assess pulse, and never palpate both carotid pulses at the same time.

Respirations
• Remember that 12 to 20 breaths/minute is normal.
• Assess respiratory rate while taking the pulse.
• Observe the number and rhythm of the breaths, symmetry of the chest, and depth of respirations.
• Assess for the use of accessory muscles, crackles, wheezing, and stridor.

Blood pressure
• Remember that normal systolic pressure is 100 to 119 mm Hg; normal diastolic pressure, 60 to 79 mm Hg.
• Use the brachial artery under normal circumstances.
• Use techniques to intensify Korotkoff sounds as needed.

Physical assessment techniques
• Use drapes, exposing only the area being examined.
• Organize your approach: Start with the same body system; proceed in the same sequence.
• Perform inspection, palpation, percussion, and auscultation in that order for most body systems. However, when examining the abdomen, use inspection, auscultation, percussion, and palpation in that order.

Inspection
• Use your vision, smell, and hearing to inspect the patient.
• Observe the patient for color, size, location, movement, texture, symmetry, odors, and sounds.

Palpation
• Always tell the patient when and why you're going to touch them.
• Use different parts of your hand to touch the patient. Always palpate tender areas last.
• Use light palpation to assess for surface abnormalities, texture, tenderness, temperature, moisture, pulsations, and masses.
• Use deep palpation to feel internal organs and masses.

Percussion
• Use direct percussion to reveal tenderness.
• Use indirect percussion to determine the makeup of the underlying tissue.
• Use indirect pressure by tapping your fingers or hands quickly and sharply against parts of the patient's body to locate organ borders, identify organ shape and position, and determine consistency.
• Listen to the sounds produced: Observe their loudness, pitch, and duration.

Auscultation
• Use a stethoscope to listen for breath, heart, and bowel sounds.
• Hold the diaphragm of the stethoscope firmly against the patient's skin to listen for high-pitched sounds.
• Hold the bell of the stethoscope lightly against the patient's skin to listen for low-pitched sounds.
• Don't auscultate over a gown. Wet excess hair on the patient's chest to eliminate interference.
• Close your eyes to focus during auscultation.
• Note the intensity and location of auscultated sounds.

Documenting findings
• Begin by documenting general information.
• Next, document information you obtained from your assessment. Record your findings by body system to organize the information.
• Use anatomic landmarks in your descriptions.

Quick quiz

1. The first technique used during the physical assessment is:
   A. palpation.
   B. auscultation.
   C. inspection.
   D. percussion.

Answer: C. It's always important to inspect surfaces for any abnormalities before progressing through the physical assessment. For example, if you saw a deep wound, you would not want to palpate that wound as the first step.

2. When auscultating the abdomen, one would expect to hear what type of sounds?
   A. Dullness
   B. Tympany
   C. Resonance
   D. Hyperresonance

Answer: B. Remember that tympany is heard with the movement of air through enclosed organs and emits a high pitch.

3. If you're auscultating the apical portion of the heart, what are you listening for?
   A. Thudlike sounds
   B. Flat sounds
   C. Booming, low-pitched sounds
   D. Hollow, low-pitched sounds

Answer: A. Solid organs emit a thudlike sound due to being solid and air not being able to move freely through the organ.

4. When measuring a blood pressure, you should first inflate the BP cuff while feeling a radial pulse until the pulse disappears. When you then check the blood pressure, how much higher should the cuff be inflated to obtain an accurate reading?
   A. 10 mm Hg
   B. 20 mm Hg
   C. 30 mm Hg
   D. 40 mm Hg

Answer: C. You should always go 30 mm Hg above the first initial reading to make sure the BP is an accurate reading.

5. In a physical assessment, which one of these is a subjective measurement?
   A. Weight
   B. Height
   C. A large lump
   D. Pain

Answer: D. Pain is subjective and can only be verified by the patient. The other examples can be observed through proper physical assessment. Remember that if subjective the patient has to state what the problem is.

Scoring

☆☆☆ If you answered all five questions correctly, hooray! You're a history-takin', physical-assessin', proudly palpatin' assessment whiz.

☆☆ If you answered four questions correctly, terrific! You're a hands-on winner.

☆ If you answered fewer than four questions correctly, it's okay. In our assessment, you have unfulfilled potential.

Chapter 3

Nutritional assessment

Just the facts

In this chapter, you'll learn:

♦ ways in which nutrition affects health
♦ questions to ask your patient during a nutritional health history
♦ methods for assessing body systems as part of a nutritional assessment
♦ the proper way to take anthropometric measurements
♦ specific laboratory tests to help identify nutritional problems
♦ abnormal findings that you may discover during a nutritional assessment.

A look at nutritional assessment

A patient's nutritional health can influence their body's response to illness and treatment. Regardless of your patient's overall condition, an evaluation of their nutritional health should be a critical part of your total assessment. A better understanding of your patient's nutritional status can help you plan their care more effectively. (See *Parts of a nutritional assessment*.)

Normal nutrition

Nutrition refers to the sum of the processes by which a living organism ingests, digests, absorbs, transports, uses, and excretes nutrients. For nutrition to be adequate, a person must receive the proper nutrients, including proteins, fats, carbohydrates, water, vitamins, and minerals. Also, their digestive system must function properly for their body to make use of nutrients.

Parts of a nutritional assessment

Remember the four parts of a nutritional assessment, shown here.

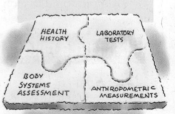

HEALTH HISTORY • LABORATORY TESTS • BODY SYSTEMS ASSESSMENT • ANTHROPOMETRIC MEASUREMENTS

Break it down

The body breaks down nutrients mechanically and chemically into simpler compounds for absorption in the stomach and intestines. The mechanical breakdown of food begins in the mouth with chewing and continues in the stomach and intestines as food is churned in the GI tract. The chemical processes start with the salivary enzymes in the mouth and continue with acid and enzyme action throughout the rest of the GI tract.

Now...or later

Nutrients can be used for the body's immediate needs, or they can be stored for later use. For example, glucose, a carbohydrate, is stored in the muscles and the liver. It can be converted quickly when the body needs energy fast. If glucose is unavailable, the body breaks down stored fat, a source of energy during periods of starvation. (See *Anabolism and catabolism*.)

Protein power

The body needs protein to ensure healthy growth and function and to maintain body tissues. Protein is stored in muscle, bone, blood, skin, cartilage, and lymph. Because the body typically preserves protein to maintain body functions, protein is used as a source of energy only when the supply of carbohydrates and fat is inadequate. Carbohydrates and fat are the primary sources of energy for the body. Vitamins, minerals, and water are also essential for healthy functioning.

Lipids on the loose

Lipids and other fats are also essential for the body's healthy functioning. To be transported throughout the body, they must combine with plasma proteins to form lipoproteins. Likewise, free fatty acids combine with albumin, whereas cholesterol, triglycerides, and phospholipids bind to globulin.

Obtaining a nutritional health history

A patient may relate various nutrition-related complaints, such as weight gain or loss; changes in energy level, appetite, or taste; dysphagia; GI tract problems, such as nausea, vomiting, and diarrhea; or other body system changes, such as skin and nail abnormalities. After establishing the patient's presenting problem, start the nutritional assessment by obtaining the patient's nutritional health history.

Anabolism and catabolism

Anabolism is a building-up process that occurs when simple substances, such as nutrients, are converted into more complex compounds to be used for tissue growth, maintenance, and repair.

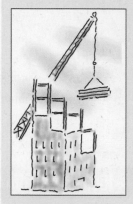

Catabolism is a breaking-down process that occurs when complex substances are converted into simple compounds and stored or used for energy.

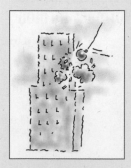

Blast from the past

During your interview, ask the patient about previous medical problems, surgical history, current medications (including over-the-counter medications, vitamins, and herbal preparations), illegal drug use, unusual physical activity, weight loss or gain, allergies, alcohol or tobacco use, eating patterns, food choices, and dietary restrictions. Also, ask about a family history of obesity, diabetes, metabolic disorders such as hypercholesterolemia, and stomach and GI disturbances. These problems have a tendency to occur in more than one family member.

A day in the life

Ask the patient to describe their typical day. This will give you important information about their routine activity level and eating habits.

Ask them to recount what and how much they ate yesterday, how the food was cooked, and who cooked it. This information not only tells you about the patient's usual intake but also gives clues about food preferences, eating patterns, and even the patient's memory and mental status. (See *Understanding differences in food intake*.)

Understanding differences in food intake

What your patient eats depends on various environmental, lifestyle, cultural, and economic influences. Understanding these influences can give you more insight into the patient's nutritional status.

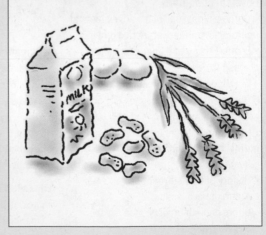

• *Socioeconomic status* may affect a patient's ability to afford healthful foods in the quantities needed to maintain proper health. Low socioeconomic status can lead to nutritional problems, especially for young children and pregnant people, who may give birth to infants with low birth weights or experience complications during labor.

• *Work schedule* can affect the amount and type of food a patient eats, especially if the patient works full time at odd hours.

• *Religion* can inform food choices. For example, some Jewish people and Muslims don't eat pork products, and many Roman Catholics avoid meat on Ash Wednesday and on Fridays during Lent.

• *Cultural background* influences food choices. For example, fish and rice are staple foods in many cultures.

Performing the assessment

After completing the health history, you'll perform a two-part nutritional physical assessment. In part one, you'll assess several key body systems. In part two, you'll take anthropometric measurements. You'll also need to evaluate laboratory studies. Remember that nutritional problems may be associated with various disorders or factors. (See *Tips for detecting nutritional problems.*)

Take a good look

Before starting your physical assessment, quickly evaluate the patient's general appearance. Does the patient look rested? Is their posture good? Is their speech clear? Are the patient's height and weight proportional to their body build? Are the patient's physical movements smooth with no apparent weaknesses? Are they free from skeletal conditions?

Tips for detecting nutritional problems

Nutritional problems may stem from physical conditions, medications, diet, or lifestyle factors. Listed below are factors that might indicate your patient is particularly susceptible to nutritional problems.

Physical conditions
• Chronic illnesses such as diabetes and neurologic, cardiac, or thyroid problems
• Family history of diabetes or heart disease
• Draining wounds or fistulas
• Obesity or a weight gain of 20% above normal body weight
• Unplanned weight loss of 20% below normal body weight
• Cystic fibrosis
• History of GI disturbances
• Anorexia or bulimia
• Depression or anxiety
• Severe trauma
• Recent chemotherapy, radiation therapy, or bone marrow transplantation

• Physical disabilities, such as paresis or paralysis
• Swallowing problems
• Recent major surgery
• Pregnancy, especially teen or multiple-birth pregnancy
• Burns
• Mouth, tooth, or denture problems

Medications, substance use, and diet
• Fad diets
• Steroid, diuretic, or antacid use
• Excessive alcohol intake
• Strict vegetarian diet
• Liquid diet or nothing by mouth for more than 3 days
• Laxative misuse

Lifestyle factors
• Lack of support from family or friends
• Financial problems
• Transportation problems
• Lack of education

Assessing each body system

Once you've assessed the patient's general appearance, you're ready to perform a head-to-toe assessment of the patient's major body systems. In addition to observing the patient's body structure, assess the following areas.

Skin, hair, and nails

When assessing the patient's skin, hair, and nails, ask yourself these questions: Is the hair shiny and full? Is the skin free from blemishes and rashes? Is it warm and dry, with normal color for that particular patient? Is the turgor normal? Are the nails firm with pink beds? Do they have a rash?

Eyes, nose, throat, and neck

Are the patient's eyes clear and shiny? Is the patient wearing contacts or glasses? Are the mucous membranes in the nose moist and pink? Is the tongue pink with papillae present? Are the gums moist and pink? Is the mouth free from ulcers or lesions? Does the patient's breath have an odor? Is the neck free from masses that would impede swallowing?

Neurologic system

Is the patient alert and responsive? Are the reflexes normal? Is the patient's behavior appropriate?

Cardiovascular system

Is the patient's heart rhythm regular? Are the heart rate and blood pressure normal for the patient's age? Are the extremities free from swelling? Are the peripheral pulses palpable?

Respiratory system

Are the patient's lungs clear? Is the patient breathing at a normal rate without effort? Is the patient's chest expansion with breathing normal?

GI system

Does the patient have normal bowel sounds? Do you see any visible scars on the abdomen? Is the abdomen free from abnormal masses on palpation? Does the patient flinch or grimace on palpation?

Urinary system

Does the patient report any trouble urinating? How much and what kind of fluid does the patient drink each day? Does the patient urinate frequently? Does the patient get up during the night to urinate? What color is the patient's urine? Does it have any odor and if so, what kind?

Musculoskeletal system

Does the patient have any evidence of muscle wasting? Can they perform the full range of motion with their extremities? Does the patient have any difficulty walking? Do you note any obvious joint conditions?

Anthropometric measurements

The second part of the physical assessment is taking anthropometric measurements. These measurements can help identify nutritional problems, especially in patients who are seriously overweight or underweight. You won't always need to take all measurements, but height and weight are usually necessary. Let the results of the patient's health history guide you.

Measuring height and weight

If your patient can stand without assistance, weigh the patient using a calibrated balance beam scale, and measure their height using the height bar on the scale. If the patient is weak or in a bed, measure their height with a measuring stick or tape and weigh them using a bed scale. (See *Overcoming problems in measuring height*.)

That elusive ideal weight

You've probably heard the term *ideal body weight*, a term that refers to standard weights associated with various heights on a reference table. Weight as a percentage of ideal body weight is obtained by dividing the patient's true weight by an ideal body weight—a number found on a table—and then multiplying that number by 100. (See *Height and weight table*.)

A body weight of 120% or more of the ideal body weight indicates obesity. Below 90% indicates underweight.

Weighty terms

Here are some weight-related definitions:
- *normal weight*—10% above or below recommended weight
- *overweight*—11% to 20% above recommended weight
- *obese*—21% or more above recommended weight
- *underweight*—11% to 20% below recommended weight
- *seriously underweight*—21% or more below recommended weight.

Overcoming problems in measuring height

Does your patient use a wheelchair? Is the patient unable to stand straight because of scoliosis? You can still get an approximate measurement of their height using the "wingspan" technique.

Have the patient hold their arms straight out from the sides of their body. Tell children to hold their arms out "like bird wings." Then measure from the tip of one middle finger to the tip of the other. That distance is the patient's approximate height.

Height and weight table

Because people of the same height may differ in muscle and bone makeup, a range of weights is normal for each height (see table at right). The higher weights in each category apply to male adults, who typically have more muscle and bone than female adults do. Height measurements are for patients not wearing shoes; weight measurements are for patients not wearing clothes.

Height	Weight	
	Ages 19–34	*Age 35 and older*
5'0"	97–128 lb	108–138 lb
5'1"	101–132 lb	111–143 lb
5'2"	104–137 lb	115–148 lb
5'3"	107–141 lb	119–152 lb
5'4"	111–146 lb	122–157 lb
5'5"	114–150 lb	126–162 lb
5'6"	118–155 lb	130–167 lb
5'7"	121–160 lb	134–172 lb
5'8"	125–164 lb	138–178 lb
5'9"	129–169 lb	142–183 lb
5'10"	132–174 lb	146–188 lb
5'11"	136–179 lb	151–194 lb
6'0"	140–184 lb	155–199 lb
6'1"	144–189 lb	159–205 lb
6'2"	148–195 lb	164–210 lb
6'3"	152–200 lb	168–216 lb
6'4"	156–205 lb	172–222 lb
6'5"	160–211 lb	177–228 lb
6'6"	164–216 lb	182–234 lb

Mass-ive formula

An alternative method of evaluating a patient's weight is by using body mass index (BMI). BMI is a measure of body fat based on height and weight. To determine a patient's BMI, consult a BMI chart or use this formula:

$$\text{BMI} = \left(\frac{\text{weight in pounds}}{(\text{height in inches}) \times (\text{height in inches})} \right) \times 703$$

Weight definitions based on BMI are the most accepted classification of weight status. (See *Interpreting BMI*, page 48.)

Anthropometric alternatives

Other anthropometric measurements include midarm circumference, midarm muscle circumference, and skinfold thickness. These measurements are used to evaluate muscle mass and subcutaneous fat, both of which relate to nutritional status. (See *Taking anthropometric arm measurements*, page 49.)

Interpreting BMI

Currently, the most widely accepted classification of weight status is the body mass index (BMI). BMI can be used as a measure of obesity and protein-calorie malnutrition as well as an indicator of health risk. All measures other than normal place the patient at a higher health risk, and nutritional needs should be assessed accordingly.

Classification	BMI
Underweight	<18.5
Normal	18.5–24.9
Overweight	25–29.9
Obesity class 1	30–34.9
Obesity class 2	35–39.9
Obesity class 3	40+

Laboratory studies

The last part of the nutritional assessment is an evaluation of the patient's laboratory test results. Below are some common biochemical tests that may be performed as part of a nutritional assessment as well as possible outcomes and interpretations. Other tests, such as thyroid function tests and serum electrolyte and vitamin levels, may also be ordered.

All about albumin

Serum albumin level is used to assess protein levels in the body. Albumin makes up more than 50% of total proteins in the serum and affects the cardiovascular system because it helps maintain plasma osmotic pressure. It also functions as a carrier protein for various substances important for nutritional health, such as iron. Keep in mind that albumin production requires functioning liver cells and an adequate supply of amino acids, which are the building blocks of proteins.

Because albumin has a long half-life (18 to 30 days), its value isn't the best indicator of current nutritional status. Prealbumin, another circulating protein with a half-life of 2 days, is a better indicator of current nutritional status.

Serum albumin level is decreased with serious protein deficiency and loss of blood protein resulting from burns, malnutrition, liver or renal disease, heart failure, major surgery, infections, or cancer.

Here's to hemoglobin!

Hemoglobin is the main component of red blood cells (RBCs), which transport oxygen. Its formation requires an adequate supply of protein in the form of amino acids.

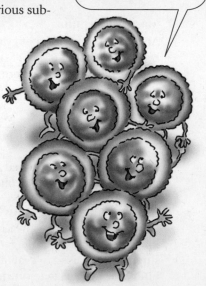

Hemoglobin values let you know how well we red blood cells are doing at our job of carrying oxygen.

Peak technique

Taking anthropometric arm measurements

Follow these steps to determine the triceps skinfold thickness, midarm circumference, and midarm muscle circumference.

Triceps skinfold thickness

1. Find the arm's midpoint circumference by placing a tape measure halfway between the axilla and the elbow. Then grasp the patient's skin with your thumb and forefinger, about ⅜″ (1 cm) above the midpoint, as shown below.

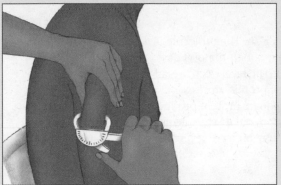

2. Place the calipers at the midpoint and squeeze for 3 seconds.
3. Record the measurement to the nearest millimeter.
4. Take two more readings and use the average.

Midarm circumference and midarm muscle circumference

1. At the midpoint, measure the midarm circumference, as shown below. Record the measurement in centimeters.

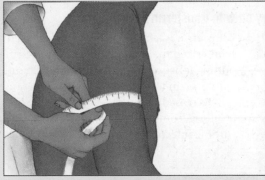

2. Calculate the midarm muscle circumference by multiplying the triceps skinfold thickness—measured in millimeters—by 3.14.
3. Subtract this number from the midarm circumference.

Recording the measurements

Record all three measurements as a percentage of the standard measurements (see chart below), using this formula:

$$\frac{\text{Actual measurement}}{\text{Standard measurement}} \times 100 = \%$$

After you've taken all the measurements, apply these rules:
• A measurement less than 90% of the standard indicates caloric deprivation.
• A measurement more than 90% indicates adequate or more than adequate energy reserves.

Measurement	Standard	90%
Triceps skinfold thickness	Men: 12.5 mm Women: 16.5 mm	Men: 11.3 mm Women: 14.9 mm
Midarm circumference	Men: 29.3 cm Women: 28.5 cm	Men: 26.4 cm Women: 25.7 cm
Midarm muscle circumference	Men: 25.3 cm Women: 23.3 cm	Men: 22.8 cm Women: 20.9 cm

Hemoglobin values help assess the blood's oxygen-carrying capacity and are useful in diagnosing anemia, protein deficiency, and hydration status.

A decreased hemoglobin level suggests iron deficiency anemia, protein deficiency, excessive blood loss, or overhydration. An increased hemoglobin level suggests dehydration or polycythemia.

Don't omit hematocrit

Hematocrit reflects the proportion of RBCs in a whole blood sample. This test helps diagnose anemia and dehydration. Decreased values suggest iron deficiency anemia, excessive fluid intake, or excessive blood loss. Increased values suggest severe dehydration or polycythemia.

Carry on with transferrin

Transferrin is a carrier protein that transports iron. The molecule is synthesized mainly in the liver. Transferrin has a half-life of 9 days, putting it between prealbumin and albumin. The level decreases along with protein levels and indicates depletion of protein stores.

Decreased values may also indicate inadequate protein production resulting from liver damage, protein loss from renal disease, acute or chronic infection, or cancer. Elevated levels may indicate severe iron deficiency.

Next comes nitrogen

A nitrogen balance test involves collecting all urine during a 24-hour period to determine the adequacy of a patient's protein intake. Proteins contain nitrogen. When proteins are broken down into amino acids, nitrogen is excreted in the urine as urea.

Nitrogen intake and excretion should be equal. Nitrogen balance is the difference between nitrogen intake (determined by a calorie count done during the same time frame as the 24-hour urine collection) and excretion. It's calculated using a formula, and the results are interpreted to determine whether the patient is receiving the appropriate amount of protein. Results may vary in patients with such conditions as burns and infection.

Trust in triglycerides

Triglycerides are the main storage form of lipids. Measuring triglyceride levels can help identify hyperlipidemia early. However, increased levels alone aren't diagnostic; further studies such as cholesterol measurements are required.

Patients who consume large amounts of sugar, soda, and refined carbohydrates commonly have elevated triglyceride levels. Decreased triglyceride levels commonly occur in those who are malnourished.

Count the cholesterol

A total cholesterol test measures circulating levels of free cholesterol and cholesterol esters. A diet high in saturated fats raises cholesterol levels by stimulating lipid absorption. Increased levels indicate an increased risk of coronary artery disease. Decreased levels are commonly associated with malnutrition.

Abnormal findings

Patients with nutritional problems may experience such signs and symptoms as excessive weight loss or gain, anorexia, or muscle wasting. Remember that clinical signs of nutritional deficiencies appear late. Also, be aware that patients hospitalized for more than 2 weeks risk developing a nutritional disorder. (See *Nutritional assessment findings*, page 52.)

Excessive weight loss

Patients with nutritional deficiencies usually experience weight loss. Weight loss may result from decreased food intake, decreased food absorption, increased metabolic requirements, or a combination of the three. Other possible causes include endocrine, neoplastic, GI, and psychiatric disorders; chronic disease; infection; and neurologic lesions that cause paralysis and dysphagia.

Excessive weight loss may also occur if the patient has a condition that prevents the patient from consuming a sufficient amount of food, such as painful oral lesions, ill-fitting dentures, or a loss of teeth. In addition, low income, fad diets, excessive exercise, or certain drugs may contribute to excessive weight loss.

Excessive weight gain

When a person consumes more calories than their body requires for energy, the body stores excess adipose tissue, resulting in weight gain. Emotional factors (such as anxiety, guilt, and depression) and social factors can trigger overeating resulting in excessive weight gain. Excessive weight gain is also a primary sign of many endocrine disorders. In addition, patients with conditions that limit activity, such as cardiovascular or respiratory disorders, may also experience excessive weight gain. (See *Overweight children*, page 53.)

Interpretation station

Nutritional assessment findings

This chart will help you interpret your nutritional assessment findings.

Body system or region	Sign or symptom	Implications
General	Weakness and fatigue	Anemia or electrolyte imbalance
	Weight loss	Decreased calorie intake, increased calorie use, or inadequate nutrient intake or absorption
Skin, hair, and nails	Dry, flaky skin	Vitamin A, vitamin B complex, or linoleic acid deficiency
	Dry skin with poor turgor	Dehydration
	Rough, scaly skin with bumps	Vitamin A or essential fatty acid deficiency
	Petechiae or ecchymoses	Vitamin C or K deficiency
	Sore that won't heal	Protein, vitamin C, or zinc deficiency
	Thinning, dry hair	Protein or zinc deficiency
	Spoon-shaped, brittle, or ridged nails	Iron deficiency
Eyes	Night blindness; corneal swelling, softening, or dryness; Bitot spots (gray triangular patches on the conjunctiva)	Vitamin A deficiency
	Red conjunctiva	Riboflavin deficiency
Throat and mouth	Cracks at corner of mouth	Riboflavin or niacin deficiency
	Magenta tongue	Riboflavin deficiency
	Beefy, red tongue	Vitamin B_{12} deficiency
	Soft, spongy, bleeding gums	Vitamin C deficiency
	Swollen neck (goiter)	Iodine deficiency
Cardiovascular	Edema	Protein deficiency
	Tachycardia and hypotension	Fluid volume deficit
GI	Ascites	Protein or vitamin B_{12} deficiency
Musculoskeletal	Bone pain and bow leg	Vitamin D or calcium deficiency
	Muscle wasting	Protein, carbohydrate, and fat deficiency
	Pain in calves and thighs	Thiamine deficiency
Neurologic	Altered mental state	Dehydration, thiamine or vitamin B_{12} deficiency, anemia, or electrolyte imbalances
	Paresthesia	Vitamin B_{12}, pyridoxine, or thiamine deficiency

Handle with care

Overweight children

Like adults, the number of children considered overweight has dramatically increased in recent years. In 2020, an estimated 39 million children under the age of 5 were overweight or obese. Over 340 million children and adolescents between the ages of 5 and 19 were overweight or obese in 2016. Most overweight children become overweight or obese adults.

More weight, more risks

Children who are overweight are more likely to develop high cholesterol levels and high blood pressure (risk factors for heart disease) as well as type 2 diabetes. They also tend to suffer from poor self-esteem and depression because of their weight.

Counting causes

During your nutritional assessment, look for these common causes of excessive weight gain in children:
- lack of exercise
- sedentary lifestyle (involving an excessive amount of watching television, using computers, or playing video games)
- unhealthy eating habits.

Healthy habits

Help the child develop an exercise plan and suggest nutritious dietary choices to prevent weight gain and promote a healthy lifestyle.

Anorexia

Defined as a lack of appetite despite a physiologic need for food, anorexia commonly occurs with GI and endocrine disorders. It can also result from anxiety, chronic pain, poor oral hygiene, and changes in taste or smell that normally accompany aging. Short-term anorexia rarely jeopardizes health, but chronic anorexia can lead to life-threatening malnutrition and other medical problems, such as cardiac, GI, and neurologic disorders. Anorexia nervosa is a psychological condition in which the patient severely restricts food intake, resulting in excessive weight loss.

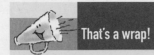

Nutritional assessment review

Evaluating nutritional status
- Nutrition is the sum of the processes by which a living organism ingests, digests, absorbs, transports, uses, and excretes nutrients.
- Nutrition includes the adequate intake of proteins, fats, carbohydrates, water, vitamins, and minerals.
- Nutrients can be used for the body's immediate needs, or they may be stored for later use.
- Proteins ensure normal growth and function and maintain body tissues.

Obtaining a nutritional health history
- Determine the patient's presenting problem.
- Obtain the patient's previous medical history, a family history, and a list of their current medications (including vitamins and herbal preparations).
- Ask the patient about their routine activity level and eating habits.
- Ask the patient about what they ate yesterday.

Performing a nutritional physical assessment
- Perform a general inspection.
- Assess key body systems: skin, hair, and nails; eyes, nose, throat, and neck; and the neurologic, cardiovascular, respiratory, GI, renal, and musculoskeletal systems.
- Obtain anthropometric measurements: height, weight, and body mass index; when needed, midarm circumference, midarm muscle circumference, and triceps skinfold thickness.

Evaluating laboratory tests
- Albumin—Decreased levels indicate protein deficiency, liver or kidney disease, heart failure, surgery, infection, or cancer.
- Hemoglobin—Decreased levels indicate iron deficiency anemia, overhydration, or excessive blood loss.
- Hematocrit—Decreased values indicate anemia; increased values, dehydration.
- Transferrin—Transferrin levels reflect protein stores; increased levels indicate iron deficiency anemia and decreased levels indicate liver disease and malnutrition.
- Nitrogen—Intake and output should be equal.
- Triglycerides—Triglyceride levels reflect lipid stores.
- Cholesterol—High levels indicate an increased risk of coronary artery disease.

Abnormal nutritional findings
- *Weight loss* reflects decreased food intake, decreased food absorption, increased metabolic requirements, or a combination of the three.
- *Weight gain* occurs when ingested calories exceed body requirements for energy, causing increased adipose tissue storage.
- *Anorexia* refers to a lack of appetite despite the physiologic need for food.
- *Muscle wasting* occurs when muscle fibers lose bulk and length, causing a visible loss of muscle size and contour.

Muscle wasting

Usually a result of chronic protein deficiency, muscle wasting, or *atrophy* results when muscle fibers lose bulk and length. The muscles involved shrink and lose their normal contour, appearing emaciated or even deformed. Associated symptoms include chronic fatigue, apathy, anorexia, dry skin, peripheral edema, and dull, sparse, dry hair.

Quick quiz

1. Lipids and other fats are also essential for the body's normal functioning. They must combine with plasma proteins to form lipoproteins. Which of the following binds to albumin to transport around the body?
  A. Cholesterol
  B. Triglycerides
  C. Free fatty acids
  D. Phospholipids

Answer: C. Free fatty acids combine with albumin, whereas cholesterol, triglycerides, and phospholipids bind to globulin.

2. A patient presents with recent weight loss and the provider would like to access the patient's current nutritional status. Which lab test would be the best option?
  A. Prealbumin
  B. Albumin
  C. Hemoglobin
  D. Cholesterol

Answer: A. A serum prealbumin test assesses protein levels in the body. Prealbumin, with a half-life of 2 days, is a better indicator of current nutritional status than albumin. Cholesterol and hemoglobin will not assess nutritional status.

3. A patient has come into the clinic for their annual physical. They are 5′6″ tall and 187 lb (85 kg). What is their body mass index?
  A. 13.71
  B. 30.18
  C. 33.72
  D. 36.51

Answer: B.

$$\text{BMI} = \left(\frac{\text{weight in pounds}}{(\text{height in inches}) \times (\text{height in inches})} \right) \times 703$$

For this patient, BMI = [187/(66*66)]*703 = 30.18. The patient is in obesity class 1 (30 to 34.9).

4.   A patient presents to the floor after suffering injuries from a motor vehicle collision. They do not have any burns or signs on infection. What lab test would assess if the patient is receiving the appropriate amount of protein to help them recover?
  A.   Transferrin
  B.   Albumin
  C.   Nitrogen balance test
  D.   Prealbumin

Answer: C. This 24-hour urine test is used to determine whether the patient is receiving the appropriate amount of protein. Results may vary in patients with such conditions as burns and infection.

Scoring

☆☆☆   If you answered all four questions correctly, congratulations! Your hunger for nutritional knowledge has been truly satisfied.

☆☆   If you answered three questions correctly, way to go! We're impressed with how you sunk your teeth into this chapter.

☆   If you answered fewer than three questions correctly, don't lose weight over it. Just feast on the facts in this chapter and then take the quiz again.

Chapter 4

Mental health assessment

Just the facts

In this chapter, you'll learn:

♦ methods for establishing a therapeutic relationship with a patient

♦ ways to obtain important information during the patient interview

♦ techniques for assessing mental status

♦ abnormal findings that may be revealed by a mental health assessment

♦ ways to identify mental health disorders.

A look at mental health assessment

Effective patient care requires consideration of the psychological as well as the physiologic aspects of health. A patient who seeks medical help for chest pain, for example, may also need to be assessed for anxiety and depression. Knowing the brain's basic function and structures will help you perform a comprehensive mental health assessment and recognize abnormalities. (See Chapter 6, Neurologic system, for a quick review.)

Obtaining a health history

Your assessment begins with a health history. For this assessment to be effective, you need to establish a therapeutic relationship with the patient that's built on trust. You must communicate to them that their thoughts and behaviors are important. Effective communication involves not only speech but also nonverbal communication, such as eye contact, posture, facial expressions, gestures, clothing, affect, and even silence. All convey a powerful message. (See *Therapeutic communication techniques*, page 58.)

Therapeutic communication techniques

Therapeutic communication is the foundation of any good nurse-patient relationship. Here are some effective techniques for developing that relationship.

Offering self
This technique is used to offer emotional support. An example of this technique is: "I'll sit with you until your family arrives."

Listening
Listening intently to the patient enables the nurse to hear and analyze everything the patient is saying, alerting the nurse to the patient's communication patterns.

Rephrasing
Succinct rephrasing of key patient statements helps ensure that the nurse understands and emphasizes important points in the patient's message. For example, the nurse might say, "You're feeling angry and you say it's because of the way your friend treated you yesterday."

Broad openings and general statements
Using broad openings and general statements to initiate conversation encourages the patient to talk about any subject that comes to mind. These openings allow the patient to focus the conversation and demonstrate the nurse's willingness to interact. An example of this technique is: "Is there something you would like to talk about?"

Exploring
This technique helps the patient feel free to talk and examine issues in depth. For example, the nurse might say, "Tell me what happened on the date."

Clarifying
Asking the patient to clarify a confusing or vague message demonstrates the nurse's desire to understand what the patient is saying. It can also elicit precise information crucial to the patient's recovery. An example of clarification is: "I'm not sure I understood what you said."

Accepting
This technique lets the patient know the nurse understands their thoughts and feelings. For instance, the nurse might say, "I can only imagine how you feel."

Focusing
With the technique called focusing, the nurse helps the patient redirect attention toward something specific. It fosters the patient's self-control and helps avoid vague generalizations, so the patient can accept responsibility for facing problems. "Let's go back to what we were just talking about," would be one example of this technique.

Silence
Silence has several benefits: It gives the patient time to talk, think, and gain insight into problems. It also allows the nurse to gather more information. The nurse must use this technique judiciously, however, to avoid giving the impression of disinterest or judgment.

Suggesting collaboration
When used correctly, the technique of suggesting collaboration gives the patient the opportunity to explore the pros and cons of a suggested approach. It must be used carefully to avoid directing the patient. An example of this technique is: "Perhaps we can meet with your parents to discuss the matter."

Summarizing
With this technique, the nurse systematically synthesizes important ideas discussed during the patient interview. An example is: "So far, we have discussed your marriage problems and your need to decrease conflict."

Validating perceptions
This technique gives the patient a chance to correct the nurse's understanding of what's being communicated. For example, the nurse might say, "Tell me if my perception of what you're telling me agrees with yours."

Bridging the gap

Transcultural communication

Communication styles vary among cultures. Qualities viewed as desirable in one culture (such as maintaining eye contact, having a certain degree of openness, offering insight, and portraying emotional expression) may not be considered appropriate in another culture. For example:
• Direct eye contact is considered inappropriate and disrespectful in some cultures.
• Some cultures focus solely on the present; they may view the future as something to be accepted as it occurs, rather than planned.
• Some cultures strongly value harmonious interpersonal relationships. As a result, members of these cultures may nod, smile, and provide answers they feel are expected to maintain harmony rather than expressing their true feelings and concerns.
• Some cultures consider direct questions to be impolite.
     Avoid making assumptions about a patient's behavior or communication style. An individual's cultural background may explain a communication style you would otherwise deem "inappropriate" or "abnormal."

Peace and quiet

Choose a quiet, private setting for the assessment interview. Interruptions and distractions threaten confidentiality and interfere with effective listening. If you're meeting the patient for the first time, introduce yourself and explain the interview's purpose. Sit a comfortable distance from the patient and give them your undivided attention. If you're interviewing a patient who has cognitive or memory losses, you may need to reorient them before beginning the interview.

Attitude counts

During the interview, be professional but friendly and maintain eye contact. A calm, nonthreatening tone of voice encourages the patient to talk more openly. Avoid value judgments. Don't rush through the interview; building a trusting therapeutic relationship takes time. (See *Transcultural communication*.)

Guidelines for an effective mental health interview

To help make your mental health interview more productive, follow these guidelines:

• Begin the interview with a broad, empathetic statement: "You look distressed; tell me what's bothering you today."

• Explore usual behaviors before discussing unusual ones: "What do you think has enabled you to cope with the pressures of your job?"

• Phrase inquiries sensitively to lessen the patient's anxiety: "Things were going well at home and then you became depressed. Tell me about that."

• Ask the patient to clarify vague statements: "Explain to me what you mean when you say, 'They're all after me.'"

• Help the patient who rambles to focus on the most pressing problem: "You've talked about several problems. Which one bothers you the most?"

• Interrupt nonstop talkers as tactfully as possible. Use such a statement as, "Thank you for your comments. Now let's move on."

• Express empathy toward tearful, silent, or confused patients who have trouble describing their problem: "I realize that it's difficult for you to talk about this."

Patient interview

A patient interview establishes a baseline and provides clues to the underlying or precipitating cause of the patient's current problem. Remember, the patient may not be a reliable source of information, for example, if they have a mental illness or other mental or cognitive condition. If possible, verify their responses with family members, friends, or health care personnel. Also, check hospital records for previous admissions, if possible, and compare the patient's past and current behavior, symptoms, and circumstances. (See *Guidelines for an effective mental health interview.*)

Presenting problem

The patient may not directly voice their presenting problem. Instead, you or others may note that they're having difficulty coping or are exhibiting unusual behavior. If you note a problem, determine whether the patient is aware of the problem. When documenting the patient's response, write it word for word and enclose it in quotation marks.

Symptom specifics

Find out about the onset of current symptoms. Inquire about the severity and persistence of the symptoms and whether they occurred suddenly or developed over time.

History of psychiatric illnesses

Discuss past psychiatric disturbances—such as episodes of delusions, violence, attempted suicides, drug or alcohol use and misuse, or depression—and previous psychiatric treatment, if any. Also ask about any family history of psychiatric illness or substance use disorder.

Demographic data

Determine the patient's age, ethnic origin, primary language, birthplace, religion, occupation, and marital status. Use this information to establish a baseline and confirm that the patient's record is correct.

Socioeconomic data

Patients experiencing hardships are more likely to show symptoms of distress during an illness. Information about your patient's educational level, family, housing conditions, income, and employment status may provide clues to the current problem.

Cultural and religious beliefs

A patient's background and values can affect how they respond to illness and adapt to care. Certain questions and behaviors considered acceptable in one culture may be inappropriate in another.

Medication history

Certain medications can cause symptoms of mental illness. Review all medications the patient is taking, including over-the-counter and herbal preparations, and check for interactions. If they're taking a psychiatric medication, ask if their symptoms have improved, if they're taking the medication as prescribed, and if they have had any adverse reactions. Also, find out if the patient uses illegal drugs and if so, ask what they are and how often they use them.

Physical illnesses

Find out if the patient has a history of medical disorders that may cause distorted thought processes, disorientation, depression, or other symptoms of mental illness. (See *COVID-19 and its impact on mental health*.) For example, does the patient have a history of kidney or hepatic failure, infection, thyroid disease, or a neurodegenerative or metabolic disorder?

COVID-19 and its impact on mental health

COVID-19 had a large impact on the mental health of our society. Not only were patients faced with an increase in symptoms related to loss, depression, and anxiety, frontline workers faced their own mental health issues as well with a decrease in available supports. There was a noted increase in substance use diagnosis, which was perpetuated by insecurities in many areas including financial, housing, food, and health. Given all the stressors people have experienced during and after the COVID-19 pandemic, including forced isolation due to work and school closures, there will likely be years of lingering mental health crisis that will add strain to our already stressed mental health care system.

Assessing mental status

Most of a mental status assessment can be done during an interview. While talking to the patient, assess appearance, behavior, mood, thought processes and cognitive function, coping mechanisms, and potential for self-destructive behavior. Record your findings.

Initial observations

Much about a patient's mental state can be determined simply by observing their appearance and how they handle themselves in your presence.

Appearance

The patient's appearance helps to indicate their emotional and mental status. Specifically, note their dress and grooming. Is their appearance clean and appropriate for their environment and situation? Is the patient's posture erect or slouched? Is their head lowered? Observe their gait—is it brisk, slow, shuffling, or unsteady? Do they walk normally? Note their facial expression. Do they look alert, or do they stare blankly? Do they appear sad or angry? Does the patient maintain eye contact? Do they stare at you for long periods? Are their arms crossed? Do they face you or turn away while you are talking?

Behavior

Note the patient's demeanor and overall attitude as well as any unexpected behavior such as speaking to a person who isn't present. Also, record the patient's mannerisms. Do they bite their nails, fidget, or pace? Do they display any tics or tremors? How do they respond to you? Are they cooperative, friendly, hostile, or indifferent?

Mood

Does the patient appear anxious or depressed? Are they crying, sweating, breathing heavily, or trembling? Ask them to describe their current feelings in concrete terms and to suggest possible reasons for these feelings. Note inconsistencies between body language and mood (such as smiling when discussing an anger-provoking situation).

Thought processes and cognitive function

Evaluate the patient's orientation to time, place, and person, noting any confusion or disorientation. Listen for any indication that the patient might be having delusions, hallucinations, obsessions, compulsions, fantasies, or daydreams.

Attention, please!

Assess the patient's attention span and ability to recall events in both the distant and recent past. For example, to assess immediate recall, ask them to repeat a series of five or six objects.

Hypothetically speaking

Test their intellectual functioning by asking them to add a series of numbers and test their sensory perception and coordination by having them copy a simple drawing. Inappropriate responses to a hypothetical situation—such as "What would you do if you won the lottery?"—can indicate impaired judgment. Keep in mind that the patient's cultural background can influence their answer.

Speech specifics

Note any speech characteristics that may indicate altered thought processes, including monosyllabic responses, irrelevant or illogical replies to questions, convoluted or excessively detailed speech, slurred speech, repetitious speech patterns, a flight of ideas, and sudden silence without obvious reason.

Onsite insight

Assess the patient's insight by asking if they understand the significance of their illness, the treatment plan, and the effect the illness will have on their life.

Coping mechanisms

The patient who's faced with a stressful situation may adopt coping, or defense, mechanisms—behaviors that operate on an unconscious level to protect the ego. Examples include denial, displacement, fantasy, identification, projection, and repression. Listen for an excessive reliance on these coping mechanisms. (See *Exploring coping mechanisms*, page 64.)

Exploring coping mechanisms

The use of coping, or defense, mechanisms helps to relieve anxiety. Common coping strategies include:

• *denial*—the refusal to admit truth or reality

• *displacement*—transferring an emotion from its original object to a substitute

• *fantasy*—the creation of unrealistic or improbable images to escape from daily pressures and responsibilities

• *identification*—the unconscious adoption of another person's personality characteristics, attitudes, values, and behaviors

• *projection*—the displacement of negative feelings onto another person

• *rationalization*—the substitution of acceptable reasons for the real or actual reasons that are motivating behavior

• *reaction formation*—behaving in a manner opposite from the way the person feels

• *regression*—the return to behavior of an earlier, more comfortable time

• *repression*—the exclusion of unacceptable thoughts and feelings from the conscious mind, leaving them to operate in the subconscious.

Potential for self-destructive behavior

Mentally healthy people may intentionally take death-defying risks such as participating in dangerous sports. The risks that self-destructive patients take, however, aren't death defying—they're death seeking.

Self-harm

Not all self-destructive behavior is suicidal in intent. Some patients engage in self-destructive behavior as a coping mechanism for emotional distress. A patient may cut or mutilate body parts to focus on physical pain, which may be less overwhelming than emotional distress.

Higher risk when they're low

Assess the patient for suicidal tendencies or ideations, particularly if they report symptoms of depression. Not all such patients want to die; however, the incidence of suicide is higher in depressed patients than in patients with other diagnoses. If the patient is actively planning suicide, be prepared to take immediate action to prevent the act from occurring. (See *Recognizing and responding to patients who are suicidal*.)

Recognizing and responding to patients who are suicidal

Throughout the assessment process, you'll want to watch for these warning signs of impending suicide:
- withdrawing from life
- avoiding any social situation
- displaying signs of depression, which may include constipation, crying, fatigue, helplessness, hopelessness, poor concentration, reduced interest in sex and other activities, sadness, weight loss or gain, and changes in sleep pattern
- bidding farewell to friends and family
- putting affairs in order
- giving away prized possessions
- expressing covert suicide messages and death wishes
- voicing obvious suicide messages such as "I'd be better off dead."

Answering a suicidal threat

If a patient shows signs of impending suicide, you'll need to assess the seriousness of the intent and the immediacy of the risk. For example, a patient who has chosen a suicide method and who plans to attempt suicide in the next 48 to 72 hours is a high-risk patient.

First, tell the patient that you're concerned and urge them to avoid self-destructive behavior until the staff has an opportunity to help them. You may specify a time for the patient to seek help.

Next, consult with the health care treatment team about arranging for psychiatric hospitalization or a safe equivalent such as having someone watch the patient at home. Initiate the following safety precautions for those with high suicide risk:
- Provide a safe environment. Check and correct conditions that could be dangerous for the patient. Look for exposed pipes, windows without safety glass, and access to the roof or open balconies.
- Remove dangerous objects, including belts, razors, suspenders, light cords, glass, knives, nail files, and clippers.
- Make the patient's specific restrictions clear to staff members. Plan for observation of the patient, and clarify the responsibilities of both day and night staff members.

The patient may ask you to keep their suicidal thoughts confidential. Remember, such a request is ambivalent; the patient wants to escape the pain of life, but they also want to live. A part of them may want you to tell other staff members so that they can be kept alive. Tell the patient that you can't keep secrets that will endanger their life or conflict with their treatment. You have a duty to keep them safe and to ensure they receive the best care.

Be alert when the patient is shaving, taking medication, or using the bathroom. These normal activities could be dangerous for the patient who is suicidal. In addition to observing the patient, maintain personal contact with them. Encourage continuity of care and consistency of health care providers. Helping the patient build emotional ties to others is the ultimate technique for preventing suicide.

After the patient's safety is assured, make sure to document the situation and intervention appropriately.

Psychological and mental status testing

Although most of a mental status assessment can be done during an interview, you'll also need to evaluate other aspects of your patient's mental status. These aspects can be assessed using psychological and mental status tests. (See *Testing older adult patients.*) Commonly used tests include:

- *Mini-Mental Status Examination*—measures orientation, registration, recall, calculation, language, and graphomotor function
- *Cognitive Capacity Screening Examination*—measures orientation, memory, calculation, and language
- *Cognitive Assessment Scale*—measures orientation, general knowledge, mental ability, and psychomotor function
- *Beck Depression Inventory*—helps diagnose depression, determine its severity, and monitor the patient's response during treatment
- *Global Deterioration Scale*—assesses and stages primary degenerative dementia based on orientation, memory, and neurologic function
- *Minnesota Multiphasic Personality Inventory*—helps assess personality traits and ego function in adolescents and adults. Test results include information on coping strategies, defenses, strengths, gender identification, and self-esteem; the test pattern may strongly suggest a diagnostic category, point to a suicide risk, or indicate potential violence.

Other specific tests are frequently used to assess older adult and pediatric populations. Specific questionnaires are also available to assess the patient for substance use and misuse.

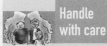

Handle with care

Testing older adult patients

Although older adult patients typically do well on the entire mental health examination, they may display functional impairment as they age. Older patients tend to retrieve and process data more slowly, and they take more time to learn new material. They also may have slower motor responses and an impaired ability to perform complex tasks. Understanding the effects of aging will help keep you from confusing these age-related impairments with mental illness.

Classifying mental disorders

Mental status disorders are classified according to the American Psychiatric Association's *Diagnostic and Statistical Manual of Mental Disorders, Fifth Edition, Text Revision* (*DSM-5-TR*). The manual provides a standardized interdisciplinary system for all members of the mental health team to use. Its classification system emphasizes observational data and de-emphasizes subjective and theoretical impressions. The *DSM-5-TR* includes a complete description of psychiatric disorders and other conditions and spells out the criteria that must be met for each diagnosis. (See *Understanding the DSM-5-TR.*)

Understanding the *DSM-5-TR*

The *DSM-5* provides clear, highly detailed definitions of mental health and brain-related conditions. It also provides details and examples of the signs and symptoms of those conditions.

In addition to defining and explaining conditions, the *DSM-5* organizes those conditions into groups. This makes it easier for health care providers to accurately diagnose conditions and tell them apart from conditions with similar signs and symptoms. This is done through clinical criteria that need to be met in order for the diagnosis to be chosen correctly.

Abnormal findings

During a mental health assessment, you may detect abnormalities in thought processes, thought content, and perception. (See *Mental health assessment findings*, pages 67 and 68.)

Interpretation station

Mental health assessment findings

Certain findings obtained from your mental health assessment may lead you to suspect a psychiatric disorder. This chart shows assessment findings associated with common psychiatric disorders.

Disorder	Assessment findings
Schizophrenia	• Delusions • Hallucinations • Disorganized speech • Grossly disorganized or catatonic behavior • Flat affect • Inability to speak • Limited eye contact • Distant and unresponsive facial expression • Limited body language
Major depressive disorder	• Severe fatigue • Inability to concentrate or make decisions • Feelings of sadness, worthlessness, or extreme guilt • Appetite changes with either weight loss or gain • Sleep disturbances • Decreased libido

(Continued)

Mental health assessment findings *(continued)*

Disorder	Assessment findings
Bipolar I disorder	• Signs and symptoms of major depressive disorder (listed above) • Manic findings, such as euphoria or irritability, delusions of grandeur, flight of ideas, extreme talkativeness, being easily distracted, spending money recklessly
Paranoid personality disorder	• Feelings of being deceived • Hostility • Major distortions of reality • Social isolation • Suspiciousness, mistrust of friends and relatives
Borderline personality disorder	• Destructive behavior • Impulsive behavior • Inability to develop a sense of self • Inability to maintain relationships • Moodiness • Self-mutilation
Delirium	• Alerted psychomotor activity, such as apathy, withdrawal, and agitation • Poor impulse control • Unusual, destructive behavior that worsens at night • Disorganized thinking • Distractibility • Impaired decision making • Inability to complete tasks • Insomnia or daytime sleepiness • Rambling, unusual, or incoherent speech
Posttraumatic stress disorder	• Anxiety • Flashbacks of the traumatic experience • Nightmares about the traumatic experience • Poor impulse control • Social isolation • Survivor guilt

Abnormal thought processes

During the interview, you may identify some of these abnormalities in your patient's thought processes:

- *derailment*—Speech vacillates from one subject to another. (The subjects are unrelated; ideas slip off track between clauses.)
- *flight of ideas*—The patient jumps abruptly from topic to topic in a continuous flow of speech.

- *neologisms*—Words are distorted or invented.
- *blocking*—The patient suddenly stops speaking.
- *circumstantiality*—Unnecessary detail and irrelevant remarks delay the patient from getting to the point.
- *perseveration*—The patient persistently repeats words or ideas.
- *confabulation*—The patient fabricates facts or events to fill in the gaps where memory loss has occurred.
- *clanging*—The patient chooses a word based on the sound rather than the meaning.
- *echolalia*—The patient repeats words or phrases that others say.
- *incoherence*—The patient's speech is incomprehensible.

Abnormal thought content

With careful questioning, you may also detect abnormalities in thought content during the interview. Be sure to follow the patient's lead. For example, "You told me a few minutes ago that your mother was responsible for your illness; would you please elaborate?" With this type of questioning, you can find abnormalities in thought content, which may include:

- *obsessions*—recurrent, uncontrollable thoughts, images, or impulses that the patient considers unacceptable
- *compulsions*—repetitive behaviors that result from attempts to alleviate an obsession
- *phobia*—an irrational and disproportionate fear of objects or situations
- *depersonalization*—the feeling that one has become detached from one's mind or body or has lost one's identity
- *delusions*—false, fixed beliefs that aren't shared by others
- *poverty of content*—thoughts that give little information because of vagueness, empty repetition, or obscure phrases.

Perception abnormalities

You can assess a patient's perception abnormalities in the same way that you assess their thought content. Ask direct questions about their perceptions, such as "What did the voice say to you when you heard it speaking? How did you feel?" If the patient doesn't speak about abnormal perceptions, you can ask if they ever hear peculiar voices or frightening sounds. Perception abnormalities include:

- *illusions*—misinterpretations of external stimuli
- *hallucinations*—auditory, visual, tactile, somatic, or gustatory sensory perceptions when no external stimuli are present.

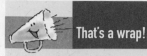

That's a wrap!

Mental health assessment review

Obtaining a mental health history
- Establish a trusting, therapeutic relationship.
- Choose a quiet, private setting.
- Maintain a calm, nonthreatening tone of voice to encourage open communication.
- Determine the patient's presenting problem, using the patient's own words to document it.
- Discuss past psychiatric disturbances and previous psychiatric treatment, if any.
- Obtain the patient's demographic and socioeconomic data.
- Discuss cultural and religious beliefs.
- Obtain a drug use history.
- Ask about a history of medical disorders; some conditions may adversely affect the patient's mental health.

Mental status checklist
- Appearance
- Demeanor and overall attitude
- Unexpected behavior
- Inconsistencies between body language and mood
- Orientation to time, place, and person
- Confusion or disorientation
- Attention span
- Ability to recall events
- Intellectual function
- Speech characteristics that indicate altered thought processes
- Insight
- Coping or defense mechanisms
- Self-destructive behavior
- Psychological and mental status test results

Abnormal mental health findings
- Abnormal thought processes—derailment, flight of ideas, neologisms, confabulation, clanging, echolalia, incoherence
- Abnormal thought content—obsessions, compulsions, phobia, depersonalization, delusions, poverty of content
- Abnormal perceptions—illusions, hallucinations

Quick quiz

1. Other sources are needed to validate data from a psychiatric patient's health history because:
    A. mental status can change abruptly in response to internal or external stimuli.
    B. personal biases might alter the interpretation of physical findings.
    C. mental illness may alter the patient's perceptions.
    D. psychiatric medications impair the patient's memory.

Answer: C. Mental illness can alter the patient's thinking, emotions, and perceptions, making the patient an unreliable source of information. If possible, verify the patient's responses with family members, friends, or health care personnel.

2. The therapeutic communication technique that involves redirecting the patient's attention toward a specific topic is called:
   A. collaboration.
   B. clarification
   C. rephrasing.
   D. focusing.

Answer: D. Focusing redirects the patient to a specific topic to prevent them from making vague generalizations.

3. Which psychological and mental status test helps assess the patient's memory?
   A. Cognitive Capacity Screening Examination
   B. Minnesota Multiphasic Personality Inventory
   C. Beck Depression Inventory
   D. Cognitive Assessment Scale

Answer: A. The Cognitive Capacity Screening Examination measures orientation, memory, calculation, and language.

4. You notice that your patient makes up events to fill in memory gaps. You identify this abnormal thought process as:
   A. derailment.
   B. echolalia.
   C. confabulation.
   D. clanging.

Answer: C. When a patient makes up events to fill in memory gaps, they're displaying confabulation.

Scoring

 If you answered all four questions correctly, fantastic! We're compelled to tell you that you're a master of mental health assessments.

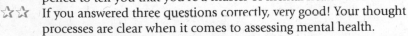 If you answered three questions correctly, very good! Your thought processes are clear when it comes to assessing mental health.

If you answered fewer than three questions correctly, try not to get too down! After a break to refresh your mental health, try reading the chapter again.

Part II

Assessing body systems

5	Skin, hair, and nails	75
6	Neurologic system	103
7	Eyes	137
8	Ears, nose, and throat	163
9	Cardiovascular system	193
10	Respiratory system	231
11	Breasts and axillae	269
12	Gastrointestinal system	287
13	Female genitourinary system	315
14	Male genitourinary system	367
15	Musculoskeletal system	389

Chapter 5

Skin, hair, and nails

Just the facts

In this chapter, you'll learn:

◆ components of skin, hair, and nails

◆ changes in skin, hair, and nails that occur normally with aging as well as those that signal a health problem

◆ questions to ask about skin, hair, and nails during the health history

◆ techniques for assessing skin, hair, and nails

◆ abnormalities of skin, hair, and nails and their causes.

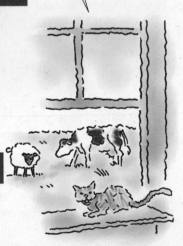

The skin, hair, and nails are like windows into a patient's health.

A look at skin, hair, and nails

The skin covers the internal structures of the body and protects them from the external world. Along with hair and nails, the skin provides a window for viewing changes taking place inside the body. As a nurse, you observe a patient's skin, hair, and nails regularly, so it's likely that you would be the first to detect abnormalities. Your sharp assessment skills will help supply a reliable picture of the patient's overall health.

Anatomy and physiology

To perform an accurate physical assessment, you'll need to understand the anatomy and physiology of the skin, hair, and nails. Let's review them one by one.

Skin

Also called the *integumentary system,* the skin is the body's largest organ and has several important functions, including:

- protecting the internal structures and tissues from trauma and bacteria
- preventing the loss of water and electrolytes from the body
- sensing temperature, pain, touch, and pressure
- regulating body temperature through sweat production and evaporation
- synthesizing vitamin D
- promoting wound repair by allowing cell replacement of surface wounds.

Layers of the skin

The skin consists of two distinct layers: the epidermis and the dermis. Subcutaneous tissue lies beneath these layers. The epidermis—the outer layer—is made of squamous epithelial tissue. It's thin and contains no blood vessels. The two major layers of the epidermis are the stratum corneum—the most superficial layer—and the deeper basal cell layer, or stratum basale. (See *A close look at skin.*)

Travel Plans

The stratum corneum is made up of cells that form in the basal cell layer, then travel to the skin's outer surface, and die as they reach the surface. However, because epidermal regeneration is continuous, new cells are constantly being produced.

The basal cell layer contains melanocytes, which produce melanin and are responsible for skin color. Hormones, the environment, and heredity influence melanocyte production. Because melanocyte production is greater in some people than in others, skin color varies considerably. Sun exposure can also increase melanocyte production.

Laying it on thick

The dermis—the thick, deeper layer of the skin—consists of connective tissue and an extracellular material called *matrix,* which contributes to the skin's strength and pliability. Blood vessels, lymphatic vessels, nerves, and hair follicles are located in the dermis, as are sweat and sebaceous glands. Because it's well supplied with blood, the dermis delivers nutrition to the epidermis. In addition, wound healing and infection control take place in the dermis.

A close look at skin

This cross section of the skin illustrates major skin structures.

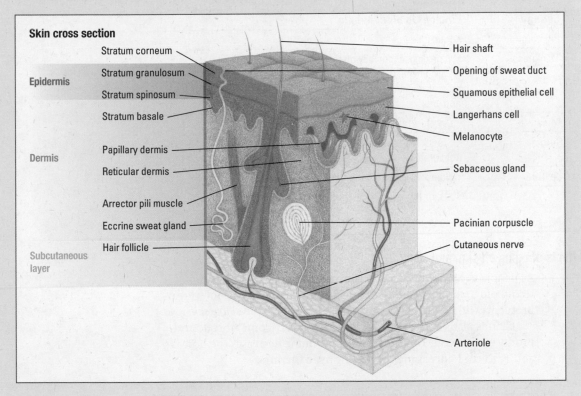

Skin cross section

Epidermis
- Stratum corneum
- Stratum granulosum
- Stratum spinosum
- Stratum basale

Dermis
- Papillary dermis
- Reticular dermis
- Arrector pili muscle
- Eccrine sweat gland

Subcutaneous layer
- Hair follicle

- Hair shaft
- Opening of sweat duct
- Squamous epithelial cell
- Langerhans cell
- Melanocyte
- Sebaceous gland
- Pacinian corpuscle
- Cutaneous nerve
- Arteriole

Give the glands a hand!

Sebaceous glands, found primarily in the skin of the scalp, face, upper body, and genital region, are part of the same structure that contains the hair follicles. Their main function is to produce sebum, which is secreted onto the skin or into the hair follicle to make the hair shiny and pliant.

There are two types of sweat glands:
- The eccrine glands, which are located over most of the body, produce a watery fluid that helps regulate body temperature.
- Apocrine glands secrete a milky substance and open into the hair follicle. They're located mainly in the axillae and the genital areas.

How skin ages

This table lists skin changes that normally occur with aging.

Change	Findings in older people
Pigmentation	• Pale color
Thickness	• Wrinkling, especially on the face, arms, and legs • Parchmentlike appearance, especially over bony prominences and on the dorsal surfaces of the hands, feet, arms, and legs
Moisture	• Dry, flaky, and rough
Turgor	• "Tents" and stands alone, especially if the patient is dehydrated
Texture	• Numerous creases and lines

Effects of aging on skin and glands

As people age, skin functions decline and normal changes occur. As a result, older adult patients are more prone to skin disease, infection, problems with wound healing, and tissue atrophy. (See *How skin ages*.)

Glands also change with age; sweat glands become fibrotic and produce less sweat. This drop in sweat volume decreases the body's ability to cool, increasing the risk for hyperthermia.

Hair

Hair is formed from keratin and produced by matrix cells in the dermal layer. Each hair lies in a hair follicle and receives nourishment from a papilla, a loop of capillaries at the base of the follicle. At the lower end of the hair shaft is the hair bulb. The hair bulb contains melanocytes, which determine hair color. (See *A close look at hair*.)

Each hair is attached at the base to a smooth muscle called the *arrector pili*. This muscle contracts during emotional stress or exposure to cold and elevates the hair, causing goose bumps.

A close look at hair

The illustration below shows a hair shaft and its associated glands.

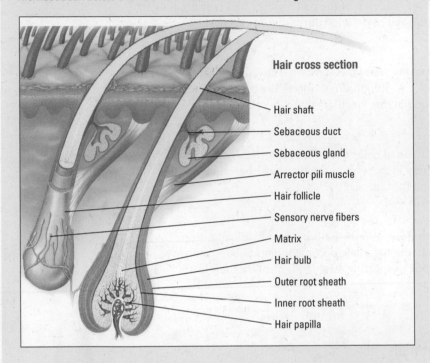

Hair cross section

- Hair shaft
- Sebaceous duct
- Sebaceous gland
- Arrector pili muscle
- Hair follicle
- Sensory nerve fibers
- Matrix
- Hair bulb
- Outer root sheath
- Inner root sheath
- Hair papilla

Hair today, gone tomorrow

A neonate's skin is covered with lanugo, a fine, downy growth of hair. Lanugo can be located over the entire body but occurs mostly on the shoulders and back. Most of the lanugo is shed within 2 weeks of birth. The amount of hair on a neonate's head varies, and all of the original hair is lost several weeks after birth. It slowly grows back, sometimes in a different color.

As a person ages, melanocyte function declines, producing light or gray hair, and the hair follicle itself becomes drier as sebaceous gland function decreases. Hair growth declines, so the amount of body hair decreases. Balding, which is genetically determined in younger individuals, occurs in many people as a normal result of aging.

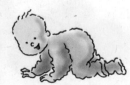

Hair changes throughout the life span.

Nails

Nails are formed when epidermal cells are converted into hard plates of keratin. The nails are made up of the nail root (or nail matrix), nail plate, nail bed, lunula, nail folds, and cuticle. (See *A close look at nails*.)

What's on your plate?

The nail plate is the visible, hardened layer that covers the fingertip. The plate is clear with fine longitudinal ridges. The pink color results from blood vessels underlying vascular epithelial cells.

What is the matrix?

The nail matrix is the site of nail growth. It's protected by the cuticle. At the end of the matrix is the white, crescent-shaped area, the lunula, which extends beyond the cuticle.

Not hard as nails anymore

With age, nail growth slows and the nails become brittle and thin. Longitudinal ridges in the nail plate become much more pronounced, making the nails prone to splitting. Also, the nails lose their luster and become yellowed.

A close look at nails

The illustration below shows the anatomic components of a fingernail.

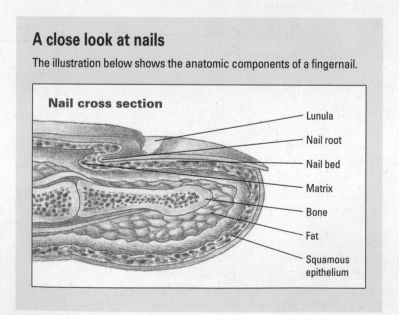

Obtaining a health history

When assessing a problem related to skin, hair, or nails, you need to thoroughly explore the patient's presenting problem, medical history, family history, psychological history, and patterns of daily living. Keep in mind that skin, hair, and nail abnormalities may result from a medical problem related to the patient's presenting problem, but the patient may overlook or minimize them.

Asking about the skin

Most skin symptoms that patients report involve itching, rashes, lesions, pigmentation abnormalities, or changes in existing lesions.

Skin deep

Typical questions to ask about changes in a patient's skin include:
- How and when did the skin changes occur?
- Are the changes in the form of a skin rash or lesion?
- Is the change confined to one area, or has the condition spread?
- Does the area bleed or have drainage?
- Does the area itch?
- How much time do you spend in the sun, and how do you protect your skin from ultraviolet rays?
- Do you have allergies?
- Do you have a family history of skin cancer or other significant diseases?
- Do you have a fever or joint pain, or have you lost weight?
- Have you had a recent insect bite?
- Do you take any drugs or herbal preparations? If so, which ones?
- What changes in your skin have you observed in the past few years?
- What skin products do you use?
- Have you recently changed or added new soaps, detergents, or dryer sheets?
  (See *Additional history questions for infants and children*, page 82.)

Asking about the hair

Most concerns about the hair refer either to hair loss or hirsutism, an increased growth and distribution of body hair. Either of these problems can be caused by such factors as skin infections, ovarian or adrenal tumors, increased stress, or systemic diseases, such as hypothyroidism and malignancies.

Getting to the root of the problem

To identify the cause of your patient's hair problem, ask:
- When did you first notice the loss (or gain) of hair? Was it sudden or gradual?
- Did the change occur in just a few spots or all over your body?
- What was happening in your life when the problem started?
- Do you take any medications or herbal preparations? If so, which ones?
- Are you experiencing itching, pain, discharge, fever, or weight loss?
- What serious illnesses, if any, have you had?
- Have you ever had hair replacements?
- Have you ever experienced hair loss (or gain) before?
- Do you use hair dye? How often?

Asking about the nails

Most concerns about the nails involves changes in growth or color. Either of these problems may result from infection, nutritional deficiencies, systemic illnesses, or stress.

Nailing down the details

Typical questions to ask about changes in a patient's nails include:
- When did you first notice the changes in your nails?
- What types of changes have you noticed (for example, nail shape, color, lines, or brittleness)?
- Were the changes sudden or gradual?
- Do you have other signs or symptoms, such as bleeding, pain, itching, or discharge?
- What's the normal condition of your nails?
- Do you have a history of serious illness?
- Do you have a history of nail problems?
- Do you bite your nails?
- Have you had nail tips attached?

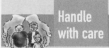

Handle with care

Additional history questions for infants and children

Remember to ask the parents these questions when obtaining a history for infants and children:
- Does the child have any birthmarks?
- When the child was a newborn, did they experience any change in skin color—for example, cyanosis or jaundice?
- Have you noted any rashes, burns, or bruises? If so, where and when, and what was the cause?
- Has the child been exposed to any contagious skin conditions—such as scabies, lice, or impetigo—or communicable diseases?

Assessing skin, hair, and nails

To assess skin, hair, and nails, you'll use the techniques of inspection and palpation. Before beginning the examination, make sure the room is well lit and comfortably warm. Wear gloves during your examination.

Skin

Before you begin your skin assessment, gather these items: a clear ruler with centimeter and millimeter markings, a tongue blade, a penlight or flashlight, a Wood's lamp, and a magnifying glass. This equipment enables you to measure and closely inspect skin lesions and other abnormalities.

The big picture

Start by observing the skin's overall appearance. Such observation can help you identify areas that need further assessment. Inspect and palpate the skin area by area, focusing on color, texture, turgor, moisture, and temperature.

Color

Look for localized areas of bruising, cyanosis, pallor, and erythema. Check for uniformity of color and hypopigmented or hyperpigmented areas. Note any scars.

A spotty record

Places exposed to the sun may show a darker pigmentation than other areas. Color changes may vary depending on skin pigmentation. (See *Detecting color variations in people with dark skin.*) Be aware that some local skin color changes are normal variations that appear in certain populations. (See *Congenital dermal melanocytosis.*)

Bridging the gap

Congenital dermal melanocytosis

Congenital dermal melanocytosis is a type of birthmark characterized by irregularly shaped areas of deep blue pigmentation. These birthmarks most commonly occur over the sacral and gluteal areas but may also appear on the shoulders, arms, abdomen, or thighs. These bluish discolored areas are normal variations of the skin in children of African, Asian, or Latin descent. In fact, 90% of Black children and 80% of Asian children have congenital dermal melanocytosis.

Congenital dermal melanocytosis is present at birth and usually remains visible into adulthood, although it may fade over time. It results from deposits of embryonic pigment in the epidermal layer left behind from fetal development.

Congenital dermal melanocytosis is completely benign and requires no treatment. When assessing children, be careful not to confuse these spots with bruises, which may cause an erroneous suspicion of child abuse.

Detecting color variations in people with dark skin

Cyanosis
Examine the conjunctivae, palms, soles, buccal mucosa, and tongue. Look for dull, dark, bluish color.

Edema
Examine the area for decreased color and palpate for tightness.

Erythema
Palpate the area for redness and/or warmth.

Jaundice
Examine the sclerae and hard palate in natural, not fluorescent, light if possible. Look for a yellow color.

Pallor
Examine the sclerae, conjunctivae, buccal mucosa, lips, tongue, nail beds, palms, and soles. Look for an ashen, grayish blue color.

Petechiae
Examine areas of lighter pigmentation such as the abdomen. Look for tiny, purplish red dots.

Rashes
Palpate the area for skin texture changes

Texture and turgor

Inspect and palpate the skin's texture, noting its thickness and mobility. It should look smooth and be intact. Rough, dry skin is common in patients with hypothyroidism, psoriasis, and excessive keratinization. Skin that isn't intact may indicate local irritation or trauma.

Turgor-nomics

Palpation also helps you evaluate the patient's hydration status. Dehydration and edema cause poor skin turgor. Note, however, that because poor skin turgor may also be caused by aging, it may not be a reliable indicator of an older adult patient's hydration status. Overhydration causes skin to appear edematous and spongy. Localized edema can also result from trauma or systemic disease. (See *Evaluating skin turgor.*)

You'll use a slightly different technique to assess skin turgor on an infant. (See *Assessing an infant's skin turgor.*)

Moisture

Observe the skin's moisture content. The skin should be relatively dry, with a minimal amount of perspiration. Skinfold areas should also be fairly dry. Overly dry skin appears red and flaky.

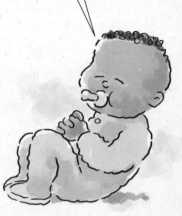

Assessing skin turgor in an infant calls for a different touch.

 Peak technique

Evaluating skin turgor

To assess skin turgor in an adult, gently squeeze the skin on the forearm or sternal area between your thumb and forefinger, as shown at right. Then release the skin.

If the skin quickly returns to its original shape, the patient has normal turgor. If it returns to its original shape slowly over 30 seconds or maintains a tented position, as shown at right, the skin has poor turgor.

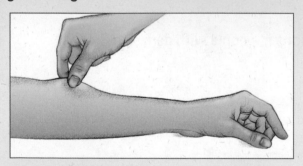

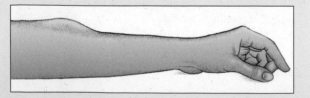

 Handle with care

Assessing an infant's skin turgor

To assess an infant's skin turgor, you'll grasp a fold of loosely adherent abdominal skin between your thumb and forefinger instead of skin on the forearm or sternal area, as you would for an adult. Pull the skin taut and then release it. The skin should return quickly to its normal position. If the skin stays tented, the infant has poor turgor and may be dehydrated.

All in a sweat

Overly moist skin can be caused by anxiety, obesity, or an environment that's too warm. Heavy sweating, or diaphoresis, usually accompanies fever; strenuous activity; cardiac, pulmonary, and other diseases; and any activity or illness that elevates metabolic rate.

Temperature

Palpate the skin bilaterally for temperature, which can range from cool to warm. Warm skin suggests normal circulation; cool skin, a possible underlying disorder. Distinguish between generalized and localized coolness and warmth. Localized skin coolness can result from vasoconstriction associated with cold environments or impaired arterial circulation to a limb. General coolness can result from such conditions as shock or hypothyroidism. (See *Assessing skin temperature*.)

Hot and bothered

Localized warmth occurs in areas that are infected, inflamed, or burned. Generalized warmth occurs with fever or systemic diseases such as hyperthyroidism. Be sure to check skin temperature bilaterally.

Lesions

During your inspection, you may see normal variations in the skin's texture and pigmentation.

Denoting disease

Red lesions caused by vascular changes include hemangiomas, scars, telangiectases, petechiae, purpura, and ecchymoses and may indicate disease.

Stamp of approval

Normal variations include birthmarks, freckles, and nevi, or moles. Birthmarks are generally flat and range in color from tan to red or brown. They can be found on all areas of the body. Freckles are small, flat macules located primarily on the face, arms, and back. They're usually red brown to brown. Nevi are either flat or raised and may be pink, tan, or dark brown. Like birthmarks, they can be found on all areas of the body.

New or not?

When investigating a lesion, start by classifying it as primary or secondary. A primary lesion is new. Changes in a primary lesion constitute a secondary lesion. Examples of secondary lesions include fissures, scales, crusts, scars, and excoriations. (See *Lesion distribution*.)

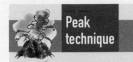

Peak technique

Assessing skin temperature

When you're trying to compare subtle temperature differences in one area of the body with those in another, use the dorsal surface of your hands and fingers. They're the most sensitive to changes in temperature.

Lesion distribution

Generalized—distributed all over the body
Regionalized—limited to one area of the body
Localized—sharply limited to a specific area
Scattered—dispersed either densely or widely
Exposed areas—limited to areas exposed to the air or sun
Intertriginous—limited to areas where skin comes in contact with itself

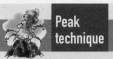

Peak technique

Illuminating lesions

Illuminating a lesion can help you see it better and learn more about its characteristics. Here are two techniques worth perfecting.

Macule or papule?
To determine whether a lesion is a macule or a papule, use this technique: Reduce the direct lighting and shine a penlight or flashlight at a right angle to the lesion. If the light casts a shadow, the lesion is a papule. Macules are flat and don't produce shadows.

Solid or fluid-filled?
To determine whether a lesion is solid or fluid-filled, use this technique: Place the tip of a flashlight or penlight against the side of the lesion. Solid lesions don't transmit light. Fluid-filled lesions transilluminate with a red glow.

It's what's inside that counts

Palpate the lesion to determine if it's solid or fluid-filled. Macules, papules, nodules, wheals, and hives are solid lesions. Vesicles, bullae, pustules, and cysts are fluid-filled lesions. You can also use a flashlight or penlight to determine whether a lesion is solid or fluid-filled. (See *Illuminating lesions*.)

Wood you light my lesion?

To identify lesions that fluoresce, use a Wood's lamp, which gives out specially filtered ultraviolet light. Darken the room and shine the light on the lesion. If the lesion looks bluish green, the patient has a fungal infection.

Lesion lowdown

After you've identified the type of lesion, you'll need to describe its characteristics, pattern, location, and distribution. A detailed description can help you determine whether the lesion is a normal or pathologic skin change. (See *Types of skin lesions*.)

Border patrol

Examine the lesion to see if it looks the same on both sides. Also, check the borders to see if they're regular or irregular. An asymmetrical lesion with an irregular border may indicate malignancy.

A horse of a different color

Lesions occur in various colors and can change color over time. Therefore, watch for such changes in your patient. For example, if a lesion such as a mole (nevus) has changed from tan or brown to multiple shades of tan, dark brown, black, or a mixture of red, white, and blue, the lesion might be malignant.

Types of skin lesions

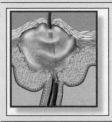

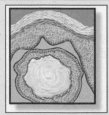

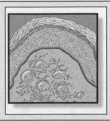

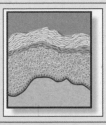

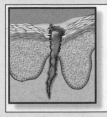

Pustule	*Cyst*	*Nodule*	*Wheal*	*Fissure*
A small, pus-filled lesion (called a *follicular pustule* if it contains a hair)	A closed sac in or under the skin that contains fluid or semisolid material	A raised lesion detectable by touch that's usually 1 cm or more in diameter	A raised, reddish area that's commonly itchy and lasts 24 hours or less	A painful, cracklike lesion of the skin that extends at least into the dermis

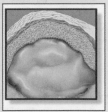

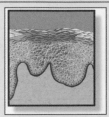

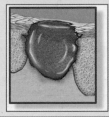

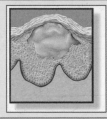

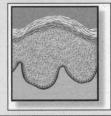

Bulla	*Macule*	*Ulcer*	*Vesicle*	*Papule*
A large, fluid-filled blister that's usually 1 cm or more in diameter	A small, discolored spot or patch on the skin	A craterlike lesion of the skin that usually extends at least into the dermis	A small, fluid-filled blister that's usually 1 cm or less in diameter	A solid, raised lesion that's usually less than 1 cm in diameter

Follow the pattern

Pay close attention as well to the shape, configuration, and distribution of the lesions. Many skin diseases have typical configuration patterns. Identifying those patterns can help you determine the cause of the problem. (See *Recognizing common lesion configurations*.)

Sizing up the situation

Measure the diameter of the lesion using a millimeter-centimeter ruler. If you estimate the diameter, you may not be able to determine subtle changes in size. An increase in the size or elevation of a mole over many years is common and probably normal. Still, be sure to take note of moles that rapidly change size, especially moles that are 6 mm or larger.

Recognizing common lesion configurations

Identify the configuration of your patient's skin lesion by matching it to one of these diagrams.

Discrete
Individual lesions are separate and distinct.

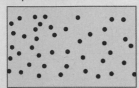

Grouped
Lesions are clustered together.

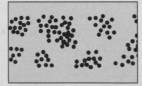

Confluent
Lesions merge so that individual lesions aren't visible or palpable.

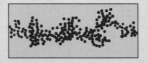

Linear
Lesions form a line.

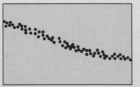

Annular
Lesions are arranged in a single ring or circle.

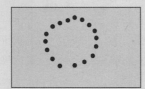

Polycyclic
Lesions are arranged in multiple circles.

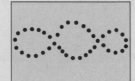

Arciform
Lesions form arcs or curves.

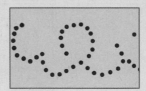

Reticular
Lesions form a meshlike network.

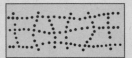

If you note drainage, document the type, color, and amount. Also note if the lesion has a foul odor, which can indicate a superimposed infection.

Hair

Start by inspecting and palpating the hair over the patient's entire body, not just on the head. Note the distribution, quantity, texture, and color. The quantity and distribution of head and body hair vary between patients. However, hair should be evenly distributed over the entire body.

Too much or too little?

Check for patterns of hair loss and growth. If you notice patchy hair loss, look for regrowth. Also, examine the scalp for erythema, scaling, and encrustation. Excessive hair loss with scalp crusting may indicate ringworm infestation. The only way to detect scalp crusting is by using a Wood's lamp. Also, note areas of excessive hair growth, which may indicate a hormone imbalance or be a sign of a systemic disorder such as Cushing syndrome.

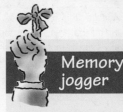

Memory jogger

To remember what to assess when evaluating a lesion, think of the letters **ABCDE**:

Asymmetry

Border

Color and Configuration

Diameter and Drainage

Evolution or progression of the lesion.

Having a bad hair day?

The texture of scalp hair also varies between patients. As a rule, hair should be shiny and smooth, not dry or brittle. Differences in grooming and use of hair products may affect the hair's texture and quality. Dryness or brittleness can result from the use of harsh hair treatments or hair care products or can be caused by a systemic illness. Extreme oiliness is usually related to excessive sebum production or poor grooming habits.

Nails

Assessing the nails is vital for two reasons: The appearance of the nails can be a critical indicator of systemic illness, and their overall condition tells you a lot about the patient's grooming habits and ability to care for themselves. Examine the nails for color, shape, thickness, consistency, and contour.

Nail that color

First, look at the color of the nails. People with light skin generally have pinkish nails. People with dark skin generally have brown nails. Brown-pigmented bands in the nail beds are normal in people with dark skin and abnormal in people with light skin. Yellow nails may occur in people who smoke as a result of nicotine stains.

Circulation check

Nail beds can be used to assess a patient's peripheral circulation. Press on the nail bed and then release, noting how long the color takes to return. It should return immediately, or at least within 3 seconds.

What shapely nails!

Next, inspect the shape and contour of the nails. The surface of the nail bed should be either slightly curved or flat. The edges of the nail should be smooth, rounded, and clean.

What's the angle?

The angle of the nail base is normally less than 180°. An increase in the nail angle suggests clubbing. Curved nails are a normal variation. They may appear to be clubbed until you notice that the nail angle is still less than 180°.

Thick and strong?

Finally, palpate the nail bed to check the thickness of the nail and the strength of its attachment to the bed.

Abnormal findings

Various abnormalities may be found when assessing the skin, hair, and nails. Because these abnormalities may be visible to others, the patient may experience some degree of emotional stress. Carefully document all abnormal findings, pertinent health history, and as much information as possible from the physical examination. (See *Skin, hair, and nail abnormalities*, pages 91 and 92.)

Skin abnormalities

The signs and symptoms you detect during your assessment may be caused by a wide variety of disorders. This section and the chart *Skin color variations* on page 93 describe the most common skin abnormalities. (See also *Recognizing common skin disorders*, page 94.)

Café-au-lait spots

Café-au-lait spots appear as flat, light brown, uniformly hyperpigmented macules or patches on the skin surface. They usually appear during the first 3 years of life but may develop at any age.

Coffee, anyone?

Café-au-lait spots can be differentiated from freckles and other benign birthmarks by their larger size and irregular shape. They usually have no significance; however, six or more café-au-lait spots may be associated with an underlying neurologic disorder such as neurofibromatosis.

Cherry angiomas

Cherry angiomas are tiny, bright red, round papules that may become brown over time. These clinically insignificant lesions occur in virtually everyone older than age 30 and increase in number with age.

Hemangiomas

Hemangiomas, commonly called *port-wine stains* or *birthmarks,* are red skin lesions in the top layer of the skin (capillary hemangiomas). They are usually present at birth and commonly appear on the face and upper body as flat purple marks. Cavernous hemangiomas occur deeper in the skin and eventually distort the skin.

Papular rash

A papular rash consists of small, raised, circumscribed—and perhaps discolored (red to purple)—lesions known as *papules.* It may erupt anywhere on the body in various configurations and may be acute or chronic. Papular rashes characterize skin disorders; they may also result from allergies or from infectious, neoplastic, and systemic disorders.

Interpretation station

Skin, hair, and nail abnormalities

After you assess the patient, a group of findings may lead you to suspect a particular disorder. The chart below shows common groups of findings for the abnormal signs and symptoms of the integumentary system, along with their probable causes.

Sign or symptom and findings	Probable cause
Alopecia	
• Patchy alopecia, typically on the lower extremities • Thin, shiny, atrophic skin • Thickened nails • Weak or absent peripheral pulses • Cool extremities • Paresthesia	Arterial insufficiency
• Translucent, charred or ulcerated skin • Pain	Burns
• Loss of the outer third of the eyebrows • Thin, dull, coarse, brittle hair on the face • Fatigue • Constipation • Cold intolerance • Weight gain • Puffy face, hands, and feet	Hypothyroidism
Clubbing	
• Anorexia • Malaise • Dyspnea • Tachypnea • Diminished breath sounds • Pursed-lip breathing • Barrel chest • Peripheral cyanosis	Emphysema

Sign or symptom and findings	Probable cause
• Wheezing • Dyspnea • Fatigue • Jugular vein distention • Palpitations • Unexplained weight gain • Dependent edema • Crackles on auscultation	Heart failure
• Hemoptysis • Dyspnea • Wheezing • Chest pain • Fatigue • Weight loss • Fever	Lung and pleural cancer
Pruritus	
• Intense, severe pruritus • Erythematous rash on dry skin at flexion points • Possible edema, scaling, and pustules	Atopic dermatitis
• Scalp excoriation from scratching • Matted, foul-smelling, lusterless hair • Occipital and cervical lymphadenopathy • Oval, gray-white nits on hair shafts	Pediculosis capitis (head lice)

(Continued)

Skin, hair, and nail abnormalities *(continued)*

Sign or symptom and findings	Probable cause	Sign or symptom and findings	Probable cause
• Gradual or sudden pruritus • Ammonia breath odor • Oliguria or anuria • Fatigue • Irritability • Muscle cramps	Chronic kidney failure	• Nonpitting, nonpruritic edema of an extremity or the face • Possibly acute laryngeal edema	Hereditary angioedema
Urticaria		• Erythema chronicum migrans that results in urticaria • Constant malaise and fatigue • Fever • Chills • Lymphadenopathy • Neurologic and cardiac abnormalities • Arthritis	Lyme disease
• Rapid eruption of diffuse urticaria and angioedema, with wheals ranging from pinpoint to palm size or larger • Pruritic, stinging lesions • Profound anxiety • Weakness • Shortness of breath • Nasal congestion • Dysphagia • Warm, moist skin	Anaphylaxis		

Pressure ulcers

A pressure ulcer is a localized area of skin or tissue breakdown (or both) that results from prolonged pressure, commonly over a bony prominence. The pressure compromises the area's vascular supply, leading to the development of necrotic tissue. Shear and friction also contribute to the breakdown. Any pressure ulcer detected requires assessment and documentation; many facilities also require a photograph of the affected area. (See *Staging pressure ulcers*.) Older adult patients are more susceptible to pressure injuries as a result of decreased mobility and skin alterations with age.

Pruritus

Commonly provoking scratching to obtain relief, this unpleasant itching sensation is the most common symptom of skin disorders.

I've got you under my skin

Pruritus may also result from a local or systemic disorder, drug use, emotional upset, or contact with skin irritants. Pruritus may be exacerbated by increased skin temperature, poor skin turgor, local vasodilation, dermatoses, and stress.

Interpretation station

Skin color variations

To interpret skin color variation findings faster, refer to this chart.

Color	Distribution	Possible cause
Absent	• Small, circumscribed areas • Generalized	• Vitiligo • Albinism
Blue	• Around lips, buccal mucosa, or generalized	• Cyanosis (*Note:* In Black people, blue gingivae is a normal finding.)
Deep red	• Generalized	• Polycythemia vera (increased red blood cell count)
Pink	• Local or generalized	• Erythema (superficial capillary dilation and congestion)
Tan to brown	• Facial patches	• Chloasma of pregnancy; butterfly rash of lupus erythematosus
Tan to brown-bronze	• Generalized (not related to sun exposure)	• Addison disease
Yellow to yellowish brown	• Sclera or generalized	• Jaundice from liver dysfunction (*Note:* In Black people, yellowish brown pigmentation of sclera is a normal finding.)
Yellowish orange	• Palms, soles, and face; not sclera	• Carotenemia (carotene in the blood)

Purpuric lesions

Purpuric lesions are caused by red blood cells and blood pigments in the skin, so they don't blanch under pressure.

On the spot
The three types of purpuric lesions are:
- petechiae—red or brown pinpoint lesions generally caused by capillary fragility; diseases associated with the formation of microemboli or bleeding, such as subacute bacterial endocarditis and thrombocytopenia, can cause petechiae
- ecchymoses—bluish or purplish discolorations resulting from blood accumulation in the skin after injury to the vessel walls
- hematomas—masses of blood that accumulate in a tissue, organ, or body space after a break in a blood vessel.

Cruisin' for a bruisin'
Purpuric lesions also produce deep red or reddish purple bruising that may be caused by bleeding disorders such as disseminated intravascular coagulation.

Recognizing common skin disorders

When assessing your patient's skin, keep an eye out for these common skin disorders.

Psoriasis

Psoriasis is a chronic disease of marked epidermal thickening. Plaques are symmetrical and generally appear as red bases topped with silvery scales. The lesions, which may connect with one another, occur most commonly on the scalp, elbows, and knees.

Urticaria (hives)

Occurring as an allergic reaction, urticaria appears suddenly as pink, edematous papules or wheals (round elevations of the skin). Itching is intense. The lesions may become large and contain vesicles.

Tinea corporis (ringworm)

Tinea corporis is characterized by round, red, scaly lesions that are accompanied by intense itching. These lesions have slightly raised, red borders consisting of tiny vesicles. Individual rings may connect to form patches with scalloped edges. They usually appear on exposed areas of the body.

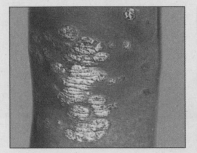

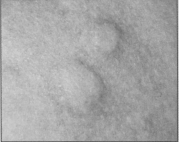

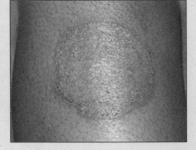

Contact dermatitis

Contact dermatitis is an inflammatory disorder that results from contact with an irritant. Primary lesions include vesicles, large oozing bullae, and red macules that appear at localized areas of redness. These lesions may itch and burn.

Herpes zoster

Herpes zoster appears as a group of vesicles or crusted lesions along a nerve root. The vesicles are usually unilateral and appear mostly on the trunk. These lesions cause pain but not a rash.

Scabies

Mites, which can be picked up from an infested person, burrow under the skin and cause scabies lesions. The lesions appear in a straight or zigzagging line about 3/8" (1 cm) long with a black dot at the end. Commonly seen between the fingers, at the bend of the elbow and knee, and around the groin, abdomen, or perineal area, scabies lesions itch and may cause a rash.

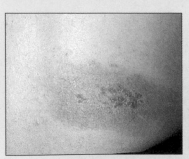

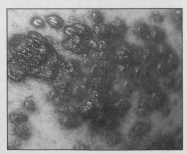

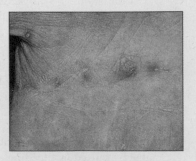

Staging pressure ulcers

You can use characteristics gained from your assessment to stage a pressure ulcer, as described here. Staging reflects the anatomic depth of exposed tissue. Keep in mind that if the wound contains necrotic tissue, you won't be able to determine the stage until you can see the wound base.

Suspected deep tissue injury
• Maroon or purple intact skin or blood-filled blister
• May be painful; mushy, firm, or boggy; and warmer or cooler than other tissue before discoloration occurs

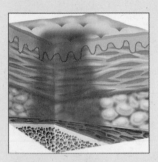

Stage I
• Intact skin that doesn't blanch
• May differ in color from surrounding area in people with darkly pigmented skin
• Usually over a bony prominence
• May be painful, firm or soft, and warmer or cooler than surrounding tissue

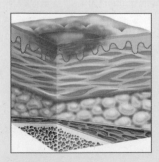

Stage II
• Superficial partial-thickness wound

• Presents as a shallow, open ulcer without slough and with a red and pink wound bed
    Note: This stage shouldn't be used to describe perineal dermatitis, maceration, tape burns, skin tears, or excoriation.

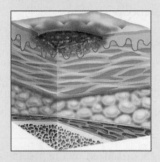

Stage III
• Involves full-thickness wound with tissue loss and possibly visible subcutaneous tissue but no exposed muscle, tendon, or bone
• May have slough but not enough to hide the depth of tissue loss
• May be accompanied by undermining and tunneling

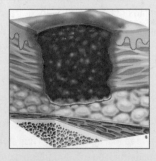

Stage IV
• Involves full-thickness skin loss, with exposed muscle, bone, and tendon

• May be accompanied by eschar, slough, undermining, and tunneling

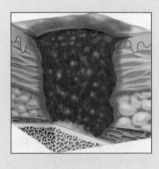

Unstageable
• Involves full-thickness tissue loss, with base of ulcer covered by slough and yellow, tan, gray, green, or brown eschar
• Can't be staged until enough slough and eschar are removed to expose the wound base

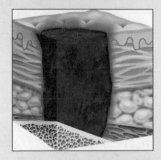

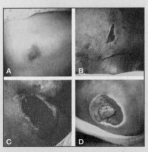

Scars

A scar consists of new collagen fibers that replace normal skin after the dermis is injured. Sweat glands and hair follicles don't grow in scar tissue. Initially, a scar may be red and raised, but it becomes flat and pale over time. How the wound heals determines a scar's shape. Overproduction of collagen tissue may result in a hypertrophic or keloid scar. (See *Types of scars*.)

Telangiectases

Telangiectases are permanently dilated, small blood vessels that typically form a weblike pattern. For example, spider hemangiomas, a type of telangiectasis, are small, red lesions arranged in a weblike configuration. They usually appear on the face, neck, and chest and may be normal or associated with pregnancy or cirrhosis.

Urticaria

Urticaria is a vascular skin reaction characterized by the eruption of transient pruritic wheals—smooth, slightly elevated patches with well-defined erythematous margins and pale centers of various shapes and sizes.

Allergy alert

Urticaria lesions, also called *hives,* are produced by the local release of histamine or other vasoactive substances as part of a hypersensitivity reaction, commonly to certain drugs, foods, insect bites, or inhalants or because of contact with certain substances. Urticaria may also result from emotional stress or environmental factors.

Types of scars

Scar tissue forms when a wound heals. It has a different texture and quality than normal tissue. Although typically a cosmetic problem, scars can still cause a patient distress. Several types of scars may form:

• *Acne scars* are pitting or sunken recesses in the skin that result from acne. They're also called *ice-pick scars* or *depressed fibrotic scars.*

• A *contracture scar* is a tightening of the skin that may impede mobility. Such scars usually result from a wound that affects muscle and nerves and commonly result from burns.

• A *hypertrophic scar* is a red, raised bump on the skin that doesn't exceed the wound boundaries. Surgery or trauma causes these scars.

• A *keloid scar* is an overgrowth of colloid tissue that results in a benign tumorous type of growth. It can result from surgery, trauma, or acne.

• *Stretch marks*—also called *striae distensae*—are reddish or purple lines that fade to a lighter color. They stem from dermal tearing during rapid growth, usually over areas where large amounts of fat are stored, such as the abdomen, hips, or buttocks.

Vesicular rash

A vesicular rash is a scattered or linear distribution of blisterlike lesions—sharply circumscribed and filled with clear, cloudy, or bloody fluid. The lesions, which are usually less than 0.5 cm in diameter, may occur singly or in groups. They sometimes occur with bullae—fluid-filled lesions larger than 0.5 cm in diameter.

A vesicular rash may be mild or severe and temporary or permanent. It can result from infection, inflammation, or allergic reactions.

Hair abnormalities

Typically stemming from other problems, hair abnormalities can cause patients emotional distress. Among the most common hair abnormalities are alopecia and hirsutism.

Alopecia

Alopecia occurs more commonly and extensively in men than in women. Diffuse hair loss, although commonly a normal part of aging, may occur as a result of pyrogenic infections, chemical trauma, ingestion of certain drugs, and endocrinopathy and other disorders. Tinea capitis, trauma, and third-degree burns can cause patchy hair loss.

Hirsutism

Excessive hairiness in women, or hirsutism, can develop on the body and face, affecting the patient's self-image. Localized hirsutism may occur on pigmented nevi. Generalized hirsutism can result from certain drug therapy or from such endocrine problems as Cushing syndrome and acromegaly.

Nail abnormalities

Although many nail abnormalities are harmless, some point to serious underlying problems. Common nail problems include Beau lines, clubbing, koilonychia, Muehrcke lines, onycholysis, and Terry nails.

Beau lines

Beau lines are transverse depressions in the nail that extend to the nail bed. These depressions occur at the same spot in most or all of the patient's nail beds. They occur with acute illness, malnutrition, anemia, and trauma that temporarily impairs nail function. A dent appears first at the cuticle and then moves forward as the nail grows.

Clubbing

With clubbed fingers, the proximal edge of the nail elevates so the angle is greater than 180°. The nail is also thickened and curved at the end, and the distal phalanx looks rounder and wider than normal. To check for clubbing, view the index finger in profile and note the angle of the nail base. (See *Evaluating clubbed fingers*.)

Koilonychia

Koilonychia refers to thin, spoon-shaped nails with lateral edges that tilt upward, forming a concave profile. The nails are white and opaque. This condition is associated with hypochromic anemia, chronic infections, Raynaud disease, and malnutrition.

Muehrcke lines

Muehrcke lines are transverse bands of white that go across the nail in pairs. They disappear when the nail bed is depressed, which compresses the vascular supply below the nail bed. The lines don't

Peak technique

Evaluating clubbed fingers

Think hypoxia when you see a patient whose fingers are clubbed. To quickly examine a patient's fingers for early clubbing, gently palpate the bases of their nails. Normally, they'll feel firm, but in early clubbing, they'll feel springy.

To evaluate late clubbing, have the patient place the first phalanges of the forefingers together. Normal nail bases are concave and create a small, diamond-shaped space when the first phalanges are opposed, as shown at top right.

In late clubbing, the now convex nail bases can touch without leaving a space (Schamroth sign), as shown at bottom right. This condition is associated with pulmonary and cardiovascular disease. When you spot clubbed fingers, think about the possible causes, such as emphysema, chronic bronchitis, lung cancer, and chronic heart failure.

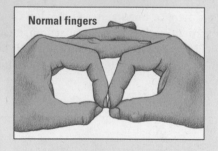

Normal fingers

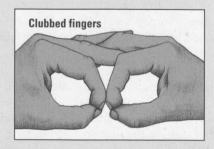

Clubbed fingers

change with nail growth because they occur within the vascular bed. Muehrcke lines are associated with hypoalbuminemia and disappear when the albumin level returns to normal.

Onycholysis

Onycholysis is the loosening of the nail plate with separation from the nail bed, which begins at the distal groove. It's associated with minor trauma to long fingernails and such disease processes as psoriasis, contact dermatitis, hyperthyroidism, and *Pseudomonas* infections.

Terry nails

In patients with Terry nails, the nail beds are white and look like ground glass. The lunula can't be seen. Terry nails may affect one or all nail beds. This finding commonly occurs with severe liver disease.

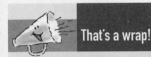

That's a wrap!

Skin, hair, and nails review

Health history
- Determine the patient's presenting problem.
- Ask the patient about skin changes, the presence of lesions, and exposure to sun.
- Ask about a family history of allergies or skin cancer.
- Ask about hair loss or gain, and about sudden or gradual nail changes.
- Ask about associated signs and symptoms, such as discharge, fever, weight loss, and joint pain.
- Determine which drugs the patient takes, including herbal preparations and illegal or recreational drugs.

Skin
Structures
- Epidermis—thin outer layer composed of epithelial tissue
- Dermis—thick, deeper layer that contains blood vessels, lymphatic vessels, nerves, hair follicles, and sweat and sebaceous glands
- Subcutaneous tissue—innermost layer

Functions
- Protects tissues
- Prevents water and electrolyte losses
- Senses temperature, pain, touch, and pressure
- Regulates body temperature
- Synthesizes vitamin D
- Promotes wound repair

Assessment
- Inspect and palpate the texture—it should be smooth and intact.
- Observe for moisture content—it should be dry with a minimal amount of perspiration.
- Palpate the skin for temperature, checking each side for localized temperature changes.
- Observe for skin lesions.

Lesion assessment
- Classify the lesion as primary or secondary.
- Determine if it's solid or fluid-filled.
- Check the borders to see if they're regular or irregular.
- Note the lesion's color as well as its pattern, location, and distribution.
- Measure the lesion's diameter using a millimeter-centimeter ruler.
- Describe any drainage, noting the type, color, amount, and odor.

Abnormal findings
- Café-au-lait spots—flat, light brown, uniformly hyperpigmented macules or patches on the skin surface
- Cherry angiomas—tiny, bright red, round papules that may become brown over time

(Continued)

Skin, hair, and nails review *(continued)*

• Hemangiomas—flat, purple marks usually present at birth that may appear on the face and upper body
• Papular rash—small, raised, circumscribed, and perhaps discolored (red to purple) lesions appearing in various configurations
• Pressure ulcers—localized areas of skin or tissue breakdown that range in severity from suspected deep tissue injury, through stages I to IV, and up to unstageable ulcers
• Pruritus—unpleasant itching sensation
• Purpuric lesions—petechiae (brown, pinpoint lesions); ecchymoses (bluish or purplish discolorations); hematomas (masses of accumulated blood)
• Scars—collagen growth that occurs after an injury to the dermis
• Telangiectases—permanently dilated, small blood vessels typically in a weblike pattern
• Urticaria—vascular skin reaction of transient pruritic wheals
• Vesicular rash—scattered or linear distribution of blisterlike lesions filled with clear, cloudy, or bloody fluid

Hair
• Formed from keratin
• Lies in a hair follicle, receiving nourishment from the papilla, and is attached at the base by the arrector pili muscle

Assessment
• Inspect and palpate the hair over the patient's entire body, noting distribution, quantity, texture, and color.
• Check for patterns of hair loss and growth.
• Inspect the scalp for erythema, scaling, and encrustations.

Abnormal findings
• Alopecia—hair loss
• Hirsutism—excessive hairiness in women

Nails
Structures
• Nail root (or nail matrix)—site of nail growth
• Nail plate—visible, hardened layer that covers the fingertip
• Lunula—white, crescent-shaped area that extends beyond the cuticle

Assessment
• Examine the nails for color, shape, thickness, and consistency.

Abnormal findings
• Beau lines—transverse depressions in the nail extending to the bed
• Clubbing—proximal end of the nail elevates so the angle is greater than 180°
• Koilonychia—thin, spoon-shaped nails with lateral edges that tilt upward
• Muehrcke lines—transverse bands of white that go across the nail
• Onycholysis—nail plate loosening with separation from the nail bed
• Terry nails—nail beds that are white and look like ground glass

Quick quiz

1. A patient with darkly pigmented skin has been admitted to the hospital with hepatitis. How does the nurse assess for jaundice in this patient?
    A. Inspect the color of the sclera.
    B. Inspect genitalia for color.
    C. Blanch the fingernails.
    D. Jaundice cannot be assessed in patients with darkly pigmented skin.

Answer: A. Inspect the sclera, the white part of the eyes. This area will appear yellow tinted with the presence of jaundice.

2. Changes in melanocyte production in what layer of skin are responsible for hair and skin color changes?
    A. Dermis
    B. Epidermis
    C. Basal
    D. Stratum corneum

Answer: C. Melanocyte production happens in the basal layer. The amount of melanocyte determines skin and hair color.

3. What is one way to assess dehydration in infants?
    A. Hair length
    B. Skin turgor
    C. Color of nail beds
    D. Skin temperature

Answer: B. When skin is grasped, pulled taut, and released, it should return to its original state quickly. If it stays tented, it could indicate dehydration.

4. Which of the following should be documented in a wound with drainage?
    A. Amount
    B. Color
    C. Odor
    D. Type
    E. All of the above
    F. Answers A, B, and D

Answer: F. Wounds with any drainage should be described with amount, color, and type of drainage, and if there is a foul odor to drainage.

5.   What is determined by pressing the nail bed and assessing the time it takes for color to return?
A.   Pain to nails
B.   Circulation to extremities
C.   Whether patient smokes
D.   Whether patient is wearing fake nails

Answer: B. Color should return to nail bed in 3 seconds or less to indicate good circulation and tissue perfusion.

Scoring

☆☆☆   If you answered all five questions correctly, fabulous! You really nailed this chapter.

☆☆   If you answered four questions correctly, good work! We aren't splitting hairs when we say your assessment skills are growing.

☆   If you answered fewer than four questions correctly, don't despair. Take a little more time to get the skinny on this topic.

 Just for fun

Match the skin assessment finding in column 1 with its general corresponding color variation in column 2.

1. Congenital dermal melanocytosis
_____

2. Erythema _____

3. Jaundice _____

4. Pallor _____

5. Cyanosis _____

6. Telangiectases _____

7. Carotenemia _____

8. Port-wine stain _____

9. Freckles _____

10. Butterfly rash _____

A. Yellow
B. Red
C. Pink
D. Purple
E. Reddish brown
F. Blue
G. Ash-white
H. Yellowish orange
I. Tan to brown

Answer: 1. F, 2. C, 3. A, 4. G, 5. F, 6. B, 7. H, 8. D, 9. E, 10. I.

Chapter 6

Neurologic system

Just the facts

In this chapter, you'll learn:

- ◆ characteristics of the organs and structures of the neurologic system
- ◆ methods to obtain a patient history of neurologic function
- ◆ techniques to conduct a physical assessment of the neurologic system
- ◆ ways to recognize neurologic abnormalities.

A look at the neurologic system

The neurologic system controls body function and is related to every other body system. Consequently, patients who have diseases of other body systems can develop neurologic impairments related to the disease. For example, a patient who has heart surgery may then have a stroke.

Because the neurologic system is so complex, evaluating it can seem overwhelming at first. Although tests for neurologic status are extensive, they're also basic and straightforward. In fact, your daily nursing care routinely includes some of these tests.

Just talking with a patient helps you assess their orientation, level of consciousness (LOC), cognitive function, and ability to formulate and produce speech. Having them perform a simple task such as walking allows you to evaluate motor ability. Your knowledge of neurologic assessment techniques will enhance your patient care and may save some patients from irreversible neurologic damage.

The neurologic system controls body function and is related to every other body system.

103

Anatomy and physiology

The neurologic system is divided into the central nervous system (CNS), the peripheral nervous system (PNS), and the autonomic nervous system (ANS). Through complex and coordinated interactions, these three parts integrate all physical, intellectual, and emotional activities. Understanding how each part works is essential to conducting an accurate neurologic assessment.

Central nervous system

The CNS includes the brain and spinal cord. These two structures collect and interpret voluntary and involuntary motor and sensory stimuli. (See *A close look at the CNS.*)

A close look at the CNS

This illustration shows a cross section of the brain and spinal cord, which together make up the central nervous system (CNS). The brain joins the spinal cord at the base of the skull and ends near the second lumbar vertebra. Note the H-shaped mass of gray matter in the spinal cord.

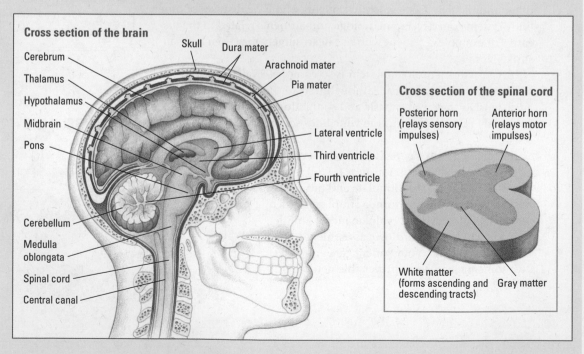

Cross section of the brain

Cerebrum
Thalamus
Hypothalamus
Midbrain
Pons
Cerebellum
Medulla oblongata
Spinal cord
Central canal

Skull   Dura mater
Arachnoid mater
Pia mater

Lateral ventricle
Third ventricle
Fourth ventricle

Cross section of the spinal cord

Posterior horn (relays sensory impulses)
Anterior horn (relays motor impulses)

White matter (forms ascending and descending tracts)   Gray matter

Brain

The brain consists of the cerebrum (or *cerebral cortex*), the brain stem, and the cerebellum. It collects, integrates, and interprets all stimuli and initiates and monitors voluntary and involuntary motor activity.

The reasons for your cerebrum

The cerebrum gives us the ability to think and reason. It's encased by the skull and enclosed by three membrane layers (the dura mater, arachnoid mater, and pia mater) called *meninges*. The space under the arachnoid layer (called the *subarachnoid space*) contains cerebrospinal fluid (CSF). If blood or fluid accumulates between these layers, pressure builds inside the skull and compromises brain function.

The cerebrum is divided into four lobes and two hemispheres. The right hemisphere controls the left side of the body, and the left hemisphere controls the right side of the body. Each lobe controls different functions. Cranial nerves I and II originate in the cerebrum. (See *A close look at the cerebrum and its functions*.)

A close look at the cerebrum and its functions

The cerebrum is divided into four lobes, based on anatomic landmarks and functional differences. The lobes—parietal, occipital, temporal, and frontal—are named for the cranial bones that lie over them.

This illustration shows the locations of the cerebral lobes and explains their functions. It also shows the location of the cerebellum.

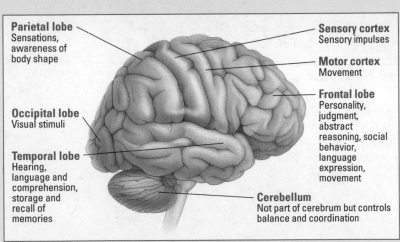

Parietal lobe
Sensations, awareness of body shape

Occipital lobe
Visual stimuli

Temporal lobe
Hearing, language and comprehension, storage and recall of memories

Sensory cortex
Sensory impulses

Motor cortex
Movement

Frontal lobe
Personality, judgment, abstract reasoning, social behavior, language expression, movement

Cerebellum
Not part of cerebrum but controls balance and coordination

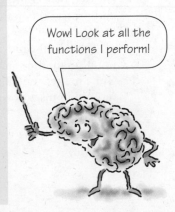

Wow! Look at all the functions I perform!

Meet the muses, Thala and Hypothala

The diencephalon, a division of the cerebrum, contains the thalamus and hypothalamus. The thalamus is a relay station for sensory impulses. The hypothalamus has many regulatory functions, including temperature control, pituitary hormone production, and water balance.

Quite the system!

The brain stem lies below the diencephalon and is divided into three parts: the midbrain, pons, and medulla. The brain stem contains cranial nerves III through XII, also known as the *nuclei*, and is a major sensory and motor pathway for impulses running to and from the cerebral cortex. It also regulates automatic body functions, such as heart rate, breathing, swallowing, and coughing.

Go to the back of the brain

The cerebellum, the most posterior part of the brain, contains the major motor and sensory pathways. It facilitates smooth, coordinated muscle movement and helps maintain equilibrium.

Spinal cord

The spinal cord is the primary pathway for messages traveling between the peripheral areas of the body and the brain. It also mediates the sensory-to-motor transmission path known as the *reflex arc*. Because the reflex arc enters and exits the spinal cord at the same level, reflex pathways don't need to travel up and down the way other stimuli do. (See *Reflex arc*.)

The spinal cord extends from the upper border of the first cervical vertebra to the lower border of the first lumbar vertebra. It's encased by a continuation of the meninges and CSF that surround and protect the brain and is also protected by the bony vertebra of the spine.

The dorsal white matter contains the ascending tracts that carry impulses up the spinal cord to higher sensory centers. The ventral white matter contains the descending motor tracts that transmit motor impulses down from the higher motor centers to the spinal cord.

Reflex arc

Spinal nerves, which have sensory and motor portions, control deep tendon and superficial reflexes. A simple reflex arc requires a sensory (or afferent) neuron and a motor (or efferent) neuron. The knee-jerk, or *patellar*, reflex illustrates the sequence of events in a normal reflex arc.

First, a sensory receptor detects the mechanical stimulus produced by the reflex hammer striking the patellar tendon. Then the sensory neuron carries the impulse along its axon by way of the spinal nerve to the dorsal root, where it enters the spinal column.

Next, in the anterior horn of the spinal cord, the sensory neuron joins with a motor neuron, which carries the impulse along its axon by way of a spinal nerve to the muscle. The motor neuron transmits the impulse to the muscle fibers through stimulation of the motor end plate. This impulse triggers the muscle to contract and the leg to extend. *Don't stand directly in front of a patient when testing this reflex!*

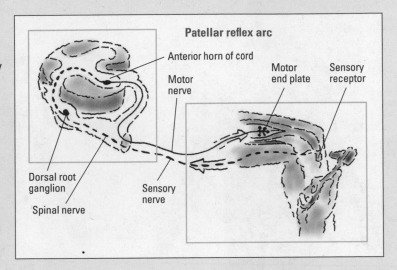

Patellar reflex arc

Anterior horn of cord

Motor nerve

Motor end plate

Sensory receptor

Dorsal root ganglion

Spinal nerve

Sensory nerve

Mapping out the body

For the purpose of documenting sensory function, the body is divided into dermatomes. Each dermatome represents an area supplied with afferent, or sensory, nerve fibers from an individual spinal root—either cervical, thoracic, lumbar, or sacral. This body map is used when testing sensation and trying to identify the source of a lesion.

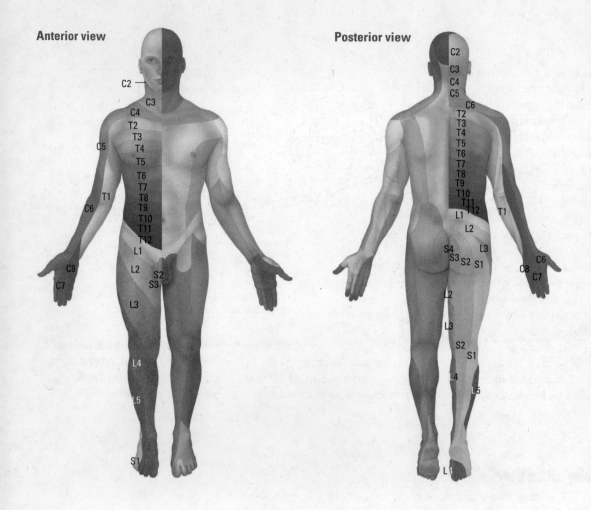

Anterior view

C2
C3
C4
T2
T3
C5
T4
T5
T6
T7
T1
T8
C6
T9
T10
T11
T12
L1
C8
L2
S2
C7
S3
L3
L4
L5
S1

Posterior view

C2
C3
C4
C5
C6
T2
T3
T4
T5
T6
T7
T8
T9
T10
T11
T12
T1
L1
L2
S4
L3
S3 S2 S1
C6
C8
C7
L2
L3
S2
S1
L4
L5
L4

Peripheral nervous system

The PNS includes the peripheral and cranial nerves. Peripheral sensory nerves transmit stimuli to the posterior horn of the spinal cord from sensory receptors located in the skin, muscles, sensory organs, and viscera. The upper motor neurons of the brain and the lower motor neurons of the cell bodies in the anterior horn of the spinal cord carry impulses that affect movement.

The 12 pairs of cranial nerves are the primary motor and sensory pathways between the brain, head, and neck. (See *Identifying cranial nerves*, page 109.)

Identifying cranial nerves

The cranial nerves have sensory function, motor function, or both. They're assigned Roman numerals and are written this way: CN I, CN II, CN III, and so forth. This illustration lists the functions of each cranial nerve.

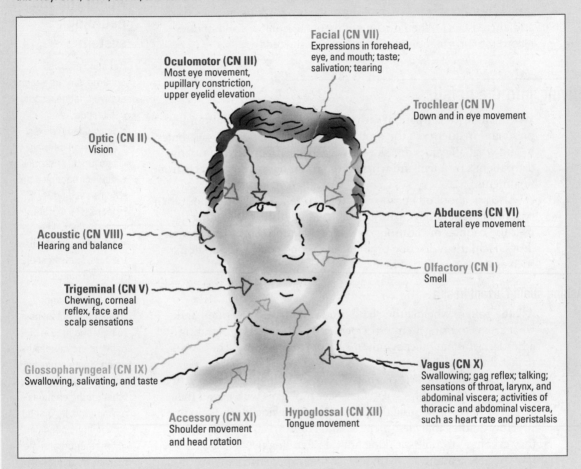

Facial (CN VII)
Expressions in forehead, eye, and mouth; taste; salivation; tearing

Oculomotor (CN III)
Most eye movement, pupillary constriction, upper eyelid elevation

Trochlear (CN IV)
Down and in eye movement

Optic (CN II)
Vision

Abducens (CN VI)
Lateral eye movement

Acoustic (CN VIII)
Hearing and balance

Olfactory (CN I)
Smell

Trigeminal (CN V)
Chewing, corneal reflex, face and scalp sensations

Glossopharyngeal (CN IX)
Swallowing, salivating, and taste

Vagus (CN X)
Swallowing; gag reflex; talking; sensations of throat, larynx, and abdominal viscera; activities of thoracic and abdominal viscera, such as heart rate and peristalsis

Accessory (CN XI)
Shoulder movement and head rotation

Hypoglossal (CN XII)
Tongue movement

Autonomic nervous system

The ANS contains motor neurons that regulate the activities of the visceral organs and affect the smooth and cardiac muscles and the glands. It consists of two subsystems:

1. sympathetic nervous system, which controls fight-or-flight reactions
2. parasympathetic nervous system, which maintains baseline body functions, such as breathing, heart rate, digestion, and metabolism.

Obtaining a health history

The most common symptoms reported about the neurologic system include headache, dizziness, faintness, confusion, impaired mental status, disturbances in balance or gait, changes in fine motor skills, and altered LOC. When documenting the reason for seeking care, record the information in the patient's own words.

Diving into the details

When you learn the patient's reason for seeking care, ask about the onset and frequency of the problem, what precipitates or exacerbates it, and what alleviates it. Ask whether other symptoms accompany the patient's problem and whether they have had adverse effects from treatments.

Also ask about other aspects of their current health and about their past health and family history. Obtain a drug history, including use of over-the-counter medications, herbal preparations, and recreational drugs. Help them describe problems by asking pertinent questions such as those mentioned here.

Asking about current health

Ask the patient whether they have headaches. If so, how often and what seems to bring them on? Does light bother their eyes during a headache? What other symptoms occur with the headache? What makes the headache better?

Does the patient have dizziness, numbness, tingling, seizures, tremors, weakness, or paralysis? Do they have problems with any of their senses or walking, keeping their balance, swallowing, or urinating?

How do they rate their memory and ability to concentrate? Do they ever have trouble speaking or understanding people? Do they have trouble reading or writing? Have they experienced any vision changes? If they have these problems, how much do they interfere with their daily activities?

Keep in mind that some neurologic changes, such as decreased reflexes, hearing, and vision, are a normal part of aging. (See *Aging and the neurologic system*.)

Asking about past health

Because many chronic diseases can affect the neurologic system, ask the patient about their past health. Inquire about major illnesses, recurrent minor illnesses, accidents or injuries, surgical procedures, and allergies.

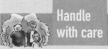
Handle with care

Aging and the neurologic system

Because neurons undergo various degenerative changes, aging can lead to:
• diminished reflexes
• decreased hearing, vision, taste, and smell
• slowed reaction time
• decreased agility
• decreased vibratory sense in the ankles
• development of muscle tremors, such as in the head and hands.

Look beyond age
Remember, not all neurologic changes in older patients are caused by aging. Some drugs can cause them as well. See whether the changes are asymmetric, indicating a pathologic condition, or whether other abnormalities need further investigation.

Considering the recent COVID-19 pandemic, research suggests neuropsychological changes that are affecting persons who contracted COVID-19 whether they were immunized or not. Although more research is needed, it is important to assess and identify all persons for any changes in their neuropsychological status from pre-COVID-19 to post-COVID-19 infection, as this could indicate conditions identified as post-COVID-19 syndrome or long COVID-19. Symptoms indicative of both long COVID-19 and post-COVID-19 syndrome include headache, fatigue, depression, anxiety, cognitive commitment, sleep and mood disorders, anosmia, and ageusia.

Asking about family history

Finally, ask about family history. Some genetic diseases are degenerative; others cause muscle weakness. For example, the incidence of seizures is higher in patients whose family history shows idiopathic epilepsy, and more than half of patients with migraine headaches have a family history of the disorder.

Assessing the neurologic system

A complete neurologic examination is so long and detailed that you probably won't ever perform one in its entirety. However, if your initial screening examination suggests a neurologic problem, you may want to perform a detailed assessment.

Order of the day

Always examine the patient's neurologic system in an orderly fashion. Begin with the highest levels of neurologic function and work down to the lowest, covering these five areas:
- mental status and speech
- cranial nerve function
- sensory function
- motor function
- reflexes.

Assessing mental status and speech

Your mental status assessment actually begins when you talk to the patient during the health history. How they respond to your questions gives clues to their orientation and memory and guides you during your physical assessment.

A quick check of mental status

To quickly screen patients for disordered thought processes, ask the questions below. An incorrect answer to any question may indicate the need for a complete mental status examination. Make sure you know the correct answers before asking the questions.

Question	Function screened
What's your name?	Orientation to person
What's your mother's name?	Orientation to other people
What year is it?	Orientation to time
Where are you now?	Orientation to place
How old are you?	Memory
Where were you born?	Remote memory
What did you have for breakfast?	Recent memory
Who's currently the US president?	General knowledge
Can you count backward from 20 to 1?	Attention span and calculation skills

Be sure to ask questions that require more than yes-or-no answers. Otherwise, confusion or disorientation may not be immediately apparent. If you have doubts about a patient's mental status, perform a screening examination. (See *A quick check of mental status*.)

Another guide during the physical assessment is the patient's reason for seeking care. For example, if the patient reports confusion or memory problems, you'll want to concentrate on the mental status part of the examination, which consists of checking:
- LOC
- appearance and behavior
- speech
- cognitive function
- constructional ability.

Level of consciousness

A change in the patient's LOC is the earliest and most sensitive indicator that their neurologic status has changed. Many terms are used to describe LOC, but their definitions may differ slightly among

practitioners. To avoid confusion, clearly describe the patient's
response to various stimuli using these guidelines:

- alert—follows commands and responds completely and appropriately to stimuli
- lethargic—is drowsy; has delayed responses to verbal stimuli; may
  drift off to sleep during examination
- stuporous—requires vigorous stimulation for a response
- comatose—doesn't respond appropriately to verbal or painful
  stimuli; can't follow commands or communicate verbally.

Perky or pooped out?

During your assessment, observe the patient's LOC. Are they alert,
or are they falling asleep? Can they focus their attention and maintain it, or are they easily distracted? If you need to use a stronger
stimulus than your voice, record what it is and how strong it needs
to be to get a response from the patient. The Glasgow Coma Scale
offers a more objective way to assess the patient's LOC. (See *Glasgow
Coma Scale*.)

Appearance and behavior

Note how the patient behaves, dresses, and grooms themselves.
Are their appearance and behavior inappropriate? Is their personal
hygiene poor? If so, discuss your findings with the family to determine whether this is a change. Even subtle changes in a patient's
behavior can signal a new onset of a chronic disease or a more acute
change that involves the frontal lobe.

Speech

Next, listen to how well the patient can express themselves. Is their
speech fluent or fragmented? Note the pace, volume, clarity, and
spontaneity of their speech. To assess for dysarthria (difficulty forming
words), ask them to repeat the phrase "No ifs, ands, or buts." Assess
comprehension by determining their ability to follow instructions and
cooperate with your examination.

Cognitive function

Assessing cognitive function involves testing the patient's memory, orientation, attention span, calculation ability, thought content, abstract
thinking, judgment, insight, and emotional status.

Telltale testing

To quickly test your patient's orientation, memory, and attention
span, use the mental status screening questions previously discussed.
Orientation to time is usually disrupted first; orientation to person,
last.

Glasgow Coma Scale

The Glasgow Coma Scale provides an easy way to describe the patient's baseline mental status and to help detect and interpret changes from baseline findings. To use the Glasgow Coma Scale, test the patient's ability to respond to verbal, motor, and sensory stimulation, and grade your findings according to the scale.

If a patient is alert, can follow simple commands, and is oriented to person, place, and time, their score will total 15 points. A decreased score in one or more categories may signal an impending neurologic crisis. A total score of seven or less indicates severe neurologic damage.

Test	Score	Patient's response
Eye-opening response		
Spontaneously	4	Opens eyes spontaneously
To speech	3	Opens eyes when told to
To pain	2	Opens eyes only on painful stimulus
None	1	Doesn't open eyes in response to stimulus
Motor response		
Obeys	6	Shows two fingers when asked
Localizes	5	Reaches toward painful stimulus and tries to remove it
Withdraws	4	Moves away from painful stimulus
Abnormal flexion	3	Assumes a decorticate posture (shown below) 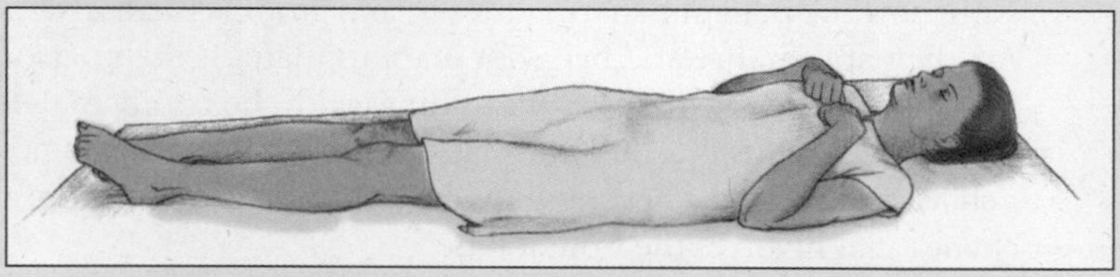

Abnormal extension	2	Assumes a decerebrate posture (shown below) 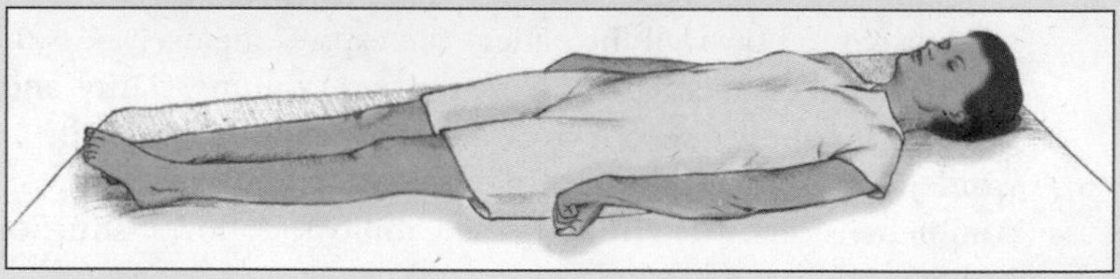

None	1	No response; just lies flaccid—an ominous sign
Verbal response		
Oriented	5	Tells current date
Confused	4	Tells incorrect year
Inappropriate words	3	Replies randomly with incorrect word
Incomprehensible	2	Moans or screams
None	1	No response
Total score		

Always consider the patient's environment and physical condition when assessing orientation. For example, an older patient admitted to the hospital for several days may not be oriented to time, especially if they have been bedridden or sedated. Also, when the person is intubated and can't speak, ask questions that require only a nod, such as "Do you know you're in the hospital?" and "Are we in Pennsylvania?"

The patient with an intact short-term memory can generally repeat five to seven nonconsecutive numbers right away and again 10 minutes later. Remember that short-term memory is commonly affected first in patients with neurologic disease.

When testing attention span and calculation skills, keep in mind that lack of mathematical ability and anxiety can affect the patient's performance. If they have difficulty with numerical computation, ask them to spell the word "world" backward. While they're performing these functions, note their ability to pay attention.

Clear and cogent?

Assess thought content by evaluating the clarity and cohesiveness of the patient's ideas. Is their conversation smooth, with logical transitions between ideas? Do they have hallucinations (sensory perceptions that lack appropriate stimuli) or delusions (beliefs not supported by reality)? Disordered thought patterns may indicate delirium or psychosis.

Extract the abstract

Test the patient's ability to think abstractly by asking them to interpret a common proverb such as "A stitch in time saves nine." A patient with dementia may interpret this proverb literally. If the patient's primary language isn't English, they'll probably have difficulty interpreting the proverb. Engage the assistance of family members when English isn't the patient's primary language. Have them ask the patient to explain a saying in their native language.

What if...?

Test the patient's judgment by asking them how they would respond to a hypothetical situation. For example, what would they do if they were in a public building and the fire alarm sounded? Evaluate the appropriateness of the answer.

Feelings, nothing more than feelings

Throughout the interview, assess the patient's emotional status. Note their mood, their emotional lability or stability, and the appropriateness of their emotional responses. Also, assess their mood by asking how they feel about themselves and their future. Keep in mind that symptoms of depression in older patients may be atypical—for example, decreased function or increased agitation rather than the usual sad affect.

Constructional ability

Constructional disorders affect the patient's ability to perform simple tasks and use various objects. They commonly occur with degenerative dementia.

Assessing cranial nerve function

There are 12 pairs of cranial nerves. These nerves transmit motor or sensory messages, or both, primarily between the brain and brain stem and the head and neck.

Something smells!

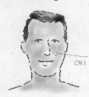

Assess cranial nerve I (the olfactory nerve) first. Before doing this, make sure the patient's nostrils are patent. Then have the patient block one nostril and inhale a familiar aromatic substance, such as coffee, cinnamon, citrus, or cloves, through the other nostril. Avoid stringent odors, such as ammonia or peppermint, which stimulate the trigeminal nerve.

Seeing eye to eye

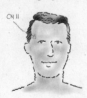

Next, assess cranial nerve II, the optic nerve. To test visual acuity quickly and informally, have the patient read a newspaper, starting with large headlines and moving to small print.

Test visual fields with a technique called *confrontation*. To do this, stand 2′ (0.6 m) in front of the patient, and have them cover one eye. Then close your eye on the side directly facing the patient's closed eye and bring your moving fingers into the patient's visual field from the periphery. Ask them to tell you when they see the object. Test each quadrant of the patient's visual field, and compare their results with your own. Chart any defects you find. (See *Visual field defects*, page 117.)

Finally, examine the fundus of the optic nerve, as described in Chapter 7. Blurring of the optic disc may indicate increased intracranial pressure (ICP).

Three real lookers

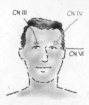

The oculomotor nerve (cranial nerve III), the trochlear nerve (cranial nerve IV), and the Abducens nerve (cranial nerve VI) all control eye movement. So assess these nerves together.

The oculomotor nerve controls most extraocular movement; it's also responsible for elevation of the eyelid and pupillary constriction. Abnormalities include ptosis, or

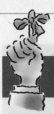

Memory jogger

Cranial nerves I, II, and VIII have sensory functions. Cranial nerves III, IV, VI, XI, and XII have motor functions. Cranial nerves V, VII, IX, and X have sensory and motor functions. How will you ever remember which does what?

Use the following mnemonic to help you remember which cranial nerves have sensory functions (**S**), motor functions (**M**), or both (**B**). The mnemonic begins with cranial nerve I and ends with cranial nerve XII:

I: **S**ome

II: **S**ay

III: **M**arry

IV: **M**oney

V: **B**ut

VI: **M**y

VII: **B**rother

VIII: **S**ays

IX: **B**ad

X: **B**usiness

XI: **M**arries

XII: **M**oney.

drooping of the upper lid, and pupil inequality. Make sure that the patient's pupils constrict when exposed to light and that their eyes accommodate to seeing objects at various distances.

To assess the oculomotor nerve, trochlear nerve (responsible for down and in eye movement), and Abducens nerve (responsible for lateral eye movement), ask the patient to follow your finger through the six cardinal positions of gaze: left superior, left lateral, left inferior, right superior, right lateral, and right inferior. Pause slightly before moving from one position to the next; this helps to assess the patient for involuntary eye movement (or nystagmus) and the ability to hold the gaze in that particular position.

"Tri" chewing without this nerve

The trigeminal nerve (cranial nerve V) is both a sensory and a motor nerve. It supplies sensation to the corneas, nasal and oral mucosa, and facial skin and supplies motor function for the jaw and all chewing muscles.

To assess the sensory component, check the patient's ability to feel light touch on their face. Ask them to close their eyes; then touch them with a wisp of cotton on their forehead, cheek, and jaw on each side. Next, test pain perception by touching the tip of a safety pin to the same three areas. Ask the patient to describe and compare both sensations.

Alternate the touches between sharp and dull to test the patient's reliability in comparing sensations. Proper assessment of the nerve requires that the patient identify sharp stimuli. To test the motor component of cranial nerve V, ask the patient to clench their teeth while you palpate the temporal and masseter muscles.

Taking a taste test

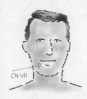

The facial nerve (cranial nerve VII) also has a sensory and a motor component. The sensory component controls taste perception on the anterior part of the tongue. You can assess taste by placing items with various tastes on the anterior portion of the patient's tongue—for example, sugar (sweet), salt, lemon juice (sour), and quinine (bitter). Simply have the patient wash away each taste with a sip of water.

The motor component is responsible for the facial muscles. Assess it by observing the patient's face for symmetry at rest and while they smile, frown, and raise their eyebrows.

If a weakness is caused by a stroke or another condition that damages the cortex, the patient will be able to raise their eyebrows and wrinkle their forehead. If the weakness is due to an interruption of the facial nerve or other peripheral nerve involvement, the entire side of the face will be immobile.

Visual field defects

Here are some examples of visual field defects. The black areas represent visual loss.

Left	Right
A: Blindness of right eye	
B: Bitemporal hemianopsia, or loss of half the visual field	
C: Left homonymous hemianopsia	
D: Left homonymous hemianopsia, superior quadrant	

Let's hear it for the acoustic nerve!

The acoustic nerve (cranial nerve VIII) is responsible for hearing and equilibrium. The cochlear division controls hearing, and the vestibular division controls balance.

To test hearing, ask the patient to cover one ear, and then stand on their opposite side and whisper a few words. See whether they can repeat what you said. Test the other ear the same way.

To test the vestibular portion of this nerve, observe the patient for nystagmus and disturbed balance, and note reports of dizziness or the room spinning.

Not so hard to swallow

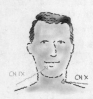

The glossopharyngeal nerve (cranial nerve IX) and the vagus nerve (cranial nerve X) are tested together because their innervation overlaps in the pharynx. The glossopharyngeal nerve is responsible for swallowing, salivation, and taste perception on the posterior one-third of the tongue. The vagus nerve controls swallowing and is also responsible for voice quality.

Start your assessment by listening to the patient's voice. Then check their gag reflex by touching the tip of a tongue blade against their posterior pharynx and asking them to open wide and say "ah." Watch for the symmetrical upward movement of the soft palate and uvula and for the midline position of the uvula.

A very important accessory

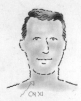

The accessory nerve (cranial nerve XI) is a motor nerve that controls the sternocleidomastoid muscles and the upper portion of the trapezius muscle. To assess this nerve, test the strength of both muscles. First, place your palm against the patient's cheek; then ask them to turn their head against your resistance.

Test the trapezius muscle by placing your hands on the patient's shoulder and asking them to shrug their shoulders against your resistance. Repeat each test on the other side, comparing muscle strength.

Speaking about the tongue

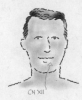

The hypoglossal nerve (cranial nerve XII) controls tongue movement involved in swallowing and speech. The tongue should be midline, without tremors or fasciculations. Test tongue strength by asking the patient to push their tongue against their cheek as you apply resistance. Observe their tongue for symmetry.

Assessing sensory function

Sensory system evaluation involves checking five areas of sensation:
- pain
- light touch
- vibration
- position
- discrimination.

This may hurt a bit

To test the patient for pain sensation, have them close their eyes; then touch all the major dermatomes, first with the sharp end of a safety pin and then with the dull end. Proceed in this order: fingers, shoulders, toes, thighs, and trunk. Ask them to identify when they feel the sharp stimulus.

If the patient has major deficits, start in the area with the least sensation, and move toward the area with the most sensation to help you determine the level of deficit.

Getting in touch

To test for the sense of light touch, follow the same routine as above but use a wisp of cotton. Lightly touch the patient's skin—don't swab or sweep the cotton, because you might miss an area of loss. A patient with a peripheral neuropathy might retain their sensation for light touch after they have lost pain sensation.

Good vibrations

To test vibratory sense, apply a tuning fork over different bony prominences while the patient keeps their eyes closed. In the lower extremities, start at the interphalangeal joint of the great toe. In the upper extremities, start at the distal interphalangeal joint of the index finger. Move proximally while testing. Test only until the patient feels the vibration, because everything above that level will be intact. (See *Evaluating vibratory sense*.) If vibratory sense is intact, you won't have to check position sense because the same pathway carries both.

Fingers and toes on the move

To assess position sense, have the patient close their eyes. Then grasp the sides of their big toe, move the toe up and down, and ask them what position it's in. To be tested for position sense, the patient needs intact vestibular and cerebellar function. To perform the same test on the patient's upper extremities, grasp the sides of their index finger and move it back and forth.

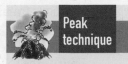

Peak technique

Evaluating vibratory sense

To evaluate vibratory sense, apply the base of a vibrating tuning fork to the interphalangeal joint of the patient's great toe, as shown below.

Ask them what they feel. If they feel the sensation, they'll typically report a feeling of buzzing or vibration. If they don't feel the sensation at the toe, try the medial malleolus. Then continue moving proximally until they feel the sensation. Note where they feel it, and then repeat the process on the other leg.

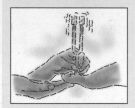

How discriminating of you!

Discrimination testing assesses the ability of the cerebral cortex to interpret and integrate information. *Stereognosis* is the ability to discriminate the shape, size, weight, texture, and form of an object by touching and manipulating it. To test this, ask the patient to close their eyes and open their hand. Then place a common object, such as a key, in their hand and ask them to identify it.

If they can't identify the object, test graphesthesia next. Have the patient keep their eyes closed and hold out their hand while you draw a large number on the palm. Ask them to identify the number. Both of these tests assess the ability of the cortex to integrate sensory input.

To test point localization, have the patient close their eyes; then touch one of their limbs, and ask them where you touched them. Test two-point discrimination by touching the patient simultaneously in two contralateral areas. They should be able to identify both touches. Failure to perceive touch on one side is called *extinction*.

Assessing motor function

Assessing the motor system includes inspecting the muscles and testing muscle tone and muscle strength. Cerebellar testing is also done because the cerebellum plays a role in smooth muscle movements, such as tics, tremors, or fasciculation.

Muscle tone

Muscle tone represents muscular resistance to passive stretching. To test arm muscle tone, move the patient's shoulder through passive range-of-motion (ROM) exercises. You should feel a slight resistance. Then let the arm drop to the patient's side. It should fall easily.

To test leg muscle tone, guide the hip through passive ROM exercises; then let the leg fall to the bed. The leg shouldn't fall into an externally rotated position; this is an abnormal finding.

Muscle strength

To perform a general examination of muscle strength, observe the patient's gait and motor activities. To evaluate muscle strength, ask the patient to move major muscles and muscle groups against resistance. For instance, to test shoulder girdle strength, have them extend their arms with their palms up and maintain this position for 30 seconds.

Strong-arm tactics

If they can't maintain this position, test further by pushing down on their outstretched arms. If they do lift both arms equally, look for pronation of the hand and downward drift of the arm on the weaker side.

Cerebellum

Cerebellar testing looks at the patient's coordination and general balance. Can they sit and stand without support? If so, observe them as they walk across the room, turn, and walk back. Note imbalances or abnormalities.

When walking wavers

With cerebellar dysfunction, the patient will have a wide-based, unsteady gait. Deviation to one side may indicate a cerebellar lesion on that side. Ask the patient to walk heel to toe, and observe their balance. Then perform Romberg test. (See *Romberg test*.)

The nose (and finger) knows

Test extremity coordination by asking the patient to touch their nose and then touch your outstretched finger as you move it. Have them do this faster and faster. Their movements should be accurate and smooth.

Quick, do these tests!

Other tests of cerebellar function assess rapid alternating movements. In these tests, the patient's movements should be accurate and smooth.

First, ask the patient to touch the thumb of their right hand to their right index finger and then to each of their remaining fingers. Observe the movements for accuracy and smoothness. Next, ask them to sit with their palms on their thighs. Tell them to turn their palms up and down, gradually increasing their speed.

A "sole"ful situation

Finally, have the patient lie in a supine position. Then stand at the foot of the table or bed and hold your palms near the soles of their feet. Ask them to alternately tap the sole of their right foot and the sole of their left foot against your palms. They should increase their speed as you observe their coordination.

Assessing reflexes

Evaluating reflexes involves testing deep tendon and superficial reflexes and observing for primitive reflexes.

Romberg test

Observe the patient's balance as they stand with their eyes open, feet together, and arms at their sides. Then ask them to close their eyes. Hold your arms out on either side of them to protect them if they sway. If they fall to one side, the result of Romberg test is positive.

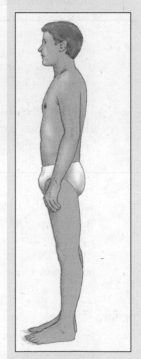

Deep tendon reflexes

The key to testing deep tendon reflexes is to make sure the patient is relaxed and the joint is flexed appropriately. First, distract the patient by asking them to focus on a point across the room. Always test deep tendon reflexes by moving from head to toe and comparing side to side. (See *Assessing deep tendon reflexes*, page 123.)

Grade deep tendon reflexes using the following scale:
- 0—absent impulses
- +1—diminished impulses
- +2—normal impulses
- +3—increased impulses (may be normal)
- +4—hyperactive impulses.

Superficial reflexes

Stimulating the skin or mucous membranes is a method of testing superficial reflexes. Because they are cutaneous reflexes, the more you try to elicit them in succession, the less of a response you'll get. So observe carefully the first time you stimulate.

Tickling the feet

Using an applicator stick, tongue blade, or key, slowly stroke the lateral side of the patient's sole from the heel to the great toe. The normal response in an adult is plantar flexion of the toes. Upward movement of the great toe and fanning of the little toes—called *Babinski reflex*—is abnormal. (See *Babinski reflex in infants*, page 124.)

Tickling the thighs

The cremasteric reflex is tested in people with testicles by using an applicator stick to stimulate the inner thigh. Normal reaction is contraction of the cremaster muscle and elevation of the testicle on the side of the stimulus.

Tickling the tummy

Test the abdominal reflexes with the patient in the supine position with their arms at their sides and their knees slightly flexed. Briskly stroke both sides of the abdomen above and below the umbilicus, moving from the periphery toward the midline. Movement of the umbilicus toward the stimulus is normal.

Primitive reflexes

Primitive reflexes are abnormal in an adult but normal in an infant, whose CNS is immature. As the neurologic system matures, these reflexes disappear. The primitive reflexes you'll assess for are the grasp, snout, sucking, and glabella reflexes.

Assessing deep tendon reflexes

Biceps reflex

Position the patient's arm so their elbow is flexed at a 45-degree angle and their arm is relaxed. Place your thumb or index finger over the biceps tendon and your remaining fingers loosely over the triceps muscle. Strike your finger with the pointed end of the reflex hammer, and watch and feel for the contraction of the biceps muscle and flexion of the forearm.

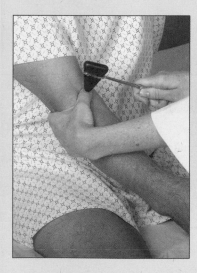

Triceps reflex

Have the patient adduct their arm and place their forearm across their chest. Strike the triceps tendon about 2″ (5 cm) above the olecranon process on the extensor surface of the upper arm. Watch for contraction of the triceps muscle and extension of the forearm.

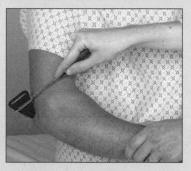

Brachioradialis reflex

Ask the patient to rest the ulnar surface of their hand on their abdomen or lap with the elbow partially flexed. Strike the radius, and watch for supination of the hand and flexion of the forearm at the elbow.

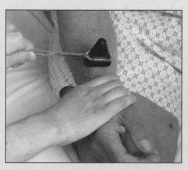

Patellar reflex

Have the patient sit with their legs dangling freely. If he can't sit up, flex their knee at a 45° angle and place your nondominant hand behind it for support. Strike the patellar tendon just below the patella, and look for contraction of the quadriceps muscle in the thigh with extension of the leg.

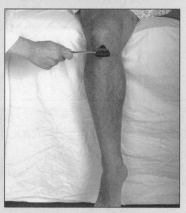

Achilles reflex

Have the patient flex their foot. Then support the plantar surface. Strike the Achilles tendon, and watch for plantar flexion of the foot at the ankle.

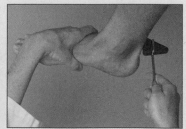

Just gotta grasp

Assess the grasp reflex by applying gentle pressure to the patient's palm with your fingers. If they grasp your fingers between their index finger and thumb, suspect cortical or premotor cortex damage.

Read my lip

The snout reflex is assessed by lightly tapping on the patient's upper lip. Pursing of the lip is a positive snout reflex that indicates frontal lobe damage.

An untimely reflex

Observe the patient while you're feeding them or if they have an oral airway or endotracheal tube in place. If you see a sucking motion, this indicates cortical damage. This reflex is commonly seen in patients with advanced dementia.

Tap, tap, blink, blink

The glabella response is elicited by repeatedly tapping the bridge of the patient's nose. The abnormal response is persistent blinking, which indicates diffuse cortical dysfunction.

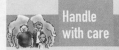

Handle with care

Babinski reflex in infants

Babinski reflex can be elicited in some healthy infants—sometimes until age 2 years. However, plantar flexion of the toes is seen in more than 90% of healthy infants.

Abnormal findings

During your assessment, you may detect abnormalities caused by neurologic dysfunction. The most common categories of abnormalities include altered LOC, cranial nerve impairment, abnormal muscle movements, and abnormal gaits. (See *Abnormal neurologic findings*, pages 125 and 126.)

Altered level of consciousness

Consciousness may be impaired by any one of several disorders that can affect the cerebral hemisphere of the brain stem. Consciousness is the most sensitive indicator of neurologic dysfunction and may be a valuable adjunct to other findings. When assessing LOC, make sure that you provide a stimulus that's strong enough to get a true picture of the patient's baseline. (See *Detecting increased ICP*, page 127.)

Interpretation station

Abnormal neurologic findings

Your assessment will reveal a group of findings that may lead you to suspect a particular disorder. The chart below shows common groups of findings for the neurologic system along with signs and symptoms and their probable causes.

Sign or symptom and findings	Probable cause
Aphasia	
• Wernicke, Broca, or global aphasia • Decreased level of consciousness (LOC) • Hemiplegia • Homonymous hemianopsia • Paresthesia and loss of sensation	Stroke
• Any type of aphasia occurring suddenly (transient or permanent) • Blurred or double vision • Headache • Cerebrospinal otorrhea and rhinorrhea • Disorientation • Behavioral changes • Signs of increased intracranial pressure	Head trauma
• Any type of aphasia occurring suddenly and resolving within 24 hours • Transient hemiparesis • Hemianopsia • Paresthesia • Dizziness and confusion	Transient ischemic attack
Decreased LOC	
• Slowly decreasing LOC, from lethargy to coma • Apathy, behavior changes • Memory loss • Decreased attention span • Morning headache • Sensorimotor disturbances	Brain tumor

Sign or symptom and findings	Probable cause
• Slowly decreasing LOC, from lethargy to possible coma • Malaise • Tachycardia • Tachypnea • Orthostatic hypotension • Hot, flushed, and diaphoretic skin	Heatstroke
• Lethargy progressing to coma • Confusion, anxiety, and restlessness • Hypotension • Tachycardia • Weak pulse with narrowing pulse pressure • Dyspnea • Oliguria • Cool, clammy skin	Shock
Tremors	
• Tremors in fingers, progressing to feet, eyelids, jaws, lips, and tongue • Characteristic pill-rolling tremor • Lead-pipe rigidity • Bradykinesia • Propulsive gait with forward-leaning posture • Masklike face • Drooling	Parkinson disease
• Intention tremor that waxes and wanes • Visual and sensory impairments • Muscle weakness, paralysis, or spasticity	Multiple sclerosis

(Continued)

Abnormal neurologic findings (continued)

Sign or symptom and findings	Probable cause	Sign or symptom and findings	Probable cause
Tremors (continued)		**Apraxia** (continued)	
• Hyperreflexia • Ataxic gait • Dysphagia		• Apathy • Aphasia	
• Intention tremor • Ataxia • Nystagmus • Muscle weakness and atrophy • Hypoactive or absent deep tendon reflexes	Cerebellar tumor	• Progressive apraxia • Decreased mental activity • Headache • Dizziness • Seizures • Pupillary changes	Brain tumor
Apraxia		• Sudden onset of apraxia • Headache • Confusion • Aphasia • Agnosia • Stupor or coma • Hemiplegia • Visual field defects	Stroke
• Gradual and irreversible apraxia • Amnesia • Anomia • Decreased attention span	Alzheimer disease		

Depressing disorders

Disorders that affect LOC include toxic encephalopathy, hemorrhage, and extensive, generalized cortical atrophy. Compression of brain stem structures by tumor or hemorrhage can also affect consciousness by depressing the reticular activating system that maintains wakefulness. In addition, sedatives and opioids can depress LOC.

Cranial nerve impairment

Damage to the cranial nerves causes many abnormalities, including olfactory, visual, auditory, and muscle problems. Vertigo and dysphagia can also indicate cranial nerve damage.

Olfactory impairment

If the patient can't detect odors with both nostrils, they may have a dysfunction in cranial nerve I. This dysfunction can result from any disease that affects the olfactory tract, such as a tumor, hemorrhage or, more commonly, a facial bone fracture that crosses the cribriform plate (portion of the ethmoid bone that separates the roof of the nose from the cranial cavity).

Detecting increased ICP

The earlier you can recognize the signs of increased intracranial pressure (ICP), the more quickly you can intervene and improve the patient's chance of recovery. By the time late signs appear, interventions may be useless.

	Early signs	Late signs
Level of consciousness	• Requires increased stimulation • Subtle orientation loss • Restlessness and anxiety • Sudden quietness	Unarousable
Pupils	• Pupil changes on side of lesion • One pupil constricts but then dilates (unilateral hippus) • Sluggish reaction of both pupils • Unequal pupils	Pupils fixed and dilated or "blown"
Motor response	• Sudden weakness • Motor changes on side opposite the lesion • Positive pronator drift; with palms up, one hand pronates	Profound weakness
Vital signs	• Intermittent increases in blood pressure	Increased systolic pressure, profound bradycardia, abnormal respirations (Cushing syndrome)

Visual impairment

Visual problems include visual field defects, pupillary changes, eye muscle impairment, and facial nerve impairment.

Far afield

Visual fields are affected by tumors or infarcts of the optic nerve head, optic chiasm, or optic tracts.

Peer at the pupils

If the patient's pupillary response to light is affected, they may have damage to the optic nerve and oculomotor nerve. Pupils are also sensitive indicators of neurologic dysfunction. Increased ICP causes dilation of the pupil ipsilateral to the mass lesion; without treatment, both pupils become fixed and dilated. (See *Understanding pupillary changes.*) Unequal pupils, or *anisocoria*, is normal in about 20% of people. In normal anisocoria, pupil size doesn't change with the amount of illumination.

Understanding pupillary changes

Use this chart as a guide to pupillary changes.

Pupillary change	Possible causes
Unilateral, dilated (4 mm), fixed, and nonreactive 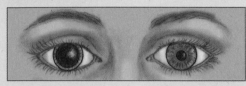	• Uncal herniation with oculomotor nerve damage • Brain stem compression • Increased intracranial pressure • Tentorial herniation • Head trauma with subdural or epidural hematoma • Normal in some people
Bilateral, dilated (4 mm), fixed, and nonreactive 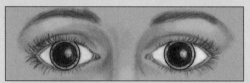	• Severe midbrain damage • Cardiopulmonary arrest (hypoxia) • Anticholinergic poisoning
Bilateral, midsize (2 mm), fixed, and nonreactive 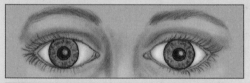	• Midbrain involvement caused by edema, hemorrhage, infarctions, lacerations, contusions
Bilateral, pinpoint (<1 mm), and usually nonreactive 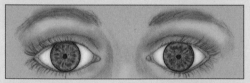	• Lesions of pons, usually after hemorrhage
Unilateral, small (1.5 mm), and nonreactive 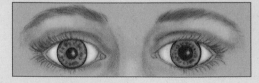	• Disruption of sympathetic nerve supply to the head caused by spinal cord lesion above the first thoracic vertebra

Don't move a muscle!

Weakness or paralysis of the eye muscles can result from cranial nerve damage. Increased ICP and intracranial lesions can affect the motor nuclei of the oculomotor, trochlear, and Abducens nerves.

The drifters

Damage to the peripheral labyrinth, brain stem, or cerebellum can cause nystagmus. The eyes drift slowly in one direction and then jerk back to the other.

Feeling droopy

Drooping of the upper eyelid, or *ptosis*, can result from a defect in the oculomotor nerve. To assess ptosis more accurately, have the patient sit upright.

Facing the pain

If the patient responds inadequately to sensory stimulation of the skin or eye, the trigeminal nerve may be affected. Trigeminal neuralgia causes severe piercing or stabbing pain over one or more of the facial dermatomes.

Auditory impairment

Sensorial hearing loss can result from lesions of the cochlear branch of the acoustic nerve or from lesions in any part of the nerve's pathway to the brain stem. A patient with this type of hearing loss may have trouble hearing high-pitched sounds, or they may have a total loss of hearing in the affected ear.

Which end is up?

Vertigo is the illusion of movement and can result from a disturbance of the vestibular centers. If it's caused by a peripheral lesion, vertigo and nystagmus will occur 10 to 20 seconds after the patient changes position, and symptoms will gradually lessen with the repetition of the position change. If the vertigo is of central origin, there's no latent period, and the symptoms won't diminish with repetition.

Speech and swallowing impairment

Aphasia is a speech disorder caused by injury to the cerebral cortex. Several types of aphasia exist, including:
- *expressive or Broca aphasia*—impaired fluency and difficulty finding words; impairment is located in the frontal lobe, the anterior speech area

- *receptive or Wernicke aphasia*—inability to understand written words or speech and the use of made-up words; impairment is located in the posterior speech cortex, which involves the temporal and parietal lobes
- *global aphasia*—lack of both expressive and receptive language; impairment of both speech areas.

  Dysphagia (difficulty swallowing) commonly occurs after a stroke but can also result from a mass lesion affecting cranial nerves IX and X.

  In *oropharyngeal dysphagia*, the mouth or throat causes the swallowing difficulty. In *esophageal dysphagia*, difficulty arises from the esophagus.

Constructional impairment

Apraxia and agnosia are two types of constructional disorders. They may occur with a stroke, dementia, or a brain lesion.

What's the purpose of this?

Apraxia is the inability to perform purposeful movements and make proper use of objects. It's commonly associated with parietal lobe dysfunction and can appear in four types:

- *ideomotor apraxia*—inability to understand the effect of motor activity; ability to perform simple activities but without awareness of performing them; inability to perform actions on command
- *conceptual apraxia*—awareness of actions that should be done in a certain order but inability to perform them that way
- *constructional apraxia*—inability to copy a design such as the face of a clock
- *dressing apraxia*—inability to understand the meaning of various articles of clothing or the sequence of actions required to get dressed.

What did you say this was?

Agnosia is the inability to identify common objects. It may indicate a lesion in the sensory cortex. Types of agnosia include:

- *visual*—inability to identify common objects without touching
- *auditory*—inability to identify common sounds
- *body image*—inability to identify body parts by sight or touch; inability to localize a stimulus; denial of existence of half the body.

Abnormal muscle movements

Neurologic disorders can cause a wide range of abnormal muscle movements from facial tics to motor restlessness. Findings may or may not indicate serious neurologic disease.

It's a tic...

Sudden, uncontrolled movements of the face, shoulders, and extremities, called *tics*, are caused by abnormal neural stimuli. Tics are normal movements that appear repetitively and inappropriately. They include blinking, shoulder shrugging, and facial twitching.

...no, a tremor...

Like tics, tremors are involuntary, repetitive movements usually seen in the fingers, wrist, eyelids, tongue, and legs. They can occur when the affected body part is at rest or with voluntary movement. For example, the patient with Parkinson disease has a characteristic pill-rolling resting tremor, and the patient with cerebellar disease has an intention tremor as they reach for an object.

...no, a fasciculation!

Fasciculations are fine twitchings in small muscle groups and are most commonly associated with lower motor neuron dysfunction.

Abnormal gaits

During your assessment, you may identify gait abnormalities. These abnormalities may result from disorders of the cerebellum, posterior columns, corticospinal tract, basal ganglia, and lower motor neurons. (See *Identifying gait abnormalities*.)

Spastic gait

Spastic gait—sometimes referred to as *paretic* or *weak gait*—is a stiff, foot-dragging walk caused by unilateral leg muscle hypertonicity. The leg doesn't swing normally at the hip or knee, so the patient's foot tends to drag or shuffle, scraping their toes on the ground. This gait indicates focal damage to the corticospinal tract and is usually permanent once it develops.

Scissors gait

Resulting from bilateral spastic paresis, scissors gait affects both legs but has little or no effect on the arms. The patient's legs flex slightly at the hips and knees, so they look as if they're crouching. With each step, their thighs adduct and their knees hit or cross in a scissorslike movement.

Propulsive gait

Propulsive gait is characterized by a stooped, rigid posture—the patient's head and neck are bent forward; their flexed, stiffened arms

Identifying gait abnormalities

The illustrations below identify five gait abnormalities.

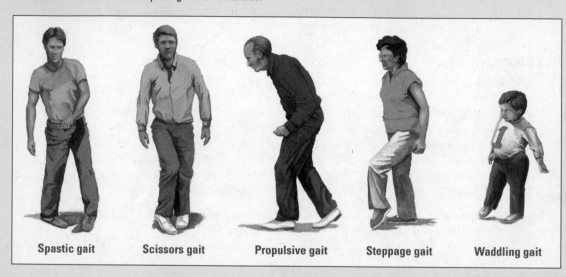

| Spastic gait | Scissors gait | Propulsive gait | Steppage gait | Waddling gait |

are held away from the body; their fingers are extended; and their knees and hips are stiffly bent. Propulsive gait is a cardinal sign of advanced Parkinson disease.

Steppage gait

Steppage gait typically results from footdrop caused by weakness or paralysis of pretibial and peroneal muscles, usually from lower motor neuron lesions. Footdrop causes the foot to hang with the toes pointing down, causing the toes to scrape the ground during ambulation. To compensate, the hip rotates outward and the hip and knee flex in an exaggerated fashion to lift the advancing leg off the ground. The foot is thrown forward and the toes hit the ground first, producing an audible slap.

Waddling gait

Waddling gait, a distinctive ducklike walk, is an important sign of muscular dystrophy, spinal muscle atrophy, or, rarely, developmental dysplasia of the hip. It may be present when the child begins to walk or may appear only later in life. The gait results from deterioration of the pelvic girdle muscles.

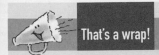

That's a wrap!

Neurologic system review

Central nervous system
Brain
- Cerebrum (cerebral cortex): enables thinking and reasoning
- Brain stem: acts as a major sensory and motor pathway for impulses to and from the cerebral cortex; regulates automatic body functions, such as heart rate and breathing
- Cerebellum: facilitates coordinated muscle movement and maintains equilibrium

Spinal cord
- Acts as the primary pathway for messages traveling between the peripheral areas of the body and the brain
- Mediates the reflex arc

Peripheral nervous system
- Peripheral nerves: serve the skin, muscles, sensory organs, and viscera
- Cranial nerves: serve the brain, head, and neck

Autonomic nervous system
- Regulates the activities of the visceral organs
- Affects smooth and cardiac muscles and glands
- Consists of the sympathetic nervous system (controls fight-or-flight reactions) and parasympathetic nervous system (maintains baseline body functions)

The health history
- Determine the patient's reason for seeking care, which may include headache, dizziness, faintness, confusion, impaired mental status, or balance or gait disturbances.
- Ask the patient about their current health, including their memory and ability to concentrate as well as their current medications.
- Ask them about their past health, including illnesses, accidents or injuries, surgeries, and allergies.
- Inquire about a family history of neurologic disorders that may have a genetic component, such as seizures and migraine headaches.

Assessment of mental status and speech
- Observe for any changes in LOC.
- Note the patient's appearance and behavior.
- Listen to how well the patient speaks and expresses themselves.
- Assess cognitive function by testing memory, orientation, attention span, calculation ability, thought content, abstract thinking, judgment, insight, and emotional status.
- Evaluate the patient's constructional ability (ability to perform simple tasks and use various objects).

Assessment of cranial nerves
- *Cranial nerve I (olfactory nerve):* Have the patient identify at least two smells.
- *Cranial nerve II (optic nerve):* Test visual acuity and visual fields with confrontation; examine the fundus of the optic nerve.
- *Cranial nerves III (oculomotor nerve), IV (trochlear nerve), and VI (Abducens nerve):* Test extraocular movement using the six cardinal positions of gaze.
- *Cranial nerve V (trigeminal nerve):* Check the patient's ability to feel light touch and pain perception over their face; have them clench their teeth to assess temporal and masseter muscles.
- *Cranial nerve VII (facial nerve):* Test taste perception; observe the patient's face for symmetry at rest and when smiling, frowning, and raising eyebrows.
- *Cranial nerve VIII (acoustic nerve):* Test hearing and check balance.
- *Cranial nerves IX (glossopharyngeal nerve) and X (vagus nerve):* Check the gag reflex.
- *Cranial nerve XI (accessory nerve):* Check the strength of the sternocleidomastoid and trapezius muscles.
- *Cranial nerve XII (hypoglossal nerve):* Assess tongue position, movement, and strength; observe for tongue symmetry.

Assessment of sensory function
- Test pain perception in all dermatomes with the sharp and dull ends of a safety pin.
- Test light touch sensation in all dermatomes using a wisp of cotton.
- Test vibratory sense with a tuning fork over bony prominences.
- Assess position sense by having the patient identify whether their toe or finger is positioned up or down as you move it.

(Continued)

Neurologic system review *(continued)*

• Assess discrimination by testing stereognosis, graphesthesia, and point localization.

Assessment of motor function

• Assess muscle tone by guiding the shoulders and hips through passive ROM exercises.
• Assess muscle strength by having the patient move major muscles and muscle groups against resistance.
• Assess cerebellar function by observing the patient's coordination and general balance, testing extremity coordination, and having the patient perform rapid alternating movements.

Assessment of reflexes

• Test deep tendon reflexes:
  – biceps reflex
  – triceps reflex
  – brachioradialis reflex
  – patellar reflex
  – Achilles reflex.
• Test superficial reflexes:
  – Babinski reflex (normally absent)
  – cremasteric reflex (in males)
  – abdominal reflexes.
• Check for primitive reflexes (shouldn't be present in an adult but are normal in infants):
  – grasp reflex
  – snout reflex
  – suck reflex
  – glabella response.

Abnormal cranial nerve findings

• Olfactory impairment: inability to detect odors
• Visual impairment: visual field defects, pupillary changes, eye muscle impairment, and facial nerve impairment
• Auditory problems: hearing loss and vertigo
• Speech and swallowing impairment: aphasia and dysphagia
• Constructional problems: apraxia and agnosia

Abnormal muscle movements

• Tics: sudden uncontrolled movements of the face, shoulders, and extremities
• Tremors: involuntary, repetitive movements in the fingers, wrists, eyelids, tongue, and legs
• Fasciculations: fine twitching in small muscle groups
• Gait: spastic, scissors, propulsive, steppage, and waddling

Quick quiz

1.   A patient who can't recognize the sound of a ringing phone probably has:
    A.   agnosia.
    B.   apraxia.
    C.   aphasia.
    D.   ataxia.

Answer: A. Agnosia, or the inability to identify common objects, occurs in three forms: visual, auditory, or body image.

2.   The most sensitive indicator of a change in a patient's neurologic status is their:
    A.   gross motor movement.
    B.   LOC.
    C.   speech pattern.
    D.   vision.

Answer: B. While gross motor movement, speech pattern, and vision may change with an alteration in neurologic status, LOC is the most sensitive and earliest indicator of a change in neurologic status.

3. Normal findings in the assessment of gross motor function include:
    A. downward drift of the arm when it's outstretched.
    B. negative Romberg test result.
    C. ability to distinguish odors.
    D. an uncoordinated gait.

Answer: B. A negative Romberg test is a normal gross motor finding as is a smooth coordinated gait.

4. One of the primitive reflexes is the:
    A. patellar reflex.
    B. sucking reflex.
    C. brachial reflex.
    D. triceps reflex.

Answer: B. The grasping, snout, sucking, and glabella are primitive reflexes that occur normally in infants, whose neurologic systems are immature. These reflexes are abnormal in adults.

5. To test sensation, you'll need a:
    A. key and tongue blade.
    B. pencil and paper.
    C. safety pin and cotton wisp.
    D. measuring tape and reflex hammer.

Answer: C. A safety pin and a cotton wisp are used to assess pain and light touch.

Scoring

☆☆☆ If you answered all five questions correctly, wow! There's obviously nothing wrong with your cerebral cortex.

☆☆ If you answered four questions correctly, fantastic! Your alert attention to the details in this chapter really paid off.

☆ If you answered fewer than four questions correctly, don't let it get on your nerves! Try reading the chapter one more time.

Chapter 7

Eyes

Just the facts

In this chapter, you'll learn:

◆ the importance of eye assessments

◆ eye structures and their functions

◆ questions to ask about the eyes during the health history

◆ techniques for assessing the eyes

◆ ways to recognize normal and abnormal variations in the eyes.

A look at the eyes

About 70% of all sensory information reaches the brain through the eyes. Disorders in vision can interfere with a patient's ability to function independently, perceive the world appropriately, and enjoy beauty.

A thorough assessment of your patient's eyes and vision can help you identify problems that can affect the patient's health and quality of life. In many cases, early detection of a problem can lead to successful, sight-saving treatment.

The eyes have it!

Fewer people lose their sight from infections or injuries today than in the past. Still, the overall incidence of blindness is rising as the population ages. Primary causes of vision loss include diabetic retinopathy, glaucoma, cataracts, and macular degeneration—conditions more common in older patients than in younger ones.

Young people can lose their sight because of opportunistic infections associated with human immunodeficiency virus (HIV) and acquired immunodeficiency syndrome. The opportunistic infections toxoplasmosis and cytomegalovirus retinitis commonly cause blindness as well. Other vision disorders that may limit a person's ability to function include strabismus, amblyopia, and refractory errors.

Anatomy and physiology

In this section, we'll look at the external (extraocular) structures as well as the internal (intraocular) structures of the eye. (See *A close look at the eye*.)

Extraocular structures

The eyes are delicate sensory organs equipped with many protective structures. On the outside, the bony orbits protect the eyes from trauma. Eyelids (or *palpebrae*), lashes, and the lacrimal apparatus protect the eyes from injury, dust, and foreign bodies.

A close look at the eye

This cross section details important anatomic structures of the eye.

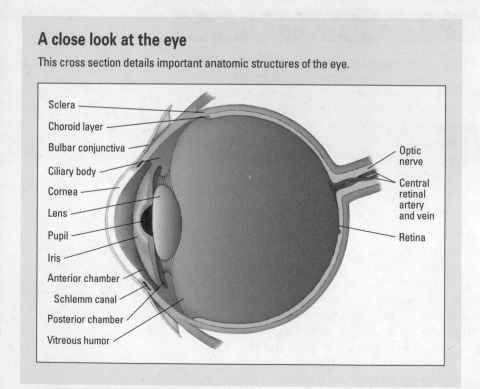

Sclera
Choroid layer
Bulbar conjunctiva
Ciliary body
Cornea
Lens
Pupil
Iris
Anterior chamber
Schlemm canal
Posterior chamber
Vitreous humor

Optic nerve
Central retinal artery and vein
Retina

Muscling in

Also included in extraocular structures are six extraocular muscles. Innervated (stimulated) by the cranial nerves, these muscles control the movement of the eyes. The coordinated actions of those muscles allow the eyes to move in tandem to provide a single image to the brain. Humans have a binocular, single vision system.

Intraocular structures

The eye contains multiple structures that function together to provide vision. Some structures are easily visible, whereas others can be viewed only with special instruments. Examining intraocular structures without the benefit of pupil dilation with ophthalmic drops is challenging. You may not be able to visualize all these structures without dilation. If you are unable to visualize these structures, and a dilated ophthalmic exam is necessary, the patient should be referred to an eye specialist. Here's a brief review of these structures.

Sclera and choroid

The white coating on the outside of the eyeball, the sclera, maintains the eye's size and shape. The choroid, which lines the recessed portion of the eyeball and lies between the sclera and the retina, contains a network of arteries and veins that maintain blood supply to the retina and helps absorb excess light.

Bulbar and palpebral conjunctivae

A thin, transparent membrane, the bulbar conjunctiva covers and protects the anterior portion of the white sclera. The palpebral conjunctiva lines the eyelid.

Cornea

The cornea is a smooth, avascular, transparent tissue that merges with the sclera at the limbus. It refracts, or bends, light rays entering the eye. Located in front of the pupil and iris, the cornea is fed by the ophthalmic branch of cranial nerve V (the trigeminal nerve). Stimulation of this nerve initiates a protective blink, the corneal reflex.

Iris

The iris is a circular, contractile diaphragm that contains smooth and radial muscles and is perforated in the center by the pupil. Varying amounts of pigment granules within the smooth muscle fibers give it color. Its posterior portion contains involuntary muscles that control pupil size and regulate the amount of light entering the eye.

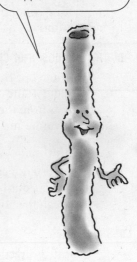

The choroid contains a network of arteries and veins that maintain blood supply to the retina.

Ciliary body

The ciliary body lies just beneath the iris. The suspensory ligaments of the ciliary body attach to the lens, controlling its shape for close and distant vision. The ciliary body also continuously produces aqueous humor.

A humorous situation

Aqueous humor is a clear, watery fluid in the front of the eye that fills the anterior and posterior chambers. It gives the front of the eye its shape and provides nourishment to the cornea and lens.

Pupil

The iris' central opening, the pupil, is normally round and equal in size to the opposite pupil. The pupil permits light to enter the eye. Depending on the patient's age, pupil diameter can range from 3 to 5 mm. Small and unresponsive to light at birth, the pupil enlarges during childhood and then progressively decreases in size throughout adulthood.

Anterior and posterior chambers

The anterior chamber is filled with clear aqueous humor. The amount of fluid in the chamber varies to maintain pressure in the eye. Fluid drains from the anterior chamber through collecting channels into Schlemm canal.

Bath time!

The posterior chamber, located between the iris and the lens, is filled with aqueous humor. This fluid bathes the lens capsule as it flows through the pupil into the anterior chamber.

Aqueous humor from the posterior chamber bathes the lens capsule as it flows through the pupil. Ah! So refreshing!

Lens

Located directly behind the iris at the pupillary opening, the lens consists of avascular, transparent fibrils in an elastic membrane called the *lens capsule.* The lens refracts and focuses light onto the retina.

Vitreous chamber

The vitreous chamber, located behind the lens, occupies four-fifths of the eyeball. This chamber is filled with vitreous humor, a thick, gelatinous substance that fills the center of the eye and maintains the placement of the retina and the shape of the eyeball.

Retina

The innermost region of eyeball, the retina receives visual stimuli and transmits images to the brain for processing.

Various vessels

There are four sets of retinal blood vessels—the superonasal, infero-nasal, superotemporal, and inferotemporal. These vessels are visible through an ophthalmoscope. Each set of vessels contains a transparent arteriole and vein. As the vessels leave the optic disk, they become progressively thinner, intertwining as they extend to the periphery of the retina.

Optic disk

A well-defined, round or oval area measuring less than ⅛″ (0.3 cm) within the retina's nasal portion, the optic disk is the opening through which the ganglion nerve axons (fibers) exit the retina to form the optic nerve. This area is called the *blind spot* because no light-sensitive cells (photoreceptors) are located there.

Cup and cover

The physiologic cup is a light-colored depression within the temporal side of the optic disk where blood vessels enter the retina. It covers about one-third of the disk but doesn't extend completely to the margin.

Photoreceptor neurons

Photoreceptor neurons make up the retina's visual receptors. Not visible through the ophthalmoscope, these receptors—some shaped like rods and some like cones—are responsible for vision. Rods respond to low-intensity light, but they don't provide sharp images or color vision. Cones respond to bright light and provide high-acuity color vision.

Macula and fovea centralis

Located laterally from the optic disk, the macula is slightly darker than the rest of the retina and contains no visible retinal vessels. Because its borders are poorly defined, the macula is difficult to see on an ophthalmologic examination. It's best identified by having the patient look straight at the ophthalmoscope's light.

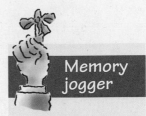

Memory jogger

To remember that cones are cells that respond to color, think of a brightly colored ice cream cone!

The fovea centralis, a slight depression in the macula, appears as a bright reflection when examined with an ophthalmoscope. Because the fovea contains the heaviest concentration of cones, it acts as the eye's clearest vision and color receptor.

Obtaining a health history

Now that you're familiar with the normal anatomy and physiology of the eyes, you're ready to obtain a health history of them. The most common eye-related symptoms that patients report are double vision (diplopia), visual floaters, photophobia (light sensitivity), vision loss, and eye pain. Other symptoms include decreased visual acuity or clarity, defects in color vision, difficulty seeing at night, and eye discharge.

Ask anyway

Even if a patient's reason for seeking care or previous diagnosis isn't eye-related, you'll need to question them about their eyes and vision. Keep in mind that poor vision can affect the patient's ability to adhere to treatment.

Asking about eyes

To obtain an accurate history, first ask the patient questions specific to their eyes:
- Do they wear corrective lenses for distance or for reading?
- Have they experienced blurred vision, blind spots, floaters, double vision, discharge, or unusual sensitivity to light?
- Do they have trouble seeing at night?
- Have they ever had an eye injury or eye surgery?
- Did they ever have a lazy eye?
- Do they have allergies?
- When was their last eye examination? Was a glaucoma test performed?
- Do they report eye pain or headaches?
- Do they squint to see objects at a distance?
- Do they hold objects close to their eyes to see them?
- Do they have a history of diabetes or high blood pressure?

Asking about general health

Now that you've asked the patient questions about their eyes, broaden your assessment to include questions about other diseases, medications, work issues, and smoking habits.

Family matters

Ask the patient if they have a history of hypertension, diabetes, stroke, multiple sclerosis, syphilis, or HIV. Find out if anyone in their family has glaucoma, cataracts, vision loss, or retinitis. Because a family history may predispose the patient to these conditions, they'll need frequent testing.

Medication connection

Ask the patient which medications they take. Some medications can affect vision. For example, digoxin (Lanoxin) overdose can cause a patient to see yellow halos around bright lights. Remember to ask about use of over-the-counter medications, herbal preparations, recreational drugs, eyedrops, and eyewashes.

All in a day's work

Ask the patient what kind of work they do and what they do for recreation. Are they exposed to chemicals, fumes, flying debris, or infectious agents? If so, do they wear eye protection? Caution all patients to wear protective eyewear when working with substances that may injure the eye. Also, find out how much time the patient spends looking at a computer.

Igniting a problem

If your patient smokes, warn them that smoking increases the risk of vascular disease, which can lead to blindness and can damage vision.

Dealing with daily living

If your patient is an older adult or has impaired vision, ask them how well they can manage activities of daily living. Assess whether they and their family need assistance in learning to use adaptive devices or a referral to an agency that helps people with impaired vision.

Kiddin' around

If your patient is a young child, the interview will vary slightly because you'll be asking the parents the questions. As a result, you may receive only objective answers, not subjective responses. (See *Seeing things differently*, page 142.)

Seeing things differently

You'll need to modify your health history for a child or an aging adult.

Children

If your patient is a child, ask the parents these questions:
• Was the child delivered vaginally or by cesarean birth? If they were delivered vaginally, did their mother have a vaginal infection at the time? (Inform the parents that infections such as chlamydia, gonorrhea, genital herpes, or candidiasis can cause eye problems in infants.)
• Did they have erythromycin ointment instilled in their eyes at birth?
• Have they passed the expected developmental milestones?
• Do they know how to hold and care for sharp objects such as scissors?

Older adults

If your patient is an aging adult, ask them these questions:
• Have you had any difficulty climbing stairs or driving or problems with night vision?
• Have you ever been tested for glaucoma? If so, when and what was the result?
• If you have glaucoma, has your doctor prescribed eye-drops for you? If so, what kind?
• How well can you instill your eyedrops?
• Do your eyes ever feel dry? Do they burn? If so, how do you treat the problem?
• Have you noticed a decrease in usual activities, such as reading or sewing?

Assessing the eyes

A complete eye assessment involves inspecting the external eye and lids, testing visual acuity, assessing visual fields, assessing eye muscle function, palpating the nasolacrimal sac, and examining intraocular structures with an ophthalmoscope.

Gather your gear

Before starting your examination, gather the necessary equipment, including a good light source, a penlight, one or two opaque cards, an ophthalmoscope, vision test cards, gloves, tissues, and cotton-tipped applicators. Make sure that the patient is seated comfortably and that you're seated at eye level with them.

Inspecting the eyes

Start your assessment by observing the patient's face. With the scalp line as the starting point, check that their eyes are in a normal position. They should be about one-third of the way down the face and about one eye's width apart from each other. Then assess the eyelid, conjunctiva, cornea, anterior chamber, iris, and pupil.

Eyelids

Each upper eyelid should cover the top quarter of the iris so the eyes look alike. Check for an excessive amount of visible sclera above the limbus (corneoscleral junction). Ask the patient to open and close their eyes to see if they close completely with spontaneous blinking every few seconds. If the downward movement of the upper eyelid in down gaze is delayed, the patient has a condition known as *lid lag*, which is a common sign of hyperthyroidism.

Assess the lids for redness, edema, inflammation, or lesions. Check for a stye, or hordeolum, a common eyelid lesion.

Eye opener

Protrusion of the eyeball, called *exophthalmos* or *proptosis*, commonly occurs in patients who have hyperthyroidism.

Crying or drying?

Inspect the eyes for excessive tearing or dryness. The eyelid margins should be pink, and the eyelashes should turn outward. Observe whether the lower eyelid turns inward toward the eyeball, called *entropion*, or outward, called *ectropion*. Examine the eyelids for lumps or lesions. Note the color and amount of any discharge.

Pressing the point

Before palpating the nasolacrimal sac, explain the procedure to the patient. Then put on examination gloves. With the patient's eyes closed, gently palpate the area below the inner canthus, noting tenderness, swelling, or discharge through the lacrimal point, which could indicate blockage of the nasolacrimal duct.

Conjunctivae

To inspect the bulbar conjunctiva, have your patient look up. Gently pull the lower eyelid down. The bulbar conjunctiva should be clear and shiny. Note excessive redness or exudate.

True colors

With the lid still secured, inspect the bulbar conjunctiva for color changes, foreign bodies, and edema. Also, observe the sclera's color, which should be white to buff. In Black patients, you may see flecks of tan. A bluish discoloration may indicate scleral thinning.

Getting an eye lift

To examine the palpebral conjunctiva, have the patient look down. Then lift the upper lid, holding the upper lashes against the eyebrow with your finger. The palpebral conjunctiva should be uniformly pink. In patients with a history of allergies, the palpebral conjunctiva may have a cobblestone appearance.

Corneas

Examine the corneas by shining a penlight first from both sides and then from straight ahead. Each cornea should be clear and without lesions. Test corneal sensitivity by lightly touching the cornea with a wisp of cotton. (See *Tips for assessing corneal sensitivity*.)

Anterior chambers and irises

The anterior chamber of the eye is bordered anteriorly by the cornea and posteriorly by the iris. The iris should appear flat, and the cornea should appear convex. Excess pressure in the eye—such as that caused by acute angle-closure glaucoma—may push the iris forward, making the anterior chamber appear very small. The irises should be the same size, color, and shape.

Pupils

Each pupil should be equal in size, round, and about one-fourth the size of the iris in normal room light. Some differences in pupil size

Peak technique

Tips for assessing corneal sensitivity

To test corneal sensitivity, touch a wisp of cotton from a cotton ball to the cornea, as shown below.

The patient should blink. If they don't, they may have suffered damage to the sensory fibers of cranial nerve V or to the motor fibers controlled by cranial nerve VI.

Keep in mind that people who wear contact lenses may have reduced sensitivity because they're accustomed to having foreign objects in their eyes.

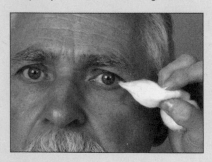

Just a wisp
Remember that a wisp of cotton is the only safe object to use for this test. Even though a 4 × 4″ gauze pad or tissue is soft, it can cause corneal abrasions and irritation.

(anisocoria) may be normal in some people. However, unequal pupils generally indicate neurologic damage, iritis, glaucoma, or therapy with certain drugs. A fixed pupil that doesn't react to light can be an ominous neurologic sign.

In perfect agreement
Test the pupils for direct and consensual response. In a slightly darkened room, hold a penlight about 20" (51 cm) from the patient's eyes, and direct the light at the eye from the side. Note the reaction of the pupil you're testing (direct response) and that of the opposite pupil (consensual response). They should both react the same way. Also, note sluggishness or inequality in the response. Repeat the test with the other pupil. *Note:* If you shine the light in a blind eye, neither pupil will respond. If you shine the light in a seeing eye, the pupils will respond consensually.

Willing to accommodate
To test the pupils for accommodation, place your finger approximately 4" (10 cm) from the bridge of the patient's nose. Ask the patient to look at a fixed object in the distance and then to look at your finger. Their pupils should constrict, and their eyes converge as they focus on your finger.

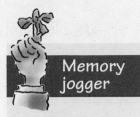

Memory jogger

To make sure that your pupil assessment is complete, think of the acronym **PERRLA**:

Pupils

Equal

Round

Reactive

Light-reacting

Accommodation.

Testing visual acuity

To test your patient's far and near vision, use a Snellen chart and a near-vision chart. To test their peripheral vision, use confrontation. Before each test, ask the patient to remove corrective lenses, if they wear them.

Snellen chart
Have the patient sit or stand 20' (6.1 m) from the chart, and then cover their left eye with an opaque object. Ask them to read the letters on one line of the chart and then to move downward to increasingly smaller lines until they can no longer discern all of the letters. Have them repeat the test covering their right eye. Finally, have them read the smallest line they can read with both eyes uncovered to test their binocular vision.

One more time
If the patient wears corrective lenses, have them repeat the test wearing them. Record the vision with and without correction.

The Big E
Use the Snellen E chart to test visual acuity in young children and other patients who can't read. Cover the patient's left eye to check the

Visual acuity charts

The most commonly used charts for testing vision are the Snellen alphabet chart (left) and the Snellen E chart (right), which is used for young children and adults who can't read. Both charts are used to test distance vision and measure visual acuity. The patient reads each chart at a distance of 20′ (6.1 m).

Recording results

Visual acuity is recorded as a fraction. The top number (20) is the distance between the patient and the chart. The bottom number is the distance from which a person with normal vision could read the line. The larger the bottom number, the poorer the patient's vision.

Age differences

In adults and children age 6 and older, normal vision is measured as 20/20. For children age 7 and younger, normal vision is 20/50; for children age 4, 20/40; and for children age 5, 20/30.

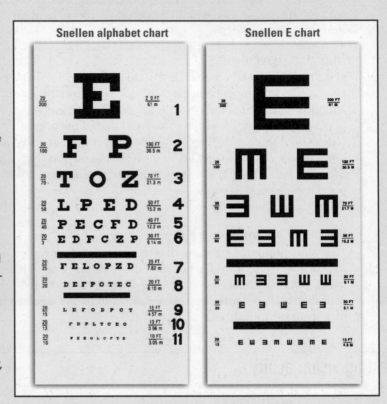

right eye, point to an E on the chart, and ask the patient to indicate which way the letter faces. Repeat the test with the left eye. (See *Visual acuity charts*.)

Eye-catching values

If the test values between the two eyes differ by two lines, such as 20/30 in one eye and 20/50 in the other, suspect an abnormality such as amblyopia (reduced vision in an eye that appears normal during ophthalmoscopic examination)—especially in children.

Near-vision chart

To test near vision, cover one of the patient's eyes with an opaque object and hold a Rosenbaum near-vision card 14″ (35.6 cm) from their eyes. Have them read the line with the smallest letters they can distinguish. Repeat the test with the other eye. If the patient wears

Using confrontation

Follow these steps to assess peripheral vision with confrontation:

• Sit directly across from the patient and have them focus their gaze on your eyes.

• Place your hands on either side of the patient's head at the level of their ears so that they're about 2′ apart (as shown).

• Tell the patient to focus their gaze on you as you gradually bring your wiggling fingers into their visual field.

• Instruct the patient to tell you as soon as they can see your wiggling fingers; they should see them at the same time you do.

• Repeat the procedure while holding your hands at the superior and inferior positions.

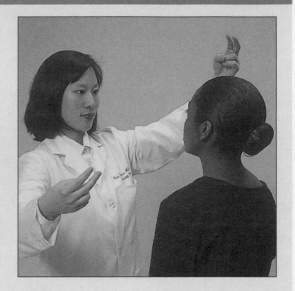

corrective lenses, have them repeat the test while wearing them. Record the visual accommodation with and without lenses.

Confrontation

To assess peripheral vision, use a method known as *confrontation*. This test can help identify abnormalities such as homonymous hemianopsia and bitemporal hemianopsia. (See *Using confrontation*.)

Assessing eye muscle function

A thorough assessment of the eyes includes an evaluation of the extraocular muscles. To evaluate these muscles, you'll need to assess the corneal light reflex and the cardinal positions of gaze, and then perform the cover-uncover test.

Corneal light reflex

To assess the corneal light reflex, ask the patient to look straight ahead; then shine a penlight on the bridge of their nose from about 12 to 15″ (30.5 to 38 cm) away. The light should fall at the same spot on each cornea. If it doesn't, the eyes aren't being held in the same plane by the extraocular muscles. This commonly occurs in a patient who lacks muscle coordination, a condition called *strabismus.*

Cardinal positions of gaze

Cardinal positions of gaze evaluate the oculomotor, trigeminal, and abducens nerves as well as the extraocular muscles. To perform this test, ask the patient to remain still while you hold a pencil or other small object directly in front of their nose at a distance of about 18″ (45.5 cm).

Eyeballs on the move

Ask them to follow the object with their eyes, without moving their head. Then move the object to each of the six cardinal positions, returning to the midpoint after each movement. The patient's eyes should remain parallel as they move. Note abnormal findings such as nystagmus and amblyopia, the failure of one eye to follow an object. (See *Cardinal positions of gaze*.)

Cover–uncover test

The cover–uncover test is done after you detect an abnormality when assessing the corneal light reflex and cardinal positions of gaze. To perform a cover–uncover test, have the patient stare at a wall on the

Cardinal positions of gaze

The illustration below identifies the six cardinal positions of gaze.

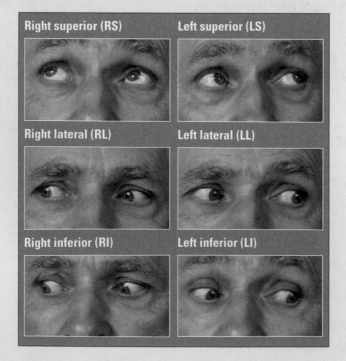

other side of the room. Cover one eye and watch for movement in the uncovered eye. Remove the eye cover and watch for movement again. Repeat the test with the other eye.

On the move

Eye movement while covering or uncovering the eye is considered abnormal. It may result from weak or paralyzed extraocular muscles, which may be caused by cranial nerve impairment.

Examining intraocular structures

The ophthalmoscope allows you to directly observe the eye's internal structures. To see those structures properly, you'll need to adjust the lens dial. Use the black, positive numbers on the dial to focus on near objects such as the patient's cornea and lens. Use the red, minus numbers to focus on more distant objects such as the retina.

Before the examination, have the patient remove their contact lenses (if they're tinted) or eyeglasses, and darken the room to dilate their pupils and make your examination easier. Ask the patient to focus on a point behind you. Tell them that you'll be moving into their visual field and blocking their view. Also, explain that you'll be shining a bright light into their eye, which may be uncomfortable but not harmful. (See *Seeing eye to eye*.)

Closing in on the cornea

Set the lens dial at zero, hold the ophthalmoscope about 4″ (10 cm) from the patient's eye, and direct the light through the pupil to elicit the red reflex, a reflection of light off the choroid. Check the red reflex for depth of color and symmetry of color between the eyes.

Now, move the ophthalmoscope closer to the eye. Adjust the lens dial so you can focus on the anterior chamber and lens. Look for clouding, foreign matter, or opacities. If the lens is opaque, indicating cataracts, you may not be able to complete the examination.

Rotating to the retinal structures

To examine the retina, start with the dial turned to zero. Rotate the lens power dial to adjust for your refractive correction and the patient's refractive error. Now, observe the vitreous body for clarity. The first retinal structures you'll see are the blood vessels. Rotating the dial into the negative numbers will bring the blood vessels into focus. The arteries will look thinner and brighter than the veins.

Follow that vessel

Follow one of the vessels along its path toward the nose until you reach the optic disk, where all vessels in the eye originate. Examine

Seeing eye to eye

This illustration shows the correct position for the examiner and the patient when an ophthalmoscope is used to examine the eye's internal structures.

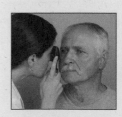

arteriovenous crossings for arteriovenous nicking (localized constrictions in the retinal vessels), which might be a sign of hypertension.

Disk details

The optic disk is a creamy pink to yellow-orange structure with clear borders and a round-to-oval shape. With practice, you'll be able to identify the physiologic cup, a small depression that occupies about one-third of the disk's diameter. The disk may fill or exceed your field of vision. If you don't see it, follow a blood vessel toward the center until you do. The nasal border of the disk may be somewhat blurred.

Riveting on the retina

Completely scan the retina by following four blood vessels from the optic disk to different peripheral areas. The retina should have a uniform color and be free from scars and pigmentation. As you scan, note any lesions or hemorrhages. (See *A close look at the retina.*)

A close look at the retina

This illustration shows the complex anatomy of the retina and its structures.

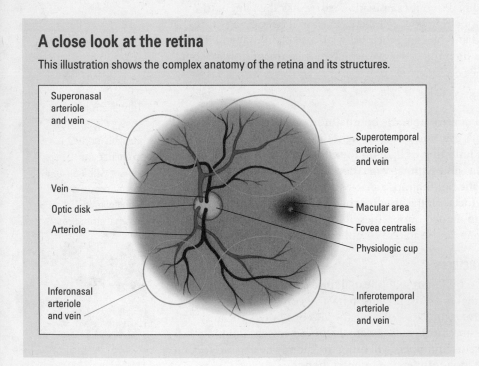

Superonasal arteriole and vein

Superotemporal arteriole and vein

Vein

Optic disk

Arteriole

Macular area

Fovea centralis

Physiologic cup

Inferonasal arteriole and vein

Inferotemporal arteriole and vein

Movin' in on the macula

Finally, move the light laterally from the optic disk to locate the macula, the part of the eye that's most sensitive to light. It appears as a dark structure, free from blood vessels. Your view may be fleeting because most patients can't tolerate having a beam of light fall on the macula. If you locate it, ask the patient to shift their gaze into the light.

Abnormal findings

Common abnormalities you may detect during an eye assessment include anisocoria, arteriolar narrowing, corneal arcus, decreased visual acuity, diplopia, ectropion and entropion, eye discharge, eye pain, jaundice, Kayser-Fleischer rings, muddy sclera, periorbital edema, pinguecula and pterygium, ptosis, strabismus, subconjunctival hemorrhage vision loss, visual floaters, and visual halos. (See *Eye abnormalities*, page 152.)

Anisocoria

Anisocoria is defined as having unequal pupils. Anisocoria can be a normal finding in up to 20% of the population. It can be caused by several pathologies including traumatic brain injury, concussion, and migraine.

Arteriolar narrowing

Typically, arterioles of the inner eye are between two-thirds and three-fourths the width of veins and have a brighter appearance. When these minute arteries narrow, they appear to be about one-half as wide as veins. Arteriolar narrowing commonly occurs in patients who have hypertension.

Corneal arcus

These whitish blueish rings surround the outside or the iris. They can be a normal finding in older adults (arcus senilis). In those under 65, it is a sign of hypercholesterolemia.

Decreased visual acuity

Decreased visual acuity—the ability to see clearly—commonly occurs with refractive errors. In nearsightedness, or myopia, the eye focuses the visual image in front of the retina, causing objects in close view to

Interpretation station

Eye abnormalities

This chart shows common groups of findings for signs and symptoms of the eyes along with their probable causes.

Sign or symptom and findings	Probable cause
Eye discharge	
• Purulent or mucopurulent, greenish white discharge that occurs unilaterally • Sticky crusts that form on the eyelids during sleep • Itching and burning • Excessive tearing • Sensation of a foreign body in the eye	Bacterial conjunctivitis
• Scant but continuous purulent discharge that's easily expressed from the tear sac • Excessive tearing • Pain and tenderness near the tear sac • Eyelid inflammation and edema noticeable around the lacrimal punctum	Dacryocystitis
• Continuous frothy discharge • Chronically red eyes with inflamed lid margins • Soft, foul-smelling, cheesy yellow discharge elicited by pressure on the meibomian glands	Meibomianitis
Decreased visual acuity	
• Gradual visual blurring • Halo vision • Visual glare in bright light • Progressive vision loss • Gray pupil that later turns milky white	Cataract

Sign or symptom and findings	Probable cause
Decreased visual acuity *(Continued)*	
• Constant morning headache that decreases in severity during the day • Possible severe, throbbing headache • Restlessness • Confusion • Nausea and vomiting • Seizures • Decreased level of consciousness	Hypertension
• Paroxysmal attacks of severe, throbbing unilateral or bilateral headache • Nausea and vomiting • Sensitivity to light and noise • Sensory or visual auras	Migraine headache
Visual floaters	
• Sudden onset of spots or flashing lights • Curtainlike loss of vision • Black retinal vessels	Retinal detachment
• Onset of spots or flashing lights • Gradual development of eye pain • Photophobia • Blurred vision • Conjunctival injection	Posterior uveitis

be seen clearly while those at a distance appear blurry. In farsighted-ness, or hyperopia, the eye focuses the visual image behind the retina, causing objects in close view to appear blurry while those at a distance seem clear. Both problems result from an abnormal shape of the eyeball.

Diplopia

When the extraocular muscles are misaligned, the visual axes aren't directed at the object of sight at the same time. This results in double vision, or diplopia.

Discharge

The excretion of any substance from the eyes other than tears is known as a *discharge*. A common finding, discharge may occur in one or both eyes and may be scant or copious. The discharge may be puru-lent, frothy, mucoid, cheesy, serous, or clear or have a stringy, white appearance. Eye discharge commonly results from inflammatory and infectious eye disorders, such as conjunctivitis, but it may also occur in certain systemic disorders.

Ectropion and entropion

Ectropion and entropion are disorders associated with age-related tis-sue relaxation. Entropion is the inversion of an eyelid. This can lead to irritation of the eye and in some cases may require surgical repair. In ectropion the lower eyelid droops down and causes a space between the lower eyelid and eye surface. This can cause both excess tearing and dry eye sensation. Topical drops can be helpful as can surgical repair.

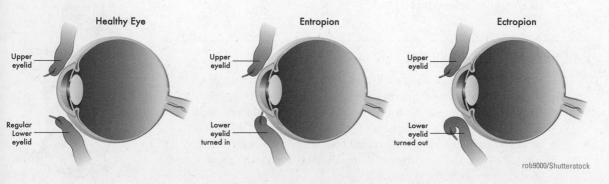

rob9000/Shutterstock

Jaundice

Jaundice of the sclera is a yellow tint to the sclera that is caused by an accumulation of bilirubin in the tissues. It can range from subtle to profound.

Kayser-Fleischer rings

These are reddish, copper-colored rings that surround the iris. They are best visualized with a Wood's lamp. They are an indicator of Wilson disease, a rare genetic disease of abnormal copper metabolism.

Muddy sclera

Not a true abnormality, muddy sclera is brown pigmentation in spots of the sclera. It can be confused with jaundice in those who are not familiar with it. It is a normal finding in patients of African descent.

Pain

Eye pain may signal an emergency and requires immediate attention. Diseases causing eye pain include acute angle-closure glaucoma and conjunctivitis. Corneal damage caused by a foreign body or abrasions as well as trauma to the eye can also cause eye pain.

Periorbital edema

Swelling around the eyes, or periorbital edema, may result from allergies, local inflammation, fluid-retaining disorders, or crying. It can also represent a very serious infection—periorbital cellulitis. This can be an ophthalmologic emergency that requires rapid evaluation and treatment by an eye specialist.

Pinguecula and pterygium

Both of these are growths on the surface of the eye. Pingueculae are fleshy, whitish-yellow growths that approach, but do not grow over, the cornea. In general, they do not affect vision and do not require any intervention. Pterygiums are similar, have more of a fleshlike appearance. Pterygiums have blood vessels and may start as a pinguecula but can cross the cornea and actually may eventually grow across it, thus impairing the visual field.

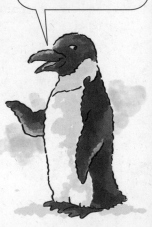

Many penguins live at the South Pole. They never "migrate" to the North Pole. Likewise, pingueculae do not migrate across the cornea.

Ptosis

Ptosis, or a drooping upper eyelid, may be caused by an interruption in sympathetic innervation to the eyelid, muscle weakness, or damage to the oculomotor nerve. (See *Recognizing periorbital edema and ptosis*.)

Strabismus

With strabismus, the eyes deviate from their normal gazing position. This condition may result from extraocular weakness or paralysis as a result of poor vision in one eye. It may also result from thyroid oph-thalmopathy. Although adults may develop strabismus, it most com-monly occurs in children. Detected early, it can be corrected without surgery. (See *Strabismus in children*.)

Subconjunctival hemorrhage

This appears as a red patch on the sclera. Although it has a shocking appearance, it is generally self-limiting, and as an isolated finding is not a cause for concern. It is caused by small broken blood vessels below the conjunctiva and provoked by minor traumas such as eye rubbing and even strong coughing or sneezing. It is painless and does not cause any visual disturbance. It is usually resolved as the blood is absorbed over a course of 1 to 2 weeks.

Recognizing periorbital edema and ptosis

During an eye examination, you may observe any of a number of abnormali-ties. These illustra-tions show periorbital edema and ptosis.

Periorbital edema

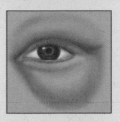

Ptosis

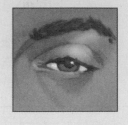

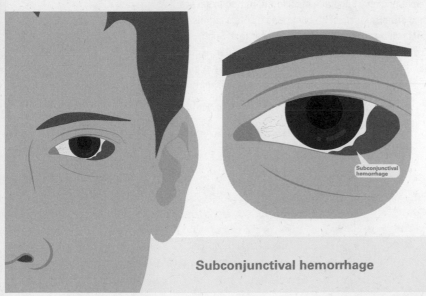

Subconjunctival hemorrhage

Vision loss

Disorders of any structure of the eye can result in vision loss. Types of vision loss include central vision loss, peripheral vision loss, or a blind spot in the middle of an area of normal vision (scotoma).

The degree and location of blindness depends on the disease causing the problem as well as the location of the lesion. The major causes of blindness in the United States include glaucoma, untreated cataracts, retinal disease, and macular degeneration.

Visual floaters

Visual floaters are specks of varying shape and size that float through the visual field and disappear when the patient tries to look at them. Caused by small cells floating in the vitreous humor, visual floaters may signal vitreous hemorrhage or retinal separation and therefore require further investigation. A large, black floater that appears suddenly may indicate retinal detachment.

Handle with care

Strabismus in children

Strabismus is the most common abnormal eye condition in children. Although severe strabismus is readily apparent, mild strabismus must be confirmed by tests for misalignment, such as the corneal light reflex test and the cover-uncover test. Such testing is crucial because early corrective measures help preserve binocular vision— which is normally achieved by age 3 to 4 months—and cosmetic appearance. Also, mild strabismus may indicate retinoblastoma, a tumor that may produce no symptoms before age two except for a characteristic whitish reflex in the pupil.

Visual halos

Increased intraocular pressure, which occurs in glaucoma, causes the patient to see halos and rainbows around bright lights. Other possible causes include corneal edema as a result of prolonged contact lens wear or a fluctuation in blood glucose levels.

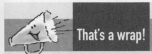

That's a wrap!

Eye review

Anatomy and physiology
- Sclera—maintains the eye's size and shape
- Choroid—maintains blood supply to the eye
- Vitreous humor—maintains the placement of the retina and the eyeball's spherical shape
- Cornea—refracts, or bends, light rays entering the eye
- Iris—contains pigment granules that give the eye its color; contains involuntary muscles that control pupil size
- Pupil—permits light to enter the eye
- Lens—refracts and focuses light onto the retina
- Retina—receives visual stimuli and transmits images to the brain for processing.

Health history
- Determine the patient's presenting problem.
- Ask if the patient wears corrective lenses.
- Obtain their past medical history. Be sure to ask about disorders that may affect vision, such as hypertension, diabetes, or stroke.

- Ask about a family history of glaucoma, cataracts, or vision loss.
- Obtain a medication history. Some medications, such as digoxin (Lanoxin), can affect vision.
- Ask a patient with vision impairment how they manage activities of daily living and assess their support system.

Assessment
- Note the position of the eyes.
- Check eyelids for closure and for redness, edema, inflammation, or lesions.
- Inspect for excessive tearing, dryness, or discharge.
- Palpate the nasolacrimal sac.
- Examine the bulbar and palpebral conjunctivae.
- Inspect the corneas and assess corneal sensitivity using a wisp of cotton.
- Evaluate each iris for size, color, and shape.
- Examine the pupils for equal size, shape, and reactivity.

Tests for visual acuity
- Snellen chart, Snellen E chart, and near-vision chart—test near and distance vision and measure visual acuity
- Confrontation—tests peripheral vision and assesses visual fields.

(Continued)

Eye review *(continued)*

Tests for extraocular muscle function

• Corneal light reflex—light should fall at the same spot on each cornea
• Cardinal positions of gaze—eyes should remain parallel and move smoothly through the six cardinal positions
• Cover-uncover test—eye shouldn't move while covering or uncovering it.

Ophthalmoscopic examination

• Have the patient remove their corrective lenses; darken the room.
• Check for the presence and depth of the red reflex.
• Examine the lens for clouding, foreign matter, or opacities.
• Examine the retina: Observe the vitreous body for clarity; note the characteristics of the blood vessels; identify the optic disk, noting color, shape, and borders; and locate the light-sensitive macula.

Abnormal findings

• Arteriolar narrowing—arterioles of the inner eye narrow to a width of about one-half that of vein width
• Decreased visual acuity—the inability to see clearly
• Diplopia—double vision
• Discharge—excretion of any substance other than tears
• Ectropion and entropion—associated with age-related tissue relaxation

• Jaundice—yellow tint to the sclera that is caused by an accumulation of bilirubin in the tissues
• Kayser-Fleischer rings—reddish, copper-colored rings that surround the iris. They are an indicator of Wilson disease.
• Muddy sclera—not a true abnormality; brown pigmentation in spots of the sclera
• Pain—may demand immediate attention
• Periorbital edema—swelling around the eyes
• Pinguecula and pterygium—both are growths on the surface of the eye
• Ptosis—a drooping upper eyelid
• Strabismus—eyes deviate from their normal gazing position
• Subconjunctival hemorrhage—appears as a red patch on the sclera; generally self-limiting, caused by broken blood vessels below the conjunctiva
• Vision loss—may be central or peripheral
• Visual floaters—specks of varying shape and size that float through the visual field but disappear when the patient tries to look at them
• Visual halos—rings or halos seen when looking at bright lights.

Quick quiz

1. The normal reaction to a corneal sensitivity test is:
   A. blinking.
   B. coughing.
   C. pupil dilation.
   D. pupil contraction.

Answer: A. The normal response to a corneal sensitivity test is blinking.

2. In addition to trauma, unequal pupils can result from:
   A. a cataract.
   B. an iridectomy.
   C. severe conjunctivitis.
   D. strabismus.

Answer: B. During an iridectomy, part of the iris is excised, resulting in an irregular pupil.

3. Cone receptors are mainly responsible for sensing:
   A. light.
   B. color.
   C. shapes.
   D. black and white.

Answer: B. Cones, which are located in the fovea centralis, aid in color recognition.

4. To determine a patient's visual acuity, you would use the:
   A. Snellen chart.
   B. cover-uncover test.
   C. corneal light reflex test.
   D. cardinal positions of gaze.

Answer: A. The Snellen chart tests visual acuity by having the patient read a series of letters. The Snellen E chart contains only the letter *E* and can be used for young children and patients who can't read.

5. The red reflex seen during an ophthalmoscopic examination is the result of:
   A. an increase in intraocular pressure.
   B. incorrect adjustment of the diopter.
   C. light from the scope reflecting back from the choroid.
   D. arteriolar narrowing.

Answer: C. The red reflex results from light reflecting off the choroid. To test for the reflex, shine the ophthalmoscope light at the patient's pupil from a distance of about 4″ (10 cm) and at a slight angle.

6. Compared with the size of a child's pupils, the size of an adult's pupils is:
    A. smaller.
    B. larger.
    C. the same throughout life.
    D. wider.

Answer: A. Pupils are small and unresponsive to light at birth. They enlarge during childhood and progressively decrease in size throughout adulthood and into old age.

7. Which item is used to test corneal sensitivity?
    A. Wisp of cotton
    B. Tissue
    C. Gauze pad
    D. Ophthalmoscope

Answer: A. A wisp of cotton is the only safe object to use for assessing corneal sensitivity. Even though a gauze pad or tissue is soft, it can cause corneal abrasions and irritation.

Scoring

⭐⭐⭐ If you answered all seven questions correctly, terrific! You're a star pupil.

⭐⭐   If you answered five or six questions correctly, good job! You really have vision.

⭐   If you answered fewer than five questions correctly, don't lose focus. Just set your eyes on the prize and move on to the next chapter.

Chapter 8

Ears, nose, and throat

Just the facts

In this chapter, you'll learn:

♦ structures of the ears, nose, and throat and their functions

♦ questions to ask about the ears, nose, and throat during the health history

♦ techniques for assessing the ears, nose, and throat

♦ ear, nose, and throat abnormalities and their causes.

A look at the ears, nose, and throat

The ability to hear, smell, and taste allows us to communicate with others, connect with the world around us, and take pleasure in life. Because these senses play such vital roles in daily life, you'll need to thoroughly assess a patient's ears, nose, and throat.

Clues for you

Besides revealing impairments in hearing, smell, and taste, your assessment also can uncover important clues to physical problems in the patient's integumentary, musculoskeletal, cardiovascular, respiratory, immune, and neurologic systems.

Anatomy and physiology

To perform an accurate physical assessment, you'll need to understand the anatomy and physiology of the ears, nose, and throat.

Ears

The ear is divided into three parts: external, middle, and inner. The anatomy and physiology of each part play separate but equally important roles in hearing. (See *A close look at the ear.*)

External ear

The flexible external ear consists mainly of elastic cartilage. This part of the ear contains the ear flap, also known as the *auricle* or *pinna,* and the auditory canal. The outer third of this canal has a bony framework. Coarse hair may be visible in the canal in male older adults. The external ear and ear canal collect sounds and transmit them to the middle ear.

A close look at the ear

Use this illustration to review the structures of the ear.

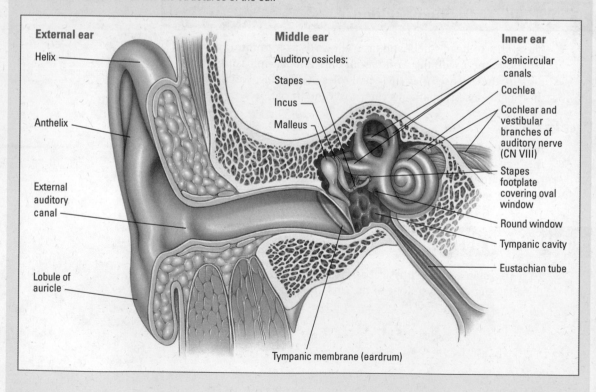

External ear

Helix

Anthelix

External auditory canal

Lobule of auricle

Middle ear

Auditory ossicles:

Stapes

Incus

Malleus

Inner ear

Semicircular canals

Cochlea

Cochlear and vestibular branches of auditory nerve (CN VIII)

Stapes footplate covering oval window

Round window

Tympanic cavity

Eustachian tube

Tympanic membrane (eardrum)

Middle ear

The tympanic membrane separates the external and middle ear. This pearl-gray structure consists of three layers: skin, fibrous tissue, and a mucous membrane. Its upper portion, the pars flaccida, has little support; its lower portion, the pars tensa, is held taut. The center, or umbo, is attached to the tip of the long process of the malleus on the other side of the tympanic membrane.

A small, air-filled structure, the middle ear performs two vital functions:

1. It transmits sound vibrations across the bony ossicle chain to the inner ear.
2. It protects the inner ear by reducing the amplitude of loud sounds.

The eustachian tube connects the middle ear to the nasopharynx and the air pressure on both sides of the tympanic membrane prevents the middle ear from rupturing.

Those bones, those bones, those ear bones

The middle ear contains three small bones of the auditory ossicles: the malleus, or hammer; the incus, or anvil; and the stapes, or stirrup. These bones are linked like a chain and vibrate in place. The long process of the malleus fits into the incus, forming a true joint, and allows the two structures to move as a single unit. The proximal end of the stapes fits into the oval window, an opening that joins the middle and inner ear.

A cleaning tube

A normally functioning eustachian tube keeps the middle ear free from contaminants from the nasopharynx. It opens during yawning or swallowing. Upper respiratory tract infections and allergies can block the tube, obstructing middle ear drainage and possibly causing otitis media or effusion.

Inner ear

The inner ear consists of closed, fluid-filled spaces within the temporal bone. It contains the bony labyrinth, which includes three connected structures: the vestibule, the semicircular canals, and the cochlea. These structures are lined with the membranous labyrinth. A fluid called *perilymph* fills the space between the bony labyrinth and the membranous labyrinth, cushioning these sensitive organs.

The vestibule and semicircular canals help maintain equilibrium. The cochlea, a spiral chamber that resembles a snail shell, is the organ of hearing. The organ of Corti, part of the membranous labyrinth, contains hair cells that receive auditory sensations.

I heard it through the...sound waves

When sound waves reach the external ear, structures there transmit the waves through the auditory canal to the tympanic membrane, where they cause a chain reaction of vibrations along the structures of the middle and inner ear. Finally, the cochlear branch of the acoustic nerve (cranial nerve VIII) transmits the vibrations to the temporal lobe of the cerebral cortex, where the brain interprets the sound.

Double duty

In addition to controlling hearing, structures in the inner ear control balance. The semicircular canals of the inner ear contain cristae—hair-like structures that respond to body movements. Endolymph fluid bathes the cristae.

Balancing act

When a person moves, the cristae bend, releasing impulses through the vestibular portion of the acoustic nerve to the brain, which controls balance. When a person is stationary, nerve impulses to the brain orient them to this position, and the pressure of gravity on the inner ear helps them maintain balance.

Nose

The nose is more than the sensory organ of smell. It also plays a key role in the respiratory system by filtering, warming, and humidifying inhaled air. When you assess the nose, you'll commonly assess the paranasal sinuses, too.

Inside and out

The lower two-thirds of the external nose consist of flexible cartilage, and the upper one-third is rigid bone. Posteriorly, the internal nose merges with the pharynx. Anteriorly, it merges with the external nose.

Dividing line

The internal and external nose are divided vertically by the nasal septum, which is straight at birth and in early life but becomes slightly deviated or deformed in almost every adult. Only the posterior end, which separates the posterior nares, remains constantly in the midline.

Nosebleed central

Kiesselbach area, the most common site of nosebleeds, is located in the anterior portion of the septum.

Just nosing around

Air entering the nose passes through the vestibule, which is lined with coarse hair that helps filter dust. Olfactory receptors lie above the vestibule in the roof of the nasal cavity and the upper one-third of the septum. Known as the *olfactory region*, this area is rich in capillaries and mucus-producing goblet cells that help warm, moisten, and clean inhaled air.

Breathe easy

Farther along the nasal passage are the superior, middle, and inferior turbinates. Separated by grooves called *meatus*, the curved bony turbinates and their mucosal covering ease breathing by further warming, filtering, and humidifying inhaled air.

Singling out the sinuses

Four pairs of paranasal sinuses open into the internal nose, including the:
- maxillary sinuses, located on the cheeks below the eyes
- frontal sinuses, located above the eyebrows
- ethmoidal and sphenoidal sinuses, located behind the eyes and nose in the head.

The sinuses serve as resonators for sound production and provide mucus. You'll be able to assess the maxillary and frontal sinuses, but the ethmoidal and sphenoidal sinuses aren't readily accessible. (See *A close look at the nose and mouth*, page 168.)

The small openings between the sinuses and the nasal cavity can easily become obstructed because they're lined with mucous membranes that can become inflamed and swollen.

Throat

The throat, or pharynx, is divided into the nasopharynx, oropharynx, and laryngopharynx. Located within the throat are the hard and soft palates, the uvula, and the tonsils. The mucous membrane lining the throat is usually smooth and bright pink to light red.

Running neck and neck

The neck is formed by the cervical vertebrae, the major neck and shoulder muscles, and their ligaments. Other important structures of the neck include the trachea, thyroid gland, and chains of lymph nodes. (See *A close look at the neck*, page 169.)

A close look at the nose and mouth

These illustrations show the anatomic structures of the nose and mouth.

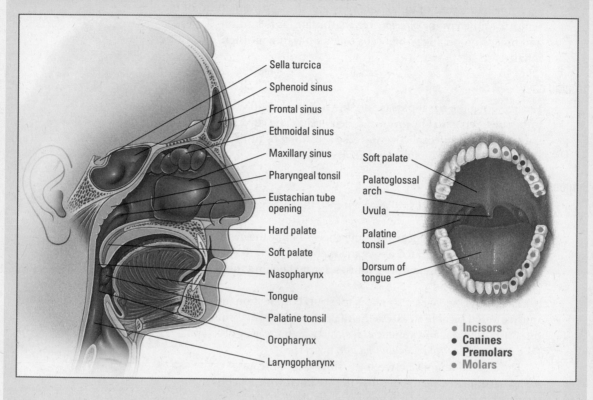

Sella turcica
Sphenoid sinus
Frontal sinus
Ethmoidal sinus
Maxillary sinus
Pharyngeal tonsil
Eustachian tube opening
Hard palate
Soft palate
Nasopharynx
Tongue
Palatine tonsil
Oropharynx
Laryngopharynx

Soft palate
Palatoglossal arch
Uvula
Palatine tonsil
Dorsum of tongue

- Incisors
- **Canines**
- **Premolars**
- Molars

Grand gland

The thyroid gland lies in the anterior neck, just below the larynx. Its two cone-shaped lobes are located on either side of the trachea and are connected by an isthmus below the cricoid cartilage, which gives the gland its butterfly shape. The largest endocrine gland, the thyroid produces the hormones triiodothyronine and thyroxine, which affect the metabolic reactions of every cell in the body.

A close look at the neck

This illustration shows the anatomic structures of the neck.

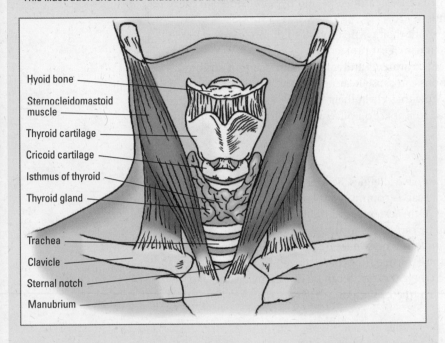

- Hyoid bone
- Sternocleidomastoid muscle
- Thyroid cartilage
- Cricoid cartilage
- Isthmus of thyroid
- Thyroid gland
- Trachea
- Clavicle
- Sternal notch
- Manubrium

Obtaining a health history

To investigate a patient's concern about the ears, nose, or throat, ask about the onset, location, duration, and characteristics of the symptom as well as what aggravates and relieves it.

Asking about the ears

The most common ear symptoms reported are hearing loss, tinnitus, pain, discharge, and dizziness. Ask the patient if they have any associated symptoms. Have them describe the color and consistency of any ear discharge, and ask about a history of head injury. Ask the patient if they have had feelings of abnormal movement or vertigo (spinning). Determine when the episodes occur, how frequently they occur, and whether they're associated with nausea, vomiting, or tinnitus.

Ask the patient if they have previously had an ear problem or injury, or if anyone in their family has ear or hearing problems. Also, ask if they have been ill recently or if they have a chronic disorder. For example, diabetes can cause hearing loss, and hypertension can cause high-pitched tinnitus.

Ask the patient about their occupation. If their job involves loud noise, ask about their use of ear protection.

Ask about current treatments and medications. Certain antibiotics and other medications can cause hearing loss and tinnitus.

Ask the patient how they clean their ears. The use of cotton-tipped applicators may lead to impaction of cerumen, which can contribute to hearing loss.

Nothing to sneeze at

Ask the patient if they have allergies. Serous otitis media, or inflammation of the middle ear, is common in people with environmental or seasonal allergies. Otitis externa, or inflammation or infection of the external ear, can be caused by an allergic reaction to hair dyes, cosmetics, perfumes, and other personal care products. It can be caused by an infection of the ear canal. It is characterized by redness of the canal and exudate in the ear canal. It can be caused by a variety of pathogens and is often treated with otic drops.

Otitis externa

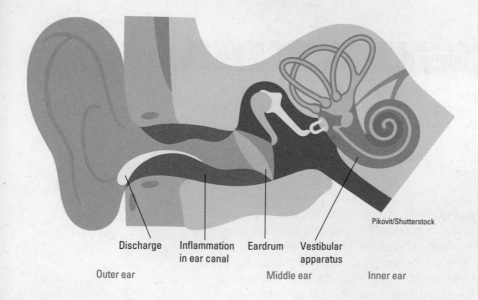

Pikovit/Shutterstock

Discharge   Inflammation   Eardrum   Vestibular
in ear canal   apparatus

Outer ear   Middle ear   Inner ear

Asking about the nose

The most common symptoms patients report about the nose include nasal stuffiness, nasal discharge, and epistaxis, or nosebleed. Ask if the patient has had any of these problems. Also ask about frequent colds, hay fever, headaches, and sinus trouble. Determine whether certain conditions or places seem to cause or aggravate the patient's problem. Ask if they have ever had nose or head trauma.

Allergens all around

Environmental allergies can cause nasal stuffiness and discharge, and stagnant nasal discharge can act as a culture medium and lead to sinusitis and other infections. Also, inquire about the color and consistency of the discharge. Ask the patient about their use of nasal sprays; stopping a nasal spray after using it for a period of time can result in rebound congestion.

Asking about the mouth, throat, and neck

Ask the patient if they have bleeding or sore gums, mouth or tongue ulcers, a bad taste in their mouth, bad breath, toothaches, loose teeth, frequent sore throats, hoarseness, or facial swelling. Also ask whether they smoke or use other types of tobacco. If the patient is having neck problems, ask if they have neck pain or tenderness, neck swelling, or trouble moving their neck.

Asking about general health

After asking specific questions about the ears, nose, mouth, throat, and neck, ask about the patient's general health. Be alert for responses that might indicate a thyroid disorder. Hyperthyroidism can cause heat intolerance, weight loss, and a short menstrual pattern with scant flow. Hypothyroidism can cause cold intolerance, weight gain, an increase in menstrual pattern and flow and, in extreme cases, bradycardia and dyspnea from low cardiac output.

Get specific

Ask the patient these questions pertaining to signs and symptoms:
- Have you noticed changes in the way you tolerate hot and cold weather?
- Has your weight changed recently? How much has it changed and over what period of time?
- Do you have breathing problems or feel as if your heart is skipping beats?
- Have you noticed a change in your menstrual pattern?
- Have you noticed any tremors, agitation, or difficulty concentrating or sleeping?

Assessing the ears, nose, and throat

Examining the ears, nose, and throat mainly involves using the techniques of inspection, palpation, and auscultation. An ear assessment also requires the use of an otoscope and the administration of hearing acuity tests.

Examining the ears

To assess your patient's ears, you'll need to inspect and palpate the external structures, perform an otoscopic examination of the ear canal, and test their hearing acuity.

External observations

Begin by observing the ears for position and symmetry. The top of the ear should line up with the outer corner of the eye, and the ears should look symmetrical, with an angle of attachment of no more than 10°. The face and ears should be the same shade and color.

Ear-y situation

Auricles that protrude from the head, or "lop" ears, are fairly common and don't affect hearing ability. However, low-set ears commonly accompany congenital disorders, including kidney problems.

An auricle oracle

Inspect the auricle for lesions, drainage, nodules, or redness. Pull the helix back and note if it's tender. If pulling the ear back hurts the patient, they may have otitis externa. Then inspect and palpate the mastoid area behind each auricle, noting tenderness, redness, or warmth, which may suggest mastoiditis.

Conclude with the canal

Finally, inspect the opening of the ear canal, noting discharge, redness, odor, or the presence of nodules or cysts. Patients normally have varying amounts of hair and cerumen (earwax) in the ear canal.

Otoscopic examination

The next part of your ear assessment involves examining the patient's auditory canal, tympanic membrane, and malleus with an otoscope. Before inserting the speculum into the patient's ear canal, check the canal for foreign bodies or discharge. (See *Using an otoscope*, page 174.)

Then palpate the tragus—the cartilaginous projection anterior to the external opening of the ear—and pull the auricle up. If this area is tender, don't insert the speculum. The patient could have otitis externa, and inserting the speculum could be painful.

Insert speculum A into ear B

To insert the speculum of the otoscope, tilt the patient's head away from you. Then grasp the superior posterior auricle with your thumb and index finger and pull it up and back to straighten the canal. Because everyone's ear canal is shaped differently, vary the angle of the speculum until you can see the tympanic membrane. If your patient is a child younger than age 3, pull the auricle down to get a good view of the membrane. Lean your hand holding the otoscope against the patient's head for steadiness.

Go gently into that good ear canal

Insert the speculum to about one-third its length when inspecting the canal. Be sure to insert it gently because the inner two-thirds of the canal are sensitive to pressure. Note the cerumen's color, amount, and consistency. (See *Cerumen variations*.) The older patient may have harder, drier cerumen because of rigid cilia in the ear canal. The external canal should be free from inflammation and scaling.

Peak technique

Using an otoscope

Here's how to use an otoscope to examine the ears.

Inserting the speculum

Before inserting the speculum into the patient's ear, straighten the ear canal by grasping the auricle and pulling it up and back, as shown at right.

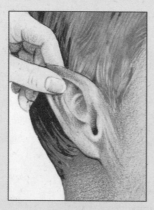

Positioning the scope

To examine the ear's external canal, hold the otoscope with the handle parallel to the patient's head, as shown below. Bracing your hand firmly against their head keeps you from hitting the canal with the speculum.

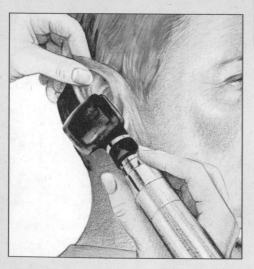

Viewing the structures

When the otoscope is positioned properly, you should see the tympanic membrane structures shown below.

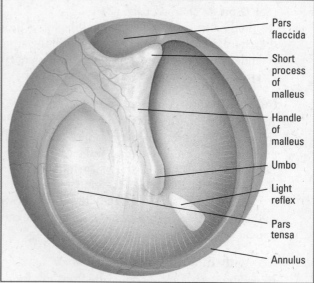

Pars flaccida

Short process of malleus

Handle of malleus

Umbo

Light reflex

Pars tensa

Annulus

Blocked view

If your view of the tympanic membrane is obstructed by excessive cerumen, don't try to remove the cerumen with an instrument because you could cause the patient excessive pain. Instead, use ceruminolytic drops and warm water irrigation as ordered.

As the speculum turns

You may need to carefully rotate the speculum for a complete view of the tympanic membrane. The membrane should be pearl gray, glistening, and transparent. The annulus should be white and denser than the rest of the membrane. Inspect the membrane carefully for bulging, retraction, bleeding, lesions, and perforations, especially at the periphery. The older patient's eardrum may appear cloudy and more prominent because of atrophy associated with aging.

"Timing" the light reflex?

Now, examine the membrane for the light reflex. The light reflex in the right ear should be at the 5 o'clock position; in the left ear, it should be at the 7 o'clock position. If the reflex is displaced or absent, the patient's tympanic membrane may be bulging, inflamed, or retracted.

Finally, look for the bony landmarks. The malleus will appear as a dense, white streak at the 12 o'clock position. At the top of the light reflex, you'll find the umbo, the inferior point of the malleus.

Hearing acuity tests

The last part of an ear assessment involves testing the patient's hearing using the whisper test, Weber test, and the Rinne test. These tests assess conduction hearing loss, impaired sound transmission to the inner ear, sensorineural hearing loss, and impaired acoustic nerve conduction or inner ear function. (See *Assessing hearing in young children*.)

Whisper test

The whisper test is a simple method for detecting hearing impairment. To perform this test, stand an arm's length (about 28 [0.6 m]) behind the patient and instruct them to place a finger over the tragus of one ear. After quietly exhaling (to help quiet your voice), whisper a number that has two or three syllables, such as 68 or 100, and then ask the patient to repeat what they heard. Repeat this procedure for the opposite ear. An inability to hear the number or an incorrect response indicates hearing impairment involving high-frequency sound.

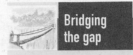

Bridging the gap

Cerumen variations

When examining your patient's ear canal, keep in mind that the presence of cerumen doesn't indicate poor hygiene. In fact, the appearance and type of cerumen is genetically determined. There are two types of cerumen:

1. *Dry cerumen*—which is gray and flaky and is mostly found in people of Asian ancestry and Native Americans (including Inuit).
2. *Wet cerumen*—which has a dark brown, moist appearance and is commonly found in people of African and European ancestry.

Weber test

Weber test is performed to distinguish between conductive and sensorineural hearing loss.

Choosing the right fork

This test uses a tuning fork to evaluate bone conduction. The tuning fork should be tuned to the frequency of normal human speech, 512 cycles/s. To perform Weber test, strike the tuning fork lightly against your hand, and then place the fork on the patient's forehead at the midline or on the top of their head.

Do you hear what I hear?

If the patient hears the tone equally well in both ears, record this as a normal Weber test. If they hear the tone better in one ear, record the result as right or left lateralization. If they hear the tone in their impaired ear, they have a conductive hearing loss. If they hear the tone in their unaffected ear, they have a sensorineural hearing loss.

Rinne test

Perform the Rinne test to compare air conduction of sound with bone conduction of sound. To administer this test, strike the tuning fork against your hand, and then place it over the patient's mastoid process. Ask them to tell you when the tone stops; note this time in seconds. Next, move the still-vibrating tuning fork to the ear's opening without touching the ear. Ask them to tell you when the tone stops. Note the time in seconds. (See *Positioning the tuning fork*, page 177.)

Air waves

The patient should hear the air-conducted tone for twice as long as they hear the bone-conducted tone. If they hear the bone-conducted tone as long as or longer than the air-conducted tone, conductive hearing loss is present. In sensorineural hearing loss, the air-conducted sound is heard longer than the bone-conducted sound.

Examining the nose and sinuses

A complete examination of the nose includes examining both the external and internal structures, evaluating the sense of smell, and checking the sinuses. To perform this examination, use the techniques of inspection, palpation, and percussion.

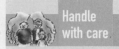
Handle with care

Assessing hearing in young children

When assessing hearing in an infant or a young child, you can't use a tuning fork. Instead, for infants younger than age 6 months, test the startle reflex. Another option in neonates, infants, and young children is to have an audiologist test brain stem evoked response. Many states now require that all neonates undergo brain stem evoked response testing before they're discharged from the hospital.

Because hearing disorders in children may lead to speech, language, and learning problems, early identification and treatment are crucial. Undiagnosed hearing disorders can also cause some children to be incorrectly diagnosed with brain damage, intellectual disabilities, or learning disabilities.

Peak technique

Positioning the tuning fork

These illustrations show how to hold a tuning fork to test a patient's hearing.

Weber test
With the tuning fork vibrating lightly, position the tip on the patient's fore-head at the midline, as shown at right. Alternatively, place the tuning fork on the top of the patient's head.

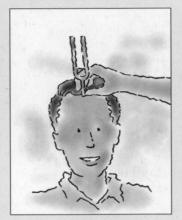

Rinne test
Strike the tuning fork against your hand, and then hold it behind the patient's ear, as shown at right. When your patient tells you the tone has stopped, move the still-vibrating tuning fork to the opening of their ear.

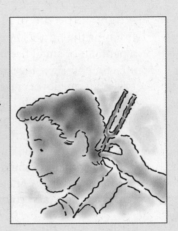

Inspecting and palpating the nose

Begin by observing the patient's nose for position, symmetry, and color. Note variations, such as discoloration, swelling, or deformity. Variations in size and shape are largely caused by differences in carti-lage and in the amount of fibroadipose tissue.

Observe for nasal discharge or flaring. If discharge is present, note the color, quantity, and consistency. If you notice nasal flaring, observe for other signs of respiratory distress.

Name that smell...

To test nasal patency and olfactory nerve (cranial nerve I) function, ask the patient to block one nostril and inhale a familiar aromatic substance through the other nostril. Possible substances include vanilla or nutmeg, soap, coffee, citrus, or tobacco. Ask them to iden-tify the aroma. Then repeat the process with the other nostril, using a different aroma.

Turn up the patient's nose

Now, inspect the nasal cavity. Ask the patient to tilt their head back slightly, and then push the tip of their nose up. Use the light from the otoscope to illuminate their nasal cavities. Check for severe deviation or perforation of the nasal septum. Examine the vestibule and turbinates for redness, softness, swelling, and discharge.

A light at the end of the speculum

Examine the nostrils by direct inspection, using a nasal speculum, a penlight or small flashlight, or an otoscope with a short, wide-tip attachment. Have the patient sit in front of you with their head tilted back. Put on gloves and insert the tip of the closed nasal speculum into one nostril to the point where the blade widens. Slowly open the speculum as wide as possible without causing discomfort. Shine the flashlight in the nostril to illuminate the area.

Observe the color and patency of the nostril, and check for exudate. The mucosa should be moist, pink to light red, and free from lesions and polyps. After inspecting one nostril, close the speculum, remove it, and inspect the other nostril. (See *Inspecting the nostrils.*)

Thumb their nose

Finally, palpate the patient's nose with your thumb and forefinger, assessing for pain, tenderness, swelling, and deformity.

Peak technique

Inspecting the nostrils

The illustration below shows the proper placement of the nasal speculum during direct inspection and the structures you should be able to see during this examination.

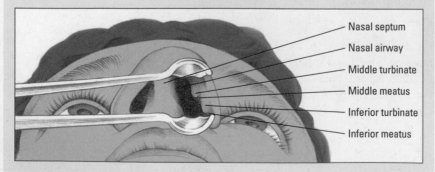

Nasal septum
Nasal airway
Middle turbinate
Middle meatus
Inferior turbinate
Inferior meatus

Examining the sinuses

Next examine the sinuses. Remember, only the frontal and maxillary sinuses are accessible; you won't be able to palpate the ethmoidal and sphenoidal sinuses. However, if the frontal and maxillary sinuses are infected, you can assume that the other sinuses are, too.

Tell me if it hurts

Begin by checking for swelling around the eyes, especially over the sinus area. Then palpate the sinuses, checking for tenderness. (See *Palpating the maxillary sinuses*, page 179.) To palpate the frontal sinuses, place your thumbs above the patient's eyes just under the bony ridges of the upper orbits, and place your fingertips on their forehead. Apply gentle pressure. Next palpate the maxillary sinuses.

Tap, tap, tap…

After palpation, percuss the frontal and maxillary sinuses by tapping them with your index and middle fingers. Note any pain or tenderness, which may indicate sinusitis.

Shed some light on the subject

If the patient reports tenderness during palpation or percussion of the sinuses, use transillumination to see if the sinuses are filled with fluid or pus. Transillumination can also help reveal tumors and obstructions. (See *Transilluminating the sinuses*, page 180.)

Peak technique

Palpating the maxillary sinuses

To palpate the maxillary sinuses, gently press your thumbs on each side of the nose just below the cheekbones, as shown at right. The illustration also shows the location of the frontal sinuses.

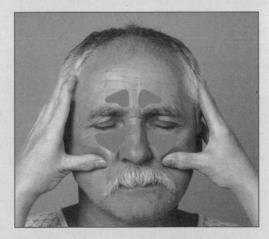

Peak technique

Transilluminating the sinuses

Transillumination of the sinuses helps detect sinus tumors and obstruction and requires only a penlight. Before you start, darken the room and have the patient close their eyes for a few seconds.

Frontal sinuses
Place the penlight on the supraorbital ring (under the eyebrow) and direct the light upward to illuminate the frontal sinuses just above the eyebrow, as shown at right.

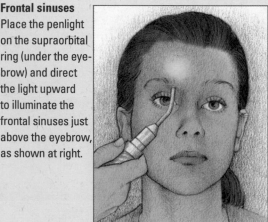

Maxillary sinuses
Place the penlight on the patient's cheekbone just below their eye and ask them to open the mouth, as shown at right. The light should transilluminate easily and equally. Upper dentures, if present, should be removed so the light isn't blocked.

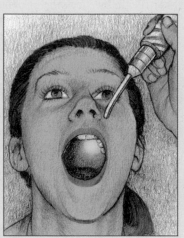

Examining the mouth, throat, and neck

Assessing the mouth and throat requires the techniques of inspection and palpation. Assessing the neck also involves auscultation.

Assessing the mouth and throat

First, inspect the patient's lips. They should be pink, moist, symmetrical, and without lesions. A bluish hue or flecked pigmentation is common in dark-skinned patients. Put on gloves and palpate the lips for lumps or surface abnormalities.

Mi casa, mucosa

Use a tongue blade and a bright light to inspect the oral mucosa. Have the patient open their mouth; then place the tongue blade on top of their tongue. The oral mucosa should be pink, smooth, moist, and free from lesions and unusual odors. Increased pigmentation is seen in dark-skinned patients.

Gums and then some

Next, observe the gingivae, or gums: They should be pink and moist and have clearly defined margins at each tooth. They shouldn't be retracted. Inspect the teeth, noting their number and condition and whether any are missing or crowded. If the patient is wearing dentures, note how they fit; then ask them to remove the dentures so you can inspect the gums underneath.

Give the tongue the once-over

Finally, inspect the tongue. It should be midline, moist, pink, and free from lesions. The posterior surface should be smooth, and the anterior surface should be slightly rough with small fissures. The tongue should move easily in all directions, and it should lie straight to the front at rest.

Ask the patient to raise the tip of their tongue and touch their palate directly behind their front teeth. Inspect the ventral surface of the tongue and the floor of the mouth. Next, wrap a piece of gauze around the tip of the tongue and move the tongue first to one side then the other to inspect the lateral borders. They should be smooth and even-textured. (See *Checking the surface*.)

Say "Ahhh"

Inspect the patient's oropharynx by asking them to open their mouth while you shine the penlight on the uvula and palate. You may need to insert a tongue blade into the mouth and depress the tongue. Place the tongue blade slightly off center to avoid eliciting the gag reflex. The uvula and oropharynx should be pink and moist, without inflammation or exudates. The tonsils should be pink and shouldn't be hypertrophied or have any exudate. Ask the patient to say "Ahhh." Observe for movement of the soft palate and uvula.

Gag order

Finally, palpate the lips, tongue, and oropharynx. Note lumps, lesions, ulcers, or edema of the lips or tongue. Assess the patient's gag reflex by gently touching the back of the pharynx with a cotton-tipped applicator or tongue blade. This should produce a bilateral response.

Inspecting and palpating the neck

First, observe the patient's neck. Both sides should be symmetrical, and the skin should be intact. Note any scars. No visible pulsations, masses, swelling, venous distention, or lymph node enlargement should be present. You may note a protruding thyroid cartilage, commonly called the *Adam's apple*. It's usually more prominent in persons

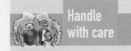
Handle with care

Checking the surface

The older patient may have varicose veins on the ventral surface of the tongue. In addition, the area underneath the tongue is a common site for the development of oral cancers. This area must be assessed thoroughly.

who were assigned male at birth than in those who were assigned female at birth. Ask the patient to move their neck through the entire range of motion and to shrug their shoulders. Also ask them to swallow. Note rising of the larynx, trachea, or thyroid. (See *Measuring the neck*, page 182.)

One lump or two?

Palpate the patient's neck to gather further data. Using the finger pads of both hands, bilaterally palpate the chain of lymph nodes under the patient's chin in the anterior cervical area; then proceed to the area under and behind the ears and then to the preauricular area. (See *Locating lymph nodes*, page 182.) Assess the nodes for size, shape, mobility, consistency, temperature, and tenderness, comparing nodes on one side with those on the other.

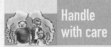

Measuring the neck

Take a little extra time when palpating the neck of an patient with obesity. A large neck may make it difficult to identify thyroid nodules, and you may need to palpate more deeply to assess lymph nodes.

Also, measure the patient's neck circumference. A neck circumference greater than 17″ (43 cm) is associated with an increased risk of obstructive sleep apnea. A thick neck may narrow the airway and excessive fatty tissue surrounding the pharynx may also contribute to sleep apnea.

Peak technique

Locating lymph nodes

This illustration shows the location of the lymph nodes in the head and neck.

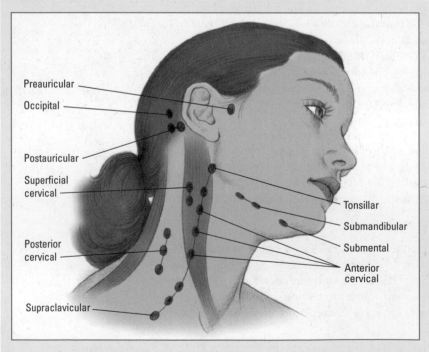

By the throat

Palpate the trachea, which is normally located midline in the neck. Place your thumbs along each side of the trachea near the lower part of the neck. Assess whether the distance between the trachea's outer edge and the sternocleidomastoid muscle is equal on both sides.

Hard to swallow

To palpate the thyroid, stand behind the patient and put your hands around their neck, with the fingers of both hands next to the cricoid cartilage. Ask them to swallow as you feel the thyroid isthmus. The isthmus should rise with swallowing because it lies across the trachea, just below the cricoid cartilage.

Displace the thyroid to the right and then to the left, palpating both lobes for enlargement, nodules, tenderness, or a gritty sensation. (See *A close look at the thyroid gland*, page 183.) Lowering the patient's chin slightly and turning toward the side you're palpating helps relax the muscle and may facilitate assessment. A normal thyroid gland isn't palpable or tender.

Auscultating the neck

Finally, auscultate the neck. Using light pressure on the bell of the stethoscope, listen over the carotid arteries. Ask the patient to hold their breath while you listen to prevent breath sounds from interfering

A close look at the thyroid gland

This illustration shows the structure and location of the thyroid gland.

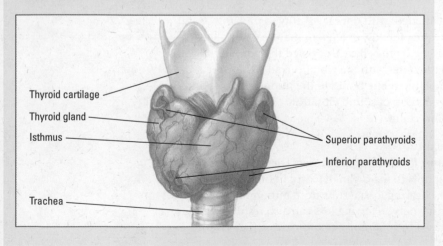

Thyroid cartilage

Thyroid gland

Isthmus

Superior parathyroids

Inferior parathyroids

Trachea

with the sounds of circulation. Listen for bruits, which signal turbulent blood flow.

If you detect an enlarged thyroid gland, also auscultate the thyroid area with the bell. Check for a bruit or a soft rushing sound, which indicates a hypermetabolic state.

Abnormal findings

As you conclude your assessment, you'll need to record your findings and evaluate any abnormalities. (See *Ear, nose, and throat abnormalities*, pages 185 and 186.)

Ear abnormalities

Common abnormalities you may find during an ear assessment include earache, hearing loss, otorrhea, and tympanosclerosis.

Earache

Earaches usually result from disorders of the external and middle ear associated with infection, obstruction, or trauma.

An earful

Earaches range in severity from a feeling of fullness or blockage to deep, boring pain. At times, it may be difficult to determine the precise location of the earache. Earaches can be intermittent or continuous and may develop suddenly or gradually.

Hearing loss

Several factors can interfere with the ear's ability to transmit sound waves. Cerumen, a foreign body, or a polyp may be obstructing the ear canal. Otitis media may have thickened the fluid in the middle ear, which interferes with the vibrations that transmit sound. Otosclerosis, a hardening of the bones in the middle ear, also interferes with the transmission of sound vibrations. Trauma can disrupt the middle ear's bony chain.

Hear today, gone tomorrow

Sensorineural hearing loss has several causes. The most common cause is loss of hair cells in the organ of Corti. In older people, presbycusis, or progressive hearing loss, results from atrophy of the organ of Corti and the acoustic nerve. Hearing loss can also result from trauma to the hair cells caused by loud noise or ototoxicity. (See *Hearing loss*, page 187.)

Interpretation station

Ear, nose, and throat abnormalities

The chart below shows common groups of findings for the signs and symptoms of the ear, nose, and throat, along with their probable causes.

Sign or symptom and findings	Probable cause
Dysphagia	
• Signs of respiratory distress, such as crowing and stridor • Oropharyngeal dysphagia with gagging and dysphonia	Airway obstruction
• Oropharyngeal and esophageal dysphagia • Rapid weight loss • Steady chest pain • Cough with hemoptysis • Hoarseness • Sore throat • Hiccups	Esophageal cancer
• Painless, progressive dysphagia • Lead line on the gums • Metallic taste • Papilledema • Ocular palsy • Footdrop or wrist drop • Mental impairment or seizures	Lead poisoning
Earache	
• Sensation of blockage or fullness in the ear • Itching • Partial hearing loss • Possible dizziness	Cerumen impaction
• Mild to moderate ear pain that occurs with tragus manipulation • Low-grade fever • Sticky yellow or purulent ear discharge • Partial hearing loss • Feeling of blockage in the ear • Swelling of the tragus, external meatus, and external canal • Lymphadenopathy	Otitis externa

Sign or symptom and findings	Probable cause
Earache (continued)	
• Severe, deep throbbing pain • Hearing loss • High fever • Bulging, fiery red eardrum	Acute otitis media
Epistaxis	
• Ecchymoses • Petechiae • Bleeding from gums, mouth, and IV puncture sites • Menorrhagia • Signs of GI bleeding, such as melena and hematemesis	Coagulation disorders
• Unilateral or bilateral epistaxis • Nasal swelling • Periorbital ecchymoses and edema • Pain • Nasal deformity • Crepitation of the nasal bones	Nasal fracture
• Oozing epistaxis • Dry cough • Abrupt onset of chills and high fever • "Rose spot" rash • Vomiting • Profound fatigue • Anorexia	Typhoid fever
Nasal obstruction	
• Watery nasal discharge • Sneezing • Temporary loss of smell and taste • Sore throat • Malaise • Arthralgia • Mild headache	Common cold

(Continued)

Ear, nose, and throat abnormalities (continued)

Sign or symptom and findings	Probable cause	Sign or symptom and findings	Probable cause
Nasal obstruction (continued)		**Throat pain** (continued)	
• Anosmia • Clear, watery nasal discharge • History of allergies, chronic sinusitis, trauma, cystic fibrosis, or asthma • Translucent, pear-shaped polyps that are unilateral or bilateral	Nasal polyps	• Mild to severe hoarseness • Temporary loss of voice • Malaise • Low-grade fever • Dysphagia • Dry cough • Tender, enlarged cervical lymph nodes	Laryngitis
• Thick, purulent drainage • Severe pain over the sinuses • Fever • Inflamed nasal mucosa with purulent mucus	Sinusitis	• Mild to severe sore throat • Pain may radiate to the ears • Dysphagia • Headache • Malaise • Fever with chills • Tender cervical lymphadenopathy	Tonsillitis, acute
Throat pain			
• Throat pain that occurs seasonally or year-round • Nasal congestion with a thin nasal discharge and postnasal drip • Paroxysmal sneezing • Decreased sense of smell • Frontal or temporal headache • Pale and glistening nasal mucosa with edematous nasal turbinates • Watery eyes	Allergic rhinitis		

Now hear this!

A toxic reaction to a drug can cause a rapid loss of hearing. If hearing loss is detected, the medication must be discontinued immediately. Drugs that may affect hearing include aspirin, aminoglycosides, loop diuretics, and several chemotherapeutic agents, including cisplatin.

Interpretation station

Hearing loss

Use this chart to review the causes, onset, and associated signs and symptoms of hearing loss.

Cause	Onset	Signs and symptoms
External ear		
Cerumen impaction	Sudden or gradual	Itching
Foreign body	Sudden	Discharge
Otitis externa	Sudden	Pain, discharge, itching
Middle ear		
Serous otitis media	Sudden or gradual	Fullness, itching
Acute otitis media	Sudden	Pain, fever, upper respiratory tract infection
Perforated tympanic membrane	Sudden	Trauma, discharge
Inner ear		
Presbycusis	Gradual	None
Drug-induced loss	Sudden or gradual	Tinnitus, other adverse drug effects
Meniere's disease	Sudden	Dizziness
Acoustic neuroma	Gradual	Vertigo

Otorrhea

Otorrhea—or drainage from the ear—may be bloody (otorrhagia), purulent, clear, or serosanguineous. Otorrhea may occur alone or with other symptoms such as ear pain. Its onset, duration, and severity provide clues to the underlying cause. Otorrhea may result from disorders that affect the external ear canal or the middle ear, including allergies, infection, neoplasms, trauma, and collagen disease.

Tympanosclerosis

Tympanosclerosis is the term for scarring of the tympanic membrane. It can be seen after surgery or after perforation due to earache. It appears as white, opaque patches on the tympanic membrane.

Nose, mouth, and throat abnormalities

During a nose, mouth, and throat assessment, you may detect epistaxis, nasal flaring, nasal stuffiness and discharge, nasal pain, dysphagia, and throat pain.

Epistaxis

A common sign, epistaxis (nosebleed) can occur spontaneously or be induced from the front or back of the nose. A rich supply of fragile blood vessels makes the nose particularly vulnerable to bleeding. Dry, irritated mucous membranes bleed easily; they're also more susceptible to infection, which may trigger epistaxis. Additional causes include trauma; septal deviation; hematologic, coagulation, kidney, and GI disorders; and certain drugs and treatments.

Nasal flaring

Some nasal flaring normally occurs during quiet breathing in adults and children. However, marked, regular nasal flaring in an adult may signal respiratory distress and calls for an immediate, rapid assessment.

Nasal stuffiness and discharge

Obstruction of the nasal mucous membranes along with a discharge of thin mucus can signal systemic disorders, nasal or sinus disorders such as a deviated septum, trauma such as a basilar skull or nasal fracture, excessive use of vasoconstricting nose drops or sprays, or allergies or exposure to irritants, such as dust, tobacco smoke, and fumes. Nasal drainage accompanied by sinus tenderness and fever suggests acute sinusitis, which usually involves the frontal or maxillary sinuses. Thick, white, yellow, or greenish drainage suggests an infection.

Take a closer look

Be sure to evaluate clear, thin drainage closely. It may simply indicate rhinitis, or it may be cerebrospinal fluid leaking from a basilar skull fracture or other defect.

Dysphagia

Dysphagia—difficulty swallowing—is the most common symptom of esophageal disorders. However, it may also result from oropharyngeal, respiratory, neurologic, and collagen disorders, or from the effects of toxins and treatments. Dysphagia increases the risk of choking and aspiration.

Throat pain

Commonly known as a *sore throat*, throat pain refers to discomfort in any part of the pharynx. This common symptom ranges from a sensation of scratchiness to severe pain. Throat pain may result from infection, trauma, allergy, cancer, or a systemic disorder. It may also follow surgery and endotracheal intubation. Additional causes include mouth breathing, alcohol consumption, inhaling smoke or chemicals such as ammonia, and vocal strain.

 That's a wrap!

Ears, nose, and throat review

Health history
- Ask about common ear symptoms, such as hearing loss, tinnitus, pain, and dizziness.
- Ask about current treatments and medications.
- Discuss past medical history, including allergies.
- Ask about common nose symptoms, such as nasal stuffiness, nasal discharge, and nosebleed.
- Ask about colds, headaches, and sinus problems.
- Ask about common mouth and throat symptoms, such as bleeding or sore gums, tooth problems, and sore throat.
- Ask the patient whether they smoke or use other types of tobacco.
- Ask about neck problems, such as neck pain, swelling, or trouble moving the neck.

Ear
External ear
- Consists mainly of elastic cartilage
- Collects sounds and transmits them to the middle ear

Middle ear
- Separated from the external ear by the tympanic membrane
- Contains three small bones: the malleus, the incus, and the stapes
- Connects to the nasopharynx via the eustachian tube
- Transmits sound vibrations to the inner ear, protects the auditory apparatus, and equalizes air pressure on both sides of the tympanic membrane

Inner ear
- Consists of closed, fluid-filled spaces
- Contains the vestibule and semicircular canals that help to maintain equilibrium, and the cochlea, the organ of hearing

Assessment
- Observe the ears for position and symmetry.
- Inspect the external ear for lesions, drainage, nodules, or redness.
- Inspect and palpate the mastoid area behind each auricle.
- Perform an otoscopic examination: examine the external canal, noting the presence and color of cerumen, and then advance the otoscope to view the tympanic membrane.
- Use the whisper test to assess hearing impairment.
- Use the Weber test to distinguish between conductive and sensorineural hearing loss.
- Use the Rinne test to compare air conduction of sound with bone conduction of sound.

Abnormal findings
- Earache—severity ranges from a feeling of fullness or blockage to deep, boring pain
- Hearing loss—can be conductive or sensorineural
- Otorrhea—drainage from the ear

Nose
- Acts as sensory organ of smell
- Filters, warms, and humidifies inhaled air
- Linked internally to four pairs of paranasal sinuses: maxillary (on the cheeks below the eyes), frontal (above the eyebrows), and ethmoidal and sphenoidal (behind the eyes and nose)

(Continued)

Ears, nose, and throat review *(continued)*

Assessment

- Observe the nose for position, symmetry, and color. Note nasal flaring or discharge.
- Test nasal patency and the olfactory nerve (cranial nerve I) by having the patient obstruct one nostril and identify a smell with the other.
- Inspect the nasal cavity using the light from the otoscope, checking the vestibule, turbinates, and nostrils.
- Palpate the nose for pain, tenderness, swelling, and deformity.
- Palpate and percuss the frontal and maxillary sinuses (the only sinuses that are accessible for examination).
- Use transillumination, if necessary, to help reveal obstructions and tumors.

Abnormal findings

- Epistaxis—nosebleed; a common sign

- Nasal flaring—may be a sign of respiratory distress
- Nasal stuffiness and discharge—obstruction of the nasal mucous membranes along with a discharge of thin mucus
- Pain or tenderness—may indicate sinusitis

Throat and neck

- Consists of nasopharynx, oropharynx, and laryngopharynx
- Contains cervical vertebrae, the major neck and shoulder muscles, and their ligaments
- Contains trachea, thyroid gland, and chains of lymph nodes

Assessment

- Inspect the lips.
- Use a tongue blade and a bright light to inspect the oral mucosa, gingivae, and teeth.

- Inspect the tongue and note the patient's ability to move it in all directions. Also inspect underneath the tongue.
- Inspect and palpate the neck.
- Assess lymph nodes.
- Palpate the trachea and thyroid gland.
- Auscultate the neck by listening over the carotid arteries and over the thyroid gland (if it's enlarged).

Abnormal findings

- Dysphagia—difficulty swallowing
- Throat pain—discomfort in any part of the pharynx; may range from a scratchy sensation to severe pain
- Swollen lymph nodes—may indicate infection

Quick quiz

1. Before inserting the otoscope into a patient's ear, the nurse should palpate the:

    A. helix.
    B. earlobe.
    C. lymph nodes.
    D. tragus.

Answer: D. Before inserting the otoscope, palpate the tragus to make sure it isn't tender. A tender tragus signals otitis externa.

2. During an otoscopic examination, the nurse should pull the superior posterior auricle of an adult patient's ear:

    A. up and back.
    B. up and forward.
    C. down and back.
    D. straight back.

Answer: A. In the adult patient, the superior posterior auricle should be pulled up and back to straighten the ear canal.

3.   To assess the frontal sinuses, the nurse should palpate and percuss:
>   A.   the forehead.
>   B.   below the cheekbones.
>   C.   over the temporal areas.
>   D.   below the ears.

Answer: A. The frontal sinuses are located in the forehead, the site of palpation and percussion for those structures.

4.   A cerumen impaction may contribute to a form of hearing loss called:
>   A.   central hearing loss.
>   B.   conductive hearing loss.
>   C.   sensorineural hearing loss.
>   D.   lateral hearing loss.

Answer: B. Conductive hearing loss occurs from abnormal function of the external or middle ear, resulting in impaired sound transmission.

5.   The patient's ability to identify a particular aroma depends on proper functioning of cranial nerve:
>   A.   I.
>   B.   II.
>   C.   IV.
>   D.   VI.

Answer: A. Nasal patency and the olfactory nerve (cranial nerve I) are tested by having the patient identify an aroma.

6.   Clear, thin nasal drainage may indicate:
>   A.   infection.
>   B.   cerebrospinal fluid leak.
>   C.   epistaxis.
>   D.   the presence of a foreign object.

Answer: B. Clear, thin nasal drainage may indicate a cerebrospinal fluid leak; therefore, you should evaluate this finding closely.

Scoring

★★★   If you answered all six questions correctly, fantastic! We wouldn't blame you if you have a lump of pride in your throat.

★★   If you answered four or five questions correctly, way to go! We heard that you've been studying, and it must be true.

★   If you answered fewer than four questions correctly, don't sniffle! Becoming an assessment whiz requires a lot of practice.

Chapter 9

Cardiovascular system

Just the facts

In this chapter, you'll learn:

- ◆ structures of the cardiovascular system and their functions
- ◆ the proper way to perform an assessment of the cardio-vascular system
- ◆ normal and abnormal findings.

A look at the cardiovascular system

The cardiovascular system plays an important role in the body. It delivers oxygenated blood to tissues and removes waste products. The heart pumps blood to all organs and tissues of the body. The autonomic nervous system controls how the heart pumps. The vascular network—the arteries and veins—carries blood throughout the body, keeps the heart filled with blood, and maintains blood pressure.

Anatomy and physiology

To make the most of your assessment of the cardiovascular system, you'll need to understand the anatomy and physiology of the heart and the vascular system.

Heart

The heart is a hollow, muscular organ encased and cushioned in its own serous membrane, the pericardium. The heart is about the size of a closed fist. Located between the lungs in the mediastinum, behind and to the left of the sternum,

> By pumping blood to all of the organs and tissues in the body, I pretty much drive the whole system!

it's about 59 (12.5 cm) long and 3½" (9 cm) in diameter at its widest point. The adult heart typically weighs 250 to 300 g (9 to 10.5 oz).

Anatomy

The heart spans the area from the second to the fifth intercostal space. The right border of the heart aligns with the right border of the sternum. The left border lines up with the left midclavicular line. The exact position of the heart may vary slightly with each patient.

Smooth sliding
Layers of the heart wall

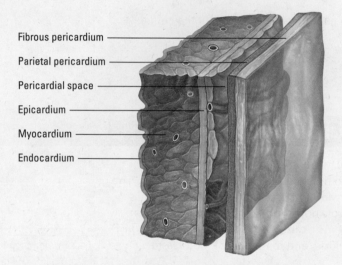

Fibrous pericardium

Parietal pericardium

Pericardial space

Epicardium

Myocardium

Endocardium

The heart is protected by a thin sac called the *pericardium*, which has an inner, or visceral, layer that forms the epicardium and an outer, or parietal, layer. The space between the two layers (also the pericardial space) contains 15 to 50 mL of serous fluid, which lubricates and cushions the surface of the heart and prevents friction between the layers as the heart pumps.

Chamber made

The heart has four chambers (two atria and two ventricles) separated by a cardiac septum. The upper atria have thin walls and serve as reservoirs for blood. They also boost the amount of blood moving into the lower ventricles, which fill primarily by gravity. The left ventricle pumps blood against a much higher pressure than does the right ventricle, so its wall is two and one-half times thicker. (See *A close look at the heart*, page 195.)

A close look at the heart

This illustration details the internal structures of the heart.

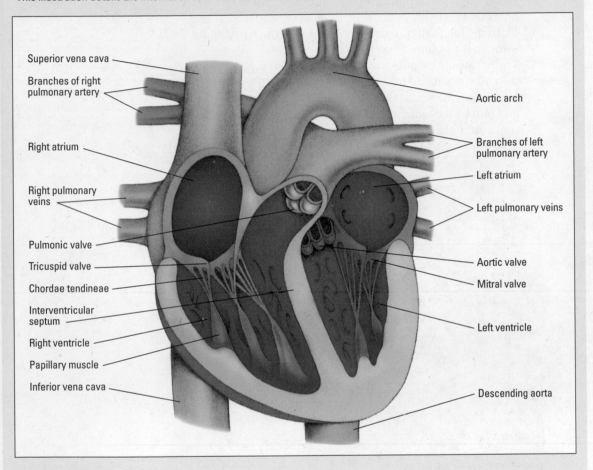

Superior vena cava

Branches of right
pulmonary artery

Right atrium

Right pulmonary
veins

Pulmonic valve

Tricuspid valve

Chordae tendineae

Interventricular
septum

Right ventricle

Papillary muscle

Inferior vena cava

Aortic arch

Branches of left
pulmonary artery

Left atrium

Left pulmonary veins

Aortic valve

Mitral valve

Left ventricle

Descending aorta

Vessels

They'rrrrrre great!

Leading into and out of the heart are the great vessels: the inferior
vena cava, the superior vena cava, the aorta, the pulmonary artery, and
four pulmonary veins.

Cardiac circulation

1. Deoxygenated venous blood returns to the right atrium through
   the superior vena cava, inferior vena cava, and coronary sinus.

2. Blood in the right atrium empties into the right ventricle passively; once the pressure in the right ventricle exceeds the pressure in the right atrium, the tricuspid valve closes. The ventricle then contracts.
3. Blood is ejected through the pulmonic valve into the pulmonary artery and then travels to the lungs to be oxygenated.
4. From the lungs, oxygenated blood travels to the left atrium through the pulmonary veins.
5. The left atrium empties the blood into the left ventricle passively; once the pressure in the left ventricle exceeds the pressure in the left atrium, the mitral valve will close. The left ventricle contracts and pumps the blood through the aortic valve into the aorta and throughout the body.

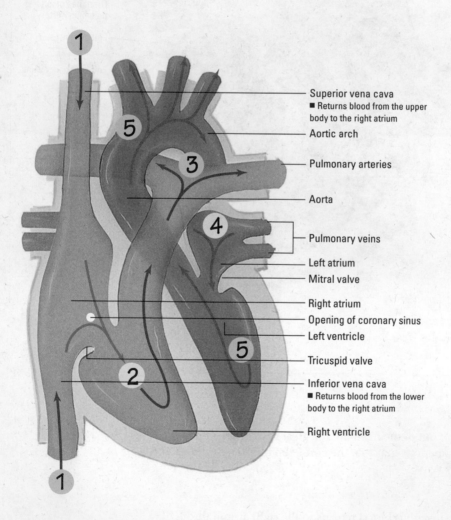

Superior vena cava
- Returns blood from the upper body to the right atrium

Aortic arch

Pulmonary arteries

Aorta

Pulmonary veins

Left atrium

Mitral valve

Right atrium

Opening of coronary sinus

Left ventricle

Tricuspid valve

Inferior vena cava
- Returns blood from the lower body to the right atrium

Right ventricle

Valves

Valvular traffic cops

Valves in the heart keep blood flowing in only one direction through the heart. Think of the valves as traffic cops at the entrances to one-way streets, preventing blood from traveling the wrong way despite great pressure to do so. Healthy valves open and close passively as a result of pressure changes within the four heart chambers.

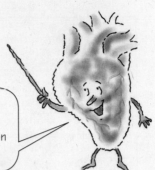

Let's take a look at the cardiac structures involved in circulation.

Which valve is where?

Valves between the atria and ventricles are called *atrioventricular valves,* often referred to as *AV valves,* and include the tricuspid valve on the right side of the heart and the mitral valve on the left. The pulmonic valve (between the right ventricle and pulmonary artery) and the aortic valve (between the left ventricle and the aorta) are called *semilunar valves.* (See *Locating the heart valves.*)

Locating the heart valves

Take a look at the illustration below to view the locations of the valves in the heart.

On the cusp

Each valve's leaflets, or cusps, are anchored to the heart wall by cords of fibrous tissue. Those cords, called *chordae tendineae,* are controlled by papillary muscles. The valves' cusps maintain tight closure. The tricuspid valve has three cusps. The mitral valve has two. The semilunar valves each have three cusps.

(Continued)

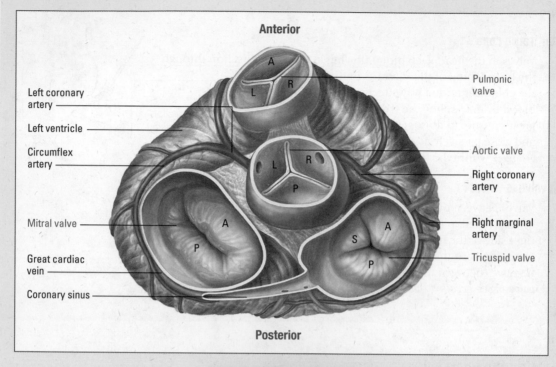

Anterior

Left coronary artery

Left ventricle

Circumflex artery

Mitral valve

Great cardiac vein

Coronary sinus

Pulmonic valve

Aortic valve

Right coronary artery

Right marginal artery

Tricuspid valve

Posterior

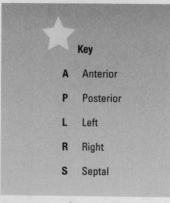

Key

A   Anterior

P   Posterior

L   Left

R   Right

S   Septal

Physiology of the heart

Contractions of the heart occur in a rhythm—the cardiac cycle—and are regulated by impulses that normally begin in the sinoatrial (SA) node, the heart's primary pacemaker. From there, it travels through the atria along Bachmann bundle and the intermodal pathways on its way to the atrioventricular (AV) node and the ventricles. After the impulses passes through the AV node, it travels to the ventricles, first down the bundle of His, then along the bundle branches, and, finally down the Purkinje fibers.

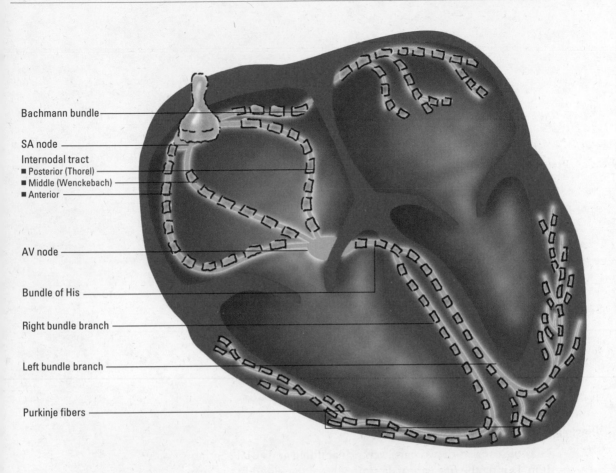

Bachmann bundle

SA node

Internodal tract
- Posterior (Thorel)
- Middle (Wenckebach)
- Anterior

AV node

Bundle of His

Right bundle branch

Left bundle branch

Purkinje fibers

A look at the cardiac cycle

The cardiac cycle consists of systole, the period when the heart contracts and sends blood on its outward journey, and diastole, the period when the heart relaxes and fills with blood.

1. **Atrial systole**

   The atria contract, emptying blood into the ventricles. As pressure within the ventricles rises, the mitral and tricuspid valves snap shut, producing the first heart sound, S_1.

2. **Ventricular systole**

   Shortly after atrial systole, the ventricles contract, ejecting blood from the heart to the lungs and the rest of the body. At the end of ventricular contraction, the aortic and pulmonic valves snap shut, producing the second heart sound, S_2.

3. **Diastole**

   Atria and ventricles relax and blood refills each chamber.

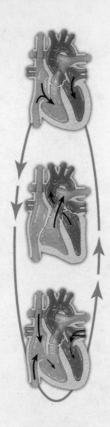

Diastole: Parts I and II

Diastole consists of two parts, ventricular filling and atrial contraction. During the first part of diastole, 70% of the blood in the atria drains into the ventricles by gravity, a passive action.

The active period of diastole, atrial contraction (also called *atrial kick*), accounts for the remaining 30% of blood that passes into the ventricles. Diastole is also when the heart muscle receives its own supply of blood, which is transported by the coronary arteries.

Snap to it

Systole is the period of ventricular contraction. As pressure within the ventricles rises, the mitral and tricuspid valves snap closed. This closure leads to the first heart sound, S_1.

Open flow

When the pressure in the ventricles rises above the pressure in the aorta and pulmonary artery, the aortic and pulmonic valves open. Blood then flows from the ventricles into the pulmonary artery to the lungs and into the aorta to the rest of the body.

Cycle of life

At the end of ventricular contraction, pressure in the ventricles drops below the pressure in the aorta and the pulmonary artery. That pressure difference forces blood to back up toward the ventricles and causes the aortic and pulmonic valves to snap shut, which produces the second heart sound, S_2. As the valves shut, the atria passively fill with blood in preparation for the next period of diastolic filling, and the cycle begins again. (See *Cardiovascular changes with aging*, page 201.)

Vascular system

The vascular system delivers oxygen, nutrients, and other substances to the body's cells and removes the waste products of cellular metabolism. The peripheral vascular system consists of a network of 60,000 miles of arteries, arterioles, capillaries, venules, and veins that are constantly filled with about 5 L of blood, which circulates to and from every functioning cell in the body. (See *A close look at arteries and veins*, page 202.)

 Handle with care

Cardiovascular changes with aging

Changes in the cardiovascular system occur as a natural part of the aging process. These changes, however, place older patients at higher risk for cardiovascular disorders than younger patients. As you assess older patients, be aware of these changes that occur with aging:
- slight decrease in heart size
- loss of cardiac contractile strength and efficiency
- decrease in cardiac output of 30% to 35% by age 70
- thickening of heart valve, causing incomplete valve closure (as well as a systolic murmur)
- increase in left ventricular wall thickness of 25% between ages 30 and 80
- fibrous tissue infiltration of sinoatrial node and internodal atrial tracts, causing arrhythmias, most commonly atrial fibrillation and flutter and premature atrial and ventricular contractions

- dilation and stretching of veins
- decline in coronary artery blood flow of 35% between ages 20 and 60
- increased aortic rigidity
- increased amount of time necessary for heart rate to return to normal after exercise
- decreased strength and elasticity of blood vessels, contributing to arterial and venous insufficiency
- decreased ability to respond to physical and emotional stress
- increase in peripheral vascular resistance, leading to increased blood pressure
- extra heart sound, S_4, more common and caused by a more rigid left ventricle
- decreased arterial wall elasticity, leading to isolated systolic hypertension.

A close look at arteries and veins

This illustration shows major arteries and veins of the body.

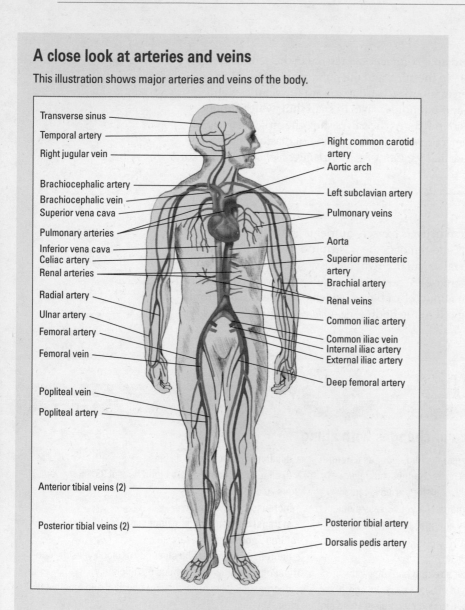

Transverse sinus
Temporal artery
Right jugular vein
Brachiocephalic artery
Brachiocephalic vein
Superior vena cava
Pulmonary arteries
Inferior vena cava
Celiac artery
Renal arteries
Radial artery
Ulnar artery
Femoral artery
Femoral vein
Popliteal vein
Popliteal artery
Anterior tibial veins (2)
Posterior tibial veins (2)

Right common carotid artery
Aortic arch
Left subclavian artery
Pulmonary veins
Aorta
Superior mesenteric artery
Brachial artery
Renal veins
Common iliac artery
Common iliac vein
Internal iliac artery
External iliac artery
Deep femoral artery
Posterior tibial artery
Dorsalis pedis artery

Arteries—Tough travelers

Arteries carry blood away from the heart. Nearly all arteries carry oxygen-rich blood from the heart throughout the rest of the body. The only exception is the pulmonary artery, which carries oxygen-depleted blood from the right ventricle to the lungs.

Arteries are thick-walled because they transport blood under high pressure. Arterial walls contain a tough, elastic layer to help propel blood through the arterial system. Arterial pulses are pressure waves of blood generated by the pumping action of the heart.

Capillaries—Thin-skinned

The exchange of fluid, nutrients, and metabolic wastes between blood and cells occurs in the capillaries. The exchange can occur because capillaries are thin-walled and highly permeable. About 5% of the circulating blood volume at any given moment is contained within the capillary network. Capillaries are connected to arteries and veins through intermediary vessels called *arterioles* and *venules*, respectively. Arterioles constrict and dilate to control blood flow to the capillaries. Venules gather blood from the capillaries.

Veins—Reservoir veins

Veins carry blood toward the heart. Nearly all veins carry oxygen-depleted blood, the sole exception being the pulmonary vein, which carries oxygenated blood from the lungs to the left atrium. Veins serve as a large reservoir for circulating blood. They can carry up to 85% of the circulating blood volume at any one time.

The wall of a vein is thinner and more pliable than the wall of an artery. That pliability allows the vein to accommodate variations in blood volume. Veins contain valves at periodic intervals to prevent blood from flowing backward.

Finger on the pulse

Arterial pulses are pressure waves of blood generated by the pumping action of the heart. All vessels in the arterial system have pulsations, but the pulsations normally can be felt only where an artery lies near the skin. You can palpate for these peripheral pulses: temporal, carotid, brachial, radial, ulnar, femoral, popliteal, posterior tibial, and dorsalis pedis.

The location of pulse points varies among individuals. In older adults, peripheral pulses may be diminished. The dorsalis pedis pulse can be absent in 2% to 5% of healthy individuals.

Obtaining a health history

To obtain a health history of a patient's cardiovascular system, begin by introducing yourself to the patient and explaining what will occur during the health history and physical examination. Then obtain the following information.

Asking about the reason for seeking care

You'll find that patients with a cardiovascular problem typically cite specific symptoms, including:

- chest or jaw pain
- pain in the extremities, such as pain that radiates to the arms or leg pain or cramps
- irregular heartbeat or palpitations
- shortness of breath on exertion, when lying down, or at night
- cough
- cyanosis or pallor
- weakness
- fatigue
- unexplained weight change
- swelling of the extremities (see *Pregnancy and vein changes*)
- dizziness
- headache
- high or low blood pressure
- peripheral skin changes, such as decreased hair distribution, skin color changes, or a thin, shiny appearance to the skin.

Pregnancy and vein changes

You might find 4+ pitting edema in the legs of a pregnant patient in the third trimester. Severe edema commonly occurs not only in the third trimester but also in pregnant patients who stand for long periods of time.

Varicose veins are another common finding during the third trimester.

Asking about personal and family health

Ask the patient for details about their family history and past medical history, including diabetes, chronic diseases of the lungs or kidneys, or liver disease. (See *At risk for cardiovascular disease*, page 205.)

Also obtain information about:

- stress and the patient's methods of coping with it
- current health habits, such as smoking, alcohol intake, caffeine intake, exercise, and dietary intake of fat and sodium
- drugs the patient is taking, including over-the-counter drugs, herbal preparations, and illegal or recreational substances
- previous operations or procedures such as a cardiac catheterization
- environmental or occupational considerations
- activities of daily living
- current weight and any recent weight gain or loss (see *How obesity affects the heart*, page 205).

Oh, the pain of it all!

Many patients with cardiovascular problems report chest pain at some point. If your patient has chest pain, ask them to rate the pain on a scale of 0 to 10, in which 0 means no pain and 10 means the worst pain imaginable. Reassess the patient's pain rating frequently during treatment to determine the effectiveness of interventions.

Handle with care

How obesity affects the heart

When you examine an patient with obesity, keep in mind that obesity affects the heart, increasing the risk of heart disease. Here's how it works: As weight increases, so does the body's total blood volume, forcing the heart to work harder to deliver oxygen and nutrients to the body. This increased workload causes the left ventricle to thicken, which affects the heart's ability to function effectively.

Obesity can also affect the heart indirectly by increasing blood pressure and total cholesterol and triglyceride levels. It can also lead to obstructive sleep apnea, which can damage the heart.

Some hearty questions

In addition to checking for pain, also ask the patient these questions:

- Are you ever short of breath? If so, what activities cause you to be short of breath?
- Do you feel dizzy or fatigued?
- Does it ever feel like your heart is racing? If so, when does it occur and what makes it better?
- Do your rings or shoes feel tight?
- Do your ankles swell?
- Have you noticed changes in color or sensation in your legs? If so, what are those changes?
- If you have sores or ulcers, how quickly do they heal?
- Do you stand or sit in one place for long periods at work?

Bridging the gap

At risk for cardiovascular disease

As you analyze a patient's problems, remember that age, sex, and race are essential considerations in identifying patients at risk for cardiovascular disorders. For example, coronary artery disease most commonly affects White males between ages 40 and 60. Hypertension occurs most often in Black people.

Female adults are also vulnerable to heart disease, especially those who are postmenopausal and those with diabetes mellitus.

Assessing the cardiovascular system

Cardiovascular disease affects people of all ages and can take many forms. A consistent, methodical approach to your assessment will help you identify abnormalities. As always, the key to accurate assessment is regular practice, which will help improve technique and efficiency.

Before you begin your physical assessment, you'll need to obtain a stethoscope with a bell and a diaphragm, an appropriate-sized blood pressure cuff, a ruler, and a penlight or other flexible light source. Make sure the room is quiet.

Ask the patient to remove all clothing except their underwear and to put on an examination gown. Have the patient lie on their back, with the head of the examination table at a 30° to 45° angle. Stand on the patient's right side if you're right-handed or their left side if you're left-handed so you can auscultate more easily.

Assessing the heart

As with assessment of other body systems, you'll inspect, palpate, percuss, and auscultate in your assessment of the heart.

Inspection

First, take a moment to assess the patient's general appearance. Are they underweight? Obese? Alert? Anxious? Note their skin color, temperature, turgor, and texture. Are their fingers clubbed? (Clubbing is a sign of chronic hypoxia caused by a lengthy cardiovascular or respiratory disorder.) If the patient is dark-skinned, inspect their mucous membranes for pallor.

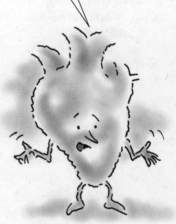

Is the patient underweight? Obese? Alert? Anxious? I'm feeling a bit anxious myself with all of these questions!

Chest check

Next, inspect the chest. Note landmarks you can use to describe your findings as well as structures underlying the chest wall. (See *Identifying cardiovascular landmarks*, page 207.)

Look for pulsations, symmetry of movement, retractions, or heaves. A heave is a strong outward thrust of the chest wall and occurs during systole.

Shed some light on the subject

Position a light source, such as a flashlight or gooseneck lamp, so that it casts a shadow on the patient's chest. Note the location of the apical impulse. This is also usually the point of maximal impulse and should be located in the fifth intercostal space at or just medial to the left midclavicular line.

The apical impulse gives an indication of how well the left ventricle is working because it corresponds to the apex of the heart. The impulse can be seen in about 50% of adults. You'll notice it more easily in children and in patients with thin chest walls. To find the apical impulse in a patient with large breasts, displace the breasts during the examination.

Palpation

Maintain a gentle touch when you palpate so that you won't obscure pulsations or similar findings. Using the ball of your hand, then your fingertips, palpate over the precordium to find the apical impulse. Note heaves, which are signs of left ventricular hypertrophy and feel like sustained outward movements. Also note thrills, palpable murmurs that feel like the purring of a cat. (See *Assessing the apical impulse*, page 208.)

Peak technique

Identifying cardiovascular landmarks

The anterior and lateral views of the thorax shown here identify where to locate critical landmarks while performing the cardiovascular assessment.

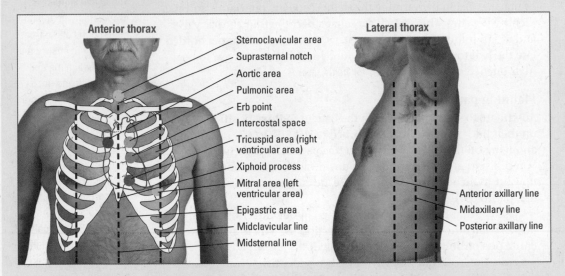

Anterior thorax

- Sternoclavicular area
- Suprasternal notch
- Aortic area
- Pulmonic area
- Erb point
- Intercostal space
- Tricuspid area (right ventricular area)
- Xiphoid process
- Mitral area (left ventricular area)
- Epigastric area
- Midclavicular line
- Midsternal line

Lateral thorax

- Anterior axillary line
- Midaxillary line
- Posterior axillary line

Try to modify

The apical impulse may be difficult to palpate in obese and pregnant patients and in patients with thick chest walls. If it's difficult to palpate with the patient lying on their back, have them lie on their left side or sit upright. It may also be helpful to have the patient exhale completely and hold their breath for a few seconds.

Plentiful places to palpate

Also palpate the sternoclavicular, aortic, pulmonic, tricuspid, and epigastric areas for abnormal pulsations. Normally, you won't feel pulsations in those areas. An aortic arch pulsation in the sternoclavicular area or an abdominal aorta pulsation in the epigastric area may be a normal finding in a thin patient.

Percussing the heart

Although percussion isn't as useful as other methods of assessment, this technique may help you locate cardiac borders. Begin percussing at the anterior axillary line and continue toward the sternum along the fifth intercostal space.

The sound changes from resonance to dullness over the left border of the heart, normally at the midclavicular line. The right border of the heart is usually aligned with the sternum and can't be percussed.

Auscultating for heart sounds

You can learn a great deal about the heart by auscultating for heart sounds. Cardiac auscultation requires a methodical approach and lots of practice. Begin by warming the stethoscope in your hands and then identify the sites where you'll auscultate: over the four cardiac valves and at Erb point, the third intercostal space at the left sternal border. Use the bell to hear low-pitched sounds and the diaphragm to hear high-pitched sounds. (See *Sites for heart sounds*, page 209.)

Planning pays off

Auscultate for heart sounds with the patient in three positions: lying on their back with the head of the bed raised 30° to 45°, sitting up, and lying on their left side. Use a zigzag pattern over the precordium. You can start at the base and work downward or at the apex and work upward. Whichever approach you use, be consistent. (See *Auscultation tips*, page 209.)

Use the diaphragm to listen as you go in one direction; use the bell as you come back in the other direction. Be sure to listen over the entire precordium, not just over the valves.

Note the heart rate and rhythm. Always identify S_1 and S_2, and then listen for adventitious sounds, such as third and fourth heart sounds (S_3 and S_4), murmurs, and rubs. (See *Cycle of heart sounds*, pages 210 and 211.)

Lub-a-dub-dub...

Start auscultating at the aortic area where S_2, the second heart sound, is loudest. S_2 is best heard at the base of the heart at the end of ventricular systole. This sound corresponds to closure of the pulmonic and aortic valves and is generally described as sounding like "dub." It's a shorter, higher-pitched, louder sound than S_1. When the pulmonic valve closes later than the aortic valve during inspiration, you'll hear a split S_2.

From the base of the heart, move to the pulmonic area and then down to the tricuspid area. Then move to the mitral area, where S_1 is the loudest. S_1 is best heard at the apex of the heart. This sound corresponds to closure of the mitral and tricuspid valves and is generally described as sounding like "lub." It's low-pitched and dull. S_1 occurs at the beginning of ventricular systole. It may be split if the mitral valve closes just before the tricuspid.

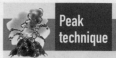

Peak technique

Assessing the apical impulse

The apical impulse is associated with the first heart sound and carotid pulsation. To ensure that you're feeling the apical impulse and not a muscle spasm or some other pulsation, use one hand to palpate the patient's carotid artery and the other to palpate the apical impulse. Then compare the timing and regularity of the impulses. The apical impulse should roughly coincide with the carotid pulsation.

Note the amplitude, size, intensity, location, and duration of the apical impulse. You should feel a gentle pulsation in an area about ¼" to ¾" (1.5 to 2 cm) in diameter.

Sites for heart sounds

When auscultating for heart sounds, place the stethoscope over the four sites illustrated below, following the numerical order shown.

Normal heart sounds indicate events in the cardiac cycle, such as the closing of heart valves, and are reflected to specific areas of the chest wall. Auscultation sites are identified by the names of heart valves but aren't located directly over the valves. Rather, these sites are located along the pathway blood takes as it flows through the heart's chambers and valves.

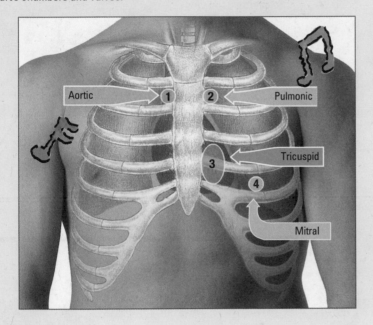

Auscultation tips

Follow these tips when you auscultate a patient's heart:
• Concentrate as you listen for each sound.
• Avoid auscultating through clothing or wound dressings because they can block sound.
• Avoid picking up extraneous sounds by keeping the stethoscope tubing off the patient's body and other surfaces.
• Until you become proficient at auscultation and can examine a patient quickly, explain to them that even though you may listen to their chest for a long period, it doesn't mean anything is wrong.
• Ask the patient to breathe normally and to hold their breath periodically to enhance sounds that may be difficult to hear.

Galloping along...

A third heart sound, S_3, is a normal finding in children and young adults. In addition, S_3 is commonly heard in patients with high cardiac output. Called *ventricular gallop* when it occurs in adults, S_3 may be a cardinal sign of heart failure.

Deep in the heart of Kentucky?

S_3 is best heard at the apex when the patient is lying on their left side. Often compared to the *y* sound in "Ken-tuck-y," S_3 is low-pitched and occurs when the ventricles fill rapidly. It follows S_2 in early

Cycle of heart sounds

When you auscultate a patient's chest and hear that familiar "lub-dub," you're hearing the first and second heart sounds, S_1 and S_2. At times, two other sounds may occur: S_3 and S_4.

Heart sounds are generated by events in the cardiac cycle. When valves close or blood fills the ventricles, vibrations of the heart muscle can be heard through the chest wall.

Varying sound patterns

The phonogram at right shows how heart sounds vary in duration and intensity. For instance, S_2 (which occurs when the semilunar valves snap shut) is a shorter-lasting sound than S_1 because the semilunar valves take less time to close than the atrioventricular valves, which cause S_1.

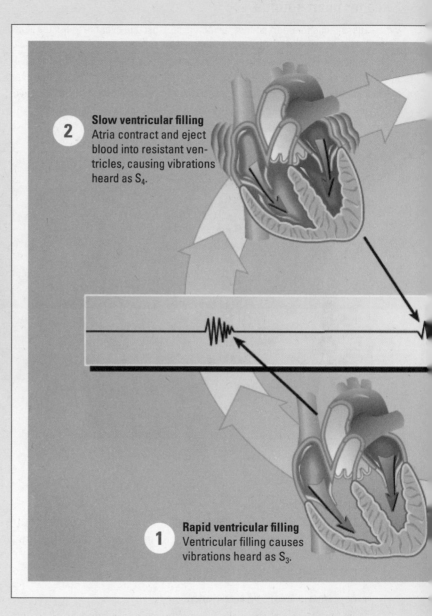

2 Slow ventricular filling
Atria contract and eject blood into resistant ventricles, causing vibrations heard as S_4.

1 Rapid ventricular filling
Ventricular filling causes vibrations heard as S_3.

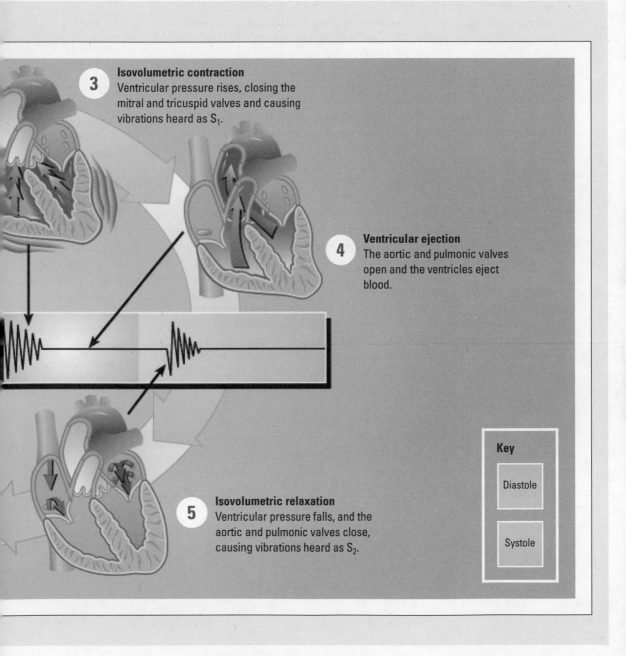

3 **Isovolumetric contraction**
Ventricular pressure rises, closing the mitral and tricuspid valves and causing vibrations heard as S_1.

4 **Ventricular ejection**
The aortic and pulmonic valves open and the ventricles eject blood.

5 **Isovolumetric relaxation**
Ventricular pressure falls, and the aortic and pulmonic valves close, causing vibrations heard as S_2.

Key

Diastole

Systole

ventricular diastole and probably results from vibrations caused by abrupt ventricular distention and resistance to filling. In addition to heart failure, S_3 may also be associated with such conditions as pulmonary edema, atrial septal defect, acute myocardial infarction (MI), and the last trimester of pregnancy.

Taking a trip to Tennessee

S_4 is an adventitious sound called an *atrial gallop* that's heard over the tricuspid or mitral area with the patient on their left side. You may hear S_4 in patients who are older or in those with hypertension, aortic stenosis, or a history of MI. S_4, commonly described as sounding like "Ten-nes-see," occurs just before S_1, after atrial contraction.

The S_4 sound indicates increased resistance to ventricular filling. It results from vibrations caused by forceful atrial ejection of blood into ventricles that are enlarged or hypertrophied and don't move or expand as much as they should.

Auscultating for murmurs

Murmurs occur when structural defects in the heart's chambers or valves cause turbulent blood flow. Turbulence may also be caused by changes in the viscosity of blood or the speed of blood flow. Listen for murmurs over the same precordial areas used in auscultation for heart sounds.

Murmur variations

Murmurs can occur during systole or diastole and are described by several criteria. (See *Tips for describing murmurs*, page 212.) Their pitch can be high, medium, or low. They can vary in intensity, growing louder or softer. (See *Grading murmurs*, page 213.) They can vary by location, sound pattern (blowing, harsh, or musical), radiation (to the neck or axillae), and period during which they occur in the cardiac cycle (systolic or diastolic).

Sit up, please

The best way to hear murmurs is with the patient sitting up and leaning forward. You can also have them lie on their left side. (See *Positioning the patient for auscultation*, page 213.)

Tips for describing murmurs

Describing murmurs can be tricky. After you've auscultated a murmur, list the terms you would use to describe it. Then check the patient's chart to see how others have described it or ask an experienced colleague to listen and describe the murmur. Compare the descriptions and then auscultate for the murmur again, if necessary, to confirm the description.

Peak technique

Positioning the patient for auscultation

If heart sounds are faint or undetectable, try listening to them with the patient seated and leaning forward or lying on their left side, which brings the heart closer to the surface of the chest. These illustrations show how to position the patient for high- and low-pitched sounds.

Left lateral recumbent
The left lateral recumbent position is best suited for hearing low-pitched sounds, such as mitral and tricuspid valve murmurs and extra heart sounds. To hear these sounds, place the bell of the stethoscope over the apical area, as shown below.

Forward-leaning
The forward-leaning position is best suited for hearing high-pitched sounds related to semilunar valve problems, such as aortic and pulmonic valve murmurs. To auscultate for these sounds, place the diaphragm of the stethoscope over the aortic and pulmonic areas in the right and left second intercostal spaces, as shown below.

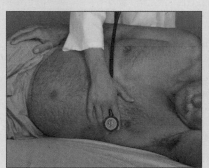

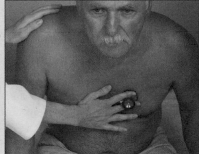

Auscultating for pericardial friction rub

To listen for a pericardial friction rub, have the patient sit upright, lean forward, and exhale. Listen with the diaphragm of the stethoscope over the third intercostal space on the left side of the chest. A pericardial friction rub has a scratchy, rubbing quality. If you suspect a rub but have trouble hearing one, ask the patient to hold their breath.

Grading murmurs

Use the system outlined below to describe the intensity of a murmur. When recording your findings, use Roman numerals as part of a fraction, always with VI as the denominator. For example, a grade III murmur would be recorded as "grade III/VI."

Making the grade
- Grade I is a barely audible murmur.
- Grade II is audible but quiet and soft.
- Grade III is moderately loud, without a thrust or thrill.
- Grade IV is loud, with a thrill.
- Grade V is very loud, and is heard with a stethoscope only partially in contact with the chest wall with a heave or a thrill.
- Grade VI is loud enough to be heard before the stethoscope comes into contact with the chest with a thrill.

Assessing the vascular system

Assessment of the vascular system is an important part of a full cardiovascular assessment. Examination of the patient's arms and legs can reveal arterial or venous disorders. Examine the patient's arms when you take their vital signs. Check the legs later during the physical examination, when the patient is lying on their back. Remember to evaluate leg veins when the patient is standing.

Inspection

Start your assessment of the vascular system the same way you start an assessment of the cardiac system—by making general observations. Are the arms equal in size? Are the legs symmetrical?

Inspect the skin color. Note how body hair is distributed. Note lesions, scars, clubbing, and edema of the extremities. If the patient is confined to bed, check the sacrum for edema. Examine the fingernails and toenails for any lesions and other abnormalities.

Assessing the neck vessels: A top-down approach

Start your inspection by observing vessels in the neck. The carotid artery should have a brisk, localized pulsation. The internal jugular vein has a softer, undulating pulsation. The carotid pulsation doesn't decrease when the patient is upright, when they inhale, or when you palpate the carotid. The internal jugular pulsation, on the other hand, changes in response to position, breathing, and palpation. The vein normally protrudes when the patient is lying down and lies flat when standing.

Check carotid artery pulsations. Are they weak or bounding? Inspect the jugular veins. Inspection of these vessels can provide information about blood volume and pressure in the right side of the heart. Assess for jugular vein distention. (See *Evaluating jugular vein distention*, page 215.)

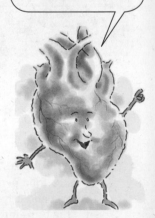

Inspecting the neck vessels can provide information about blood volume and pressure in the right side of the heart.

Palpation

The first step in palpation is to assess skin temperature, texture, and turgor. Then check capillary refill by assessing the nail beds on the fingers and toes. Refill time should be no more than 3 seconds, or long enough to say "capillary refill."

Swell scale
Palpate the patient's arms and legs for temperature and edema. Edema is graded on a four-point scale. If your finger leaves a slight imprint, the edema is recorded as +1. If your finger leaves a deep imprint that only slowly returns to normal, the edema is recorded as +4.

Evaluating jugular vein distention

With the patient in a supine position, position so that you can visualize jugular vein pulsations reflected from the right atrium.
• Elevate the head of the bed 30° to 45°.
• Locate the angle of Louis (sternal notch). To do so, palpate the clavicles where they join the sternum (the suprasternal notch). Place your first two fingers on the suprasternal notch. Then, without lifting them from the skin, slide them down the sternum until you feel a bony protuberance—this is the angle of Louis.
• Find the internal jugular vein. (It indicates venous pressure more reliably than the external jugular vein.)
• Shine a flashlight across the patient's neck to create shadows that highlight the venous pulse. Be sure to distinguish jugular vein pulsations from carotid artery pulsations. You can do this by palpating the vessel: Arterial pulsations continue, whereas venous pulsations disappear with light finger pressure. Also, venous pulsations increase or decrease with changes in body position; arterial pulsations remain constant.
• Locate the highest point along the vein where you can see pulsations.
• Using a centimeter ruler, measure the distance between the high point and the sternal notch. Record this finding as well as the angle at which the patient was lying. A finding greater than 1¼", to 1½", (3 to 4 cm) above the sternal notch, with the head of the bed at a 45° angle, indicates jugular vein distention.

Artery check!

Palpate for arterial pulses by gently pressing with the pads of your index and middle fingers. Start at the top of the patient's body at the temporal artery and work your way down. Check the carotid, brachial, radial, femoral, popliteal, posterior tibial, and dorsalis pedis pulses.

Palpate for the pulse on each side, comparing pulse volume and symmetry. *Don't palpate both carotid arteries at the same time or press too firmly. If you do, the patient may faint or become bradycardic.* If you haven't put on gloves for the examination, do so when you palpate the femoral arteries.

Making the grade

All pulses should be regular in rhythm and equal in strength. Pulses are also graded on a four-point scale: 4+ is bounding, 3+ is increased, 2+ is normal, 1+ is weak, and 0 is absent. (See *Assessing arterial pulses*, page 216.)

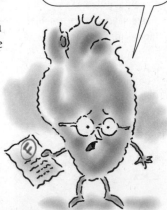

I'm afraid my pulses didn't make the grade.

Auscultation

After you palpate, use the bell of the stethoscope to begin auscultation; then follow the palpation sequence and listen over each

Peak technique

Assessing arterial pulses

To assess arterial pulses, apply pressure with your index and middle fingers. These illustrations show where to position your fingers when palpating for various pulses.

Carotid pulse

Lightly place your fingers just lateral to the trachea and below the jaw angle. Never palpate both carotid arteries at the same time. The pulse should be regular in rhythm and have equal strength in the right and left carotid arteries. You shouldn't be able to detect any palpable vibrations, known as *thrills*. Don't palpate both carotid arteries at the same time or press too firmly. If you do, the patient may faint or become bradycardic.

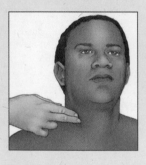

Brachial pulse

Position your fingers medial to the biceps tendon.

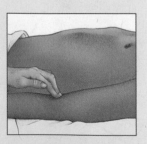

Radial pulse

Apply gentle pressure to the medial and ventral side of the wrist, just below the base of the thumb.

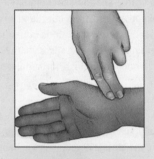

Femoral pulse

Press relatively hard at a point inferior to the inguinal ligament. For an obese patient, palpate in the crease of the groin, halfway between the pubic bone and the hip bone.

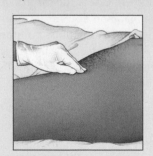

Popliteal pulse

Press firmly in the popliteal fossa at the back of the knee.

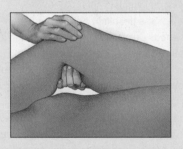

Posterior tibial pulse

Apply pressure behind and slightly below the malleolus of the ankle.

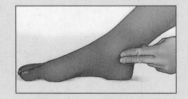

Dorsalis pedis pulse

Place your fingers on the medial dorsum of the foot while the patient points their toes down. The pulse is difficult to palpate here and may seem to be absent even in healthy patients.

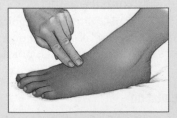

artery. Ask the patient to hold the breath while you auscultate each artery. Doing so will help eliminate respiratory sounds that may interfere with your findings. You shouldn't hear sounds over the carotid arteries. A hum or bruit sounds like buzzing or blowing and could indicate arteriosclerotic plaque formation.

Assess the upper abdomen for abnormal pulsations, which could indicate the presence of an abdominal aortic aneurysm. Finally, auscultate for the femoral and popliteal pulses, checking for a bruit or other abnormal vascular sounds.

Abnormal findings

This section outlines some of the most common cardiovascular abnormalities and their causes. (See *Cardiovascular abnormalities*, pages 217 and 218.)

Chest pain

Chest pain can arise suddenly or gradually, and its cause may be difficult to ascertain initially. The pain can radiate to the arms, neck, jaw, or back. It can be steady or intermittent, mild or acute. In addition, the pain can range in character from a sharp, shooting sensation to a feeling of heaviness, fullness, or even indigestion.

Interpretation station

Cardiovascular abnormalities

This chart shows some common groups of findings for signs and symptoms of the cardiovascular system, along with their probable causes.

Sign or symptom and findings	Probable cause	Sign or symptom and findings	Probable cause
Fatigue		• Persistent fatigue unrelated to exertion	Depression
• Fatigue following mild activity	Anemia	• Headache	
• Pallor		• Anorexia	
• Tachycardia		• Constipation	
• Dyspnea		• Sexual dysfunction	
		• Loss of concentration	
		• Irritability	

(Continued)

Cardiovascular abnormalities *(continued)*

Sign or symptom and findings	Probable cause
• Progressive fatigue • Cardiac murmur • Exertional dyspnea • Cough • Hemoptysis	Valvular heart disease
Palpitations	
• Paroxysmal palpitations • Diaphoresis • Facial flushing • Trembling • Impending sense of doom • Hyperventilation • Dizziness	Acute anxiety attack
• Paroxysmal or sustained palpitations • Dizziness • Weakness • Fatigue • Irregular, rapid, or slow pulse rate • Decreased blood pressure • Confusion • Diaphoresis	Cardiac arrhythmias
• Sustained palpitations • Fatigue • Irritability • Hunger • Cold sweats • Tremors • Anxiety	Hypoglycemia

Sign or symptom and findings	Probable cause
Peripheral edema	
• Headache • Bilateral leg edema with pitting ankle edema • Weight gain despite anorexia • Nausea • Chest tightness • Hypotension • Pallor • Palpitations • Inspiratory crackles	Heart failure
• Bilateral arm edema accompanied by facial and neck edema • Edematous areas marked by dilated veins • Headache • Vertigo • Visual disturbances	Superior vena cava syndrome
• Moderate to severe, unilateral or bilateral leg edema • Darkened skin • Stasis ulcers around the ankle	Venous insufficiency

Common culprits

Chest pain may be caused by various disorders. Common cardiovascular causes include angina, MI, and cardiomyopathy. Chest pain may be provoked or aggravated by stress, anxiety, exertion, deep breathing, or eating certain foods. (See *Chest pain*, page 219.)

Palpitations

Palpitations—defined as a conscious awareness of one's heartbeat—are usually felt over the precordium or in the throat or neck.

Interpretation station

Chest pain

Use this chart to help you more accurately assess chest pain.

What it feels like	Where it's located	What makes it worse	What causes it	What makes it better
Aching, squeezing, pressure, heaviness, or burning pain; usually subsides within 10 minutes	Substernal; may radiate to jaw, neck, arms, and back	Eating, physical effort, smoking, cold weather, stress, anger, hunger, lying down	Angina pectoris	Rest, nitroglycerin, oxygen (Note: Unstable angina appears even at rest.)
Tightness or pressure; burning, aching pain, possibly accompanied by shortness of breath, diaphoresis, weakness, fatigue, anxiety, or nausea; sudden onset; lasts 30 minutes to 2 hours	Typically across chest but may radiate to jaw, neck, arms, or back	Exertion, anxiety	Acute myocardial infarction	Opioid analgesics such as morphine sulfate, nitroglycerin, oxygen, reperfusion of blocked coronary artery
Sharp and continuous; may be accompanied by friction rub; sudden onset	Substernal; may radiate to neck or left arm	Deep breathing, supine position	Pericarditis	Sitting up, leaning forward, anti-inflammatory drugs
Excruciating, tearing pain; may be accompanied by blood pressure difference between right and left arm; sudden onset	Retrosternal, upper abdominal, or epigastric; may radiate to back, neck, or shoulders	Not applicable	Dissecting aortic aneurysm	Analgesics, surgery
Sudden, stabbing pain; may be accompanied by cyanosis, dyspnea, or cough with hemoptysis	Over lung area	Inspiration	Pulmonary embolus	Analgesics
Sudden and severe pain, sometimes accompanied by dyspnea, increased pulse rate, decreased breath sounds (especially on one side), or deviated trachea	Lateral thorax	Normal respiration	Pneumothorax	Analgesics, chest tube insertion
Dull, pressurelike, squeezing pain	Substernal, epigastric areas	Food, cold liquids, exercise	Esophageal spasm	Nitroglycerin, calcium channel blockers

(Continued)

Chest pain *(continued)*

What it feels like	Where it's located	What makes it worse	What causes it	What makes it better
Sharp, severe pain	Lower chest or upper abdomen	Eating a heavy meal, bending, lying down	Hiatal hernia	Antacids, walking, semi-Fowler position
Burning feeling after eating sometimes accompanied by hematemesis or tarry stools; sudden onset that generally subsides within 15–20 minutes	Epigastric	Lack of food or highly acidic foods	Peptic ulcer	Food, antacids
Gripping, sharp pain; possibly nausea and vomiting	Right epigastric or abdominal areas; possible radiation to shoulders	Eating fatty foods, lying down	Cholecystitis	Rest and analgesics, surgery
Continuous or intermittent sharp pain; possibly tender to touch; gradual or sudden onset	Anywhere in chest	Movement, palpation	Chest wall syndrome	Time, analgesics, heat applications
Dull or stabbing pain usually accompanied by hyperventilation or breathlessness; sudden onset; lasting less than 1 minute or as long as several days	Anywhere in chest	Increased respiratory rate, stress, or anxiety	Acute anxiety	Slowing of respiratory rate, stress relief

The patient may describe them as pounding, jumping, turning, fluttering, or flopping or as missed or skipped beats. Palpitations may be regular or irregular, fast or slow, paroxysmal or sustained.

Palpitation provokers

Although usually insignificant, palpitations may result from a cardiac or metabolic disorder or from the effects of certain drugs. Nonpathologic palpitations may occur with a newly implanted prosthetic valve because the valve's clicking sound heightens the patient's awareness of their heartbeat. Transient palpitations may accompany emotional stress (such as fright, anger, or anxiety) or physical stress (such as exercise or fever). Stimulants such as tobacco and caffeine may also cause palpitations.

Fatigue

Fatigue is a feeling of excessive tiredness, lack of energy, or exhaustion accompanied by a strong desire to rest or sleep. Fatigue is a normal and important response to physical overexertion, prolonged emotional stress, and sleep deprivation. However, it can also be a nonspecific symptom of cardiovascular disease, especially heart failure and valvular heart disease.

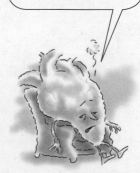

Fatigue can be a nonspecific symptom of cardiovascular disease.

Skin and hair abnormalities

Cyanosis, pallor, or cool skin may indicate decreased cardiac output and poor tissue perfusion. Conditions causing fever or increased cardiac output may make the skin warmer than is normal. Absence of body hair on the arms or legs may indicate diminished arterial blood flow to those areas. (See *Findings in arterial and venous insufficiency*, page 221.)

Findings in arterial and venous insufficiency

Assessment findings in patients with arterial insufficiency differ from those in patients with chronic venous insufficiency. The illustrations below show those differences.

Arterial insufficiency
In a patient with arterial insufficiency, pulses may be decreased or absent. The skin will be cool, pale, and shiny, with loss of hair, and the patient may have pain in the legs and feet. Ulcerations typically occur in the area around the toes, and the foot usually turns deep red when dependent. Nails may be thick and ridged.

Chronic venous insufficiency
In a patient with chronic venous insufficiency, check for ulcerations around the ankle. Pulses are present but may be difficult to find because of edema. The foot may become cyanotic when dependent. Skin discolorations, usually hyperpigmentations, are quite common.

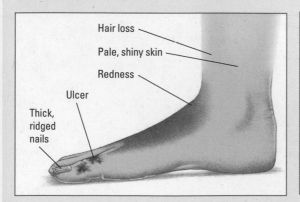

Hair loss
Pale, shiny skin
Redness
Ulcer
Thick, ridged nails

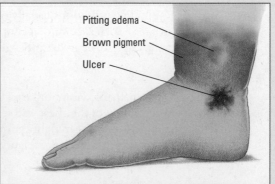

Pitting edema
Brown pigment
Ulcer

That's just swell

Swelling, or edema, may indicate heart failure or venous insufficiency. It may also result from varicosities or thrombophlebitis.

Chronic right-sided heart failure may cause ascites and generalized edema. Right-sided heart failure may cause swelling in the lower legs. If the patient has compression of a vein in a specific area, they may have localized swelling along the path of the compressed vessel.

Abnormal pulsations

A displaced apical impulse may indicate an enlarged left ventricle, which may be caused by heart failure or hypertension. A forceful apical impulse, or one lasting longer than a third of the cardiac cycle, may point to increased cardiac output. If you find a pulsation in the patient's aortic, pulmonic, or tricuspid area, their heart chamber may be enlarged or they may have valvular disease.

Pulses here, there, everywhere

Increased cardiac output or an aortic aneurysm may also produce pulsations in the aortic area. A patient with an epigastric pulsation may have early heart failure or an aortic aneurysm. A pulsation in the sternoclavicular area suggests an aortic aneurysm. A patient with anemia, anxiety, increased cardiac output, or a thin chest wall may have slight pulsations to the right and left of the sternum.

Weak ones, strong ones

A weak arterial pulse may indicate decreased cardiac output or increased peripheral vascular resistance, both of which point to arterial atherosclerotic disease. Many older patients have weak pedal pulses.

Strong or bounding pulsations usually occur in a patient with a condition that causes increased cardiac output, such as hypertension, hypoxia, anemia, exercise, or anxiety. (See *Pulse waveforms*, page 223.)

Heave–ho!

A thrill, which is a palpable vibration, usually suggests a valvular dysfunction. A heave, lifting of the chest wall felt during palpation, along the left sternal border may mean right ventricular hypertrophy; over the left ventricular area, a ventricular aneurysm.

Pulse waveforms

To identify abnormal arterial pulses, check these waveforms and see which one matches the patient's peripheral pulse.

Weak pulse
A weak pulse has a decreased amplitude with a slower upstroke and downstroke. Possible causes of a weak pulse include increased peripheral vascular resistance, as occurs in cold weather or with severe heart failure, and decreased stroke volume, as occurs with hypovolemia or aortic stenosis.

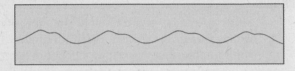

Bounding pulse
A bounding pulse has a sharp upstroke and downstroke with a pointed peak. The amplitude is elevated. Possible causes of a bounding pulse include increased stroke volume, as with aortic insufficiency, or stiffness of arterial walls, as with aging.

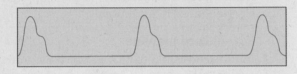

Pulsus alternans
Pulsus alternans has a regular, alternating pattern of a weak and a strong pulse. This pattern is associated with left-sided heart failure.

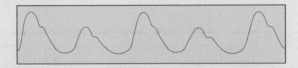

Pulsus bigeminus
Pulsus bigeminus is similar to pulsus alternans but occurs at irregular intervals. This pattern is caused by premature atrial or ventricular beats.

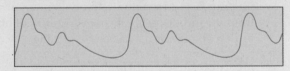

Pulsus paradoxus
Pulsus paradoxus has increases and decreases in amplitude associated with the respiratory cycle. Marked decreases occur when the patient inhales. Pulsus paradoxus is associated with pericardial tamponade, advanced heart failure, and constrictive pericarditis.

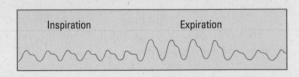

Pulsus bisferiens
Pulsus bisferiens shows an initial upstroke, a subsequent downstroke, and then another upstroke during systole. Pulsus bisferiens is caused by aortic stenosis and aortic insufficiency.

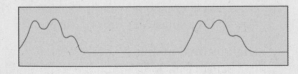

Abnormal sounds

Abnormal auscultation findings include abnormal heart sounds (see *Abnormal heart sounds*, page 225), heart murmurs, and bruits.

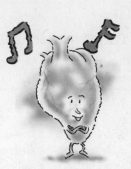

Murmurs

Murmurs can occur as a result of a number of conditions and have widely varied characteristics. Here's a rundown on some of the more common murmur types. If you identify a heart murmur, listen closely to determine its timing in the cardiac cycle. Then determine its other characteristics: quality (blowing, musical, harsh, or rumbling), pitch (medium, high, or low), and location (where the murmur sounds the loudest). Use a standard, six-level grading scale to describe the intensity (loudness) of the murmur.

Low-pitched murmur

Aortic stenosis, a condition in which the aortic valve has calcified and restricts blood flow, causes a midsystolic, low-pitched, harsh murmur that radiates from the valve to the carotid artery.

That's intense!

This murmur shifts from crescendo to decrescendo and back. *Crescendo* is a term used to describe the configuration of a murmur that increases in intensity. Likewise, a *decrescendo* murmur decreases in intensity. The crescendo-decrescendo murmur of aortic stenosis results from the turbulent, highly pressured flow of blood across stiffened leaflets and through a narrowed opening.

Medium-pitched murmur

During auscultation, listen for a murmur near the pulmonic valve. This murmur might indicate pulmonic stenosis, a condition in which the pulmonic valve has calcified and interferes with the flow of blood out of the right ventricle.

And that's so harsh…

This murmur is medium-pitched, systolic, and harsh and shifts from crescendo to decrescendo and back. It's caused by turbulent blood flow across a stiffened, narrowed valve.

High-pitched murmur

In a patient with aortic insufficiency, the blood flows backward through the aortic valve and causes a high-pitched, blowing, decrescendo, diastolic murmur. This murmur radiates from the aortic valve area to the left sternal border.

Murmur grading

Grade 1—barely audible, even to the trained ear

Grade 2—clearly audible

Grade 3—moderately loud

Grade 4—loud with palpable thrill

Grade 5—very loud with a palpable thrill; can be heard when the stethoscope has only partial contact with the chest

Grade 6—extremely loud with a palpable thrill; can be heard with the stethoscope lifted just off the chest wall

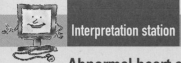

Interpretation station

Abnormal heart sounds

Whenever auscultation reveals an abnormal heart sound, try to identify the sound and its timing in the cardiac cycle. Knowing those characteristics can help you identify the possible cause of the sound. Use this chart to put all that information together.

Abnormal heart sound	Timing	Possible causes
Accentuated S_1	Beginning of systole	High-output states (fever, exercise, anemia, hyperthyroidism) or mitral stenosis
Diminished S_1	Beginning of systole	Mitral insufficiency, first-degree heart block, heart failure, increased pericardial fluid, or obesity
Split S_1	Beginning of systole	Right bundle branch block (BBB) or premature ventricular contractions (normal in children, young adults, and athletes)
Accentuated S_2	End of systole	Pulmonary or systemic hypertension
Diminished or inaudible S_2	End of systole	Aortic or pulmonic stenosis or pericardial effusion
Persistent S_2 split	End of systole	Delayed closure of the pulmonic valve, usually from overfilling of the right ventricle, causing prolonged systolic ejection time; may suggest atrial septal defect and right ventricular failure
Reversed or paradoxical S_2 split that appears during exhalation and disappears during inspiration	End of systole	Delayed ventricular stimulation, left BBB, or prolonged left ventricular ejection time
S_3 (ventricular gallop)	Early diastole	Overdistention of the ventricles during the rapid filling segment of diastole or mitral insufficiency or ventricular failure (normal in children, young adults, and pregnant patients)
S_4 (atrial or presystolic gallop)	Late diastole	Pulmonic stenosis, hypertension, coronary artery disease, aortic stenosis, or forceful atrial contraction due to resistance to ventricular filling late in diastole (resulting from left ventricular hypertrophy); normal in older adult patients
Pericardial friction rub (grating or leathery sound at the left sternal border; usually muffled, high-pitched, and transient)	Throughout systole and diastole	Pericardial inflammation

Wrong way!

In a patient with pulmonic insufficiency, the blood flows backward through the pulmonic valve, causing a blowing, diastolic, decrescendo murmur at Erb point. If the patient has a higher-than-normal pulmonary pressure, the murmur is high-pitched. If not, it will be low-pitched.

Rumbling murmur

Mitral stenosis is a condition in which the mitral valve has calcified and is impeding blood flow out of the left atrium. Listen for a low-pitched, rumbling, crescendo-decrescendo murmur in the mitral valve area. This murmur results from turbulent blood flow across the stiffened, narrowed valve.

Blowing murmur

In a patient with mitral insufficiency, blood regurgitates into the left atrium. The regurgitation produces a high-pitched, blowing murmur throughout systole (pansystolic or holosystolic). This murmur may radiate from the mitral area to the left axillary line. You can hear it best at the apex.

Low, rumbling murmur

Tricuspid stenosis is a condition in which the tricuspid valve has calcified and is impeding blood flow through the valve from the right atrium. Listen for a low, rumbling, crescendo-decrescendo murmur in the tricuspid area. This murmur results from turbulent blood flow across the stiffened, narrowed valvular leaflets.

High-pitched, blowing murmur

In a patient with tricuspid insufficiency, blood regurgitates into the right atrium. This backflow of blood through the valve causes a high-pitched, blowing murmur throughout systole in the tricuspid area. This murmur becomes louder when the patient inhales.

Bruits

A murmurlike sound of vascular (rather than cardiac) origin is called a bruit. If you hear a bruit during arterial auscultation, the patient may have occlusive arterial disease or an arteriovenous fistula. Various high cardiac output conditions—such as anemia, hyperthyroidism, and pheochromocytoma—may also cause bruits.

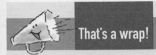
That's a wrap!

Cardiovascular system review

Anatomy and physiology
Heart
• A hollow, muscular organ that pumps blood to all organs and tissues of the body
• Protected by a thin sac called the pericardium
• Consists of four chambers: two atria and two ventricles
• Contains valves to keep blood flowing in only one direction
• Contracts to send blood out (systole), then relaxes and fills with blood (diastole)

Vascular system
• Arteries: thick-walled vessels that carry oxygenated blood away from the heart (exception: pulmonary artery)
• Veins: thin-walled vessels that carry deoxygenated blood toward the heart (exception: pulmonary vein)
• Pulses: pressure waves of blood generated by the pumping action of the heart

Blood circulation
• Deoxygenated venous blood flows from the superior vena cava, inferior vena cava, and coronary sinus into the right atrium.
• Blood flows from the right atrium through the tricuspid valve and into the right ventricle.
• Blood is then ejected through the pulmonic valve into the pulmonary artery, where it travels to the lungs for oxygenation.
• Oxygenated blood then flows through the pulmonary veins and returns to the left atrium.
• Blood passes through the mitral valve and into the left ventricle.
• Blood is pumped through the aortic valve and into the aorta for delivery to the rest of the body.

Obtaining a health history
• Ask about current and past problems, including chest pain, palpitations, shortness of breath, peripheral skin changes, and changes in extremities.
• Have the patient rate their chest pain on a scale of 0 to 10, with 0 being no pain and 10 being the worst pain imaginable.
• Ask about personal and family history of cardiovascular disease, diabetes, and chronic diseases of the lungs or kidneys.

Assessing the heart
• Inspect the patient's general appearance, noting skin color, temperature, turgor, and texture.
• Inspect the chest, noting the location of the apical impulse.
• Palpate over the precordium to find the apical impulse.
• Palpate the sternoclavicular, aortic, pulmonic, tricuspid, and epigastric areas for abnormal pulsations.
• Percuss the chest wall to locate cardiac borders.
• Auscultate for heart sounds with the patient lying on their back with the head of the bed raised 30° to 45°, with them sitting up, and with them lying on their left side.
• Auscultate for murmurs by asking the patient to sit up and lean forward or having them lie on their left side.
• Auscultate for a pericardial friction rub by asking the patient to sit upright, lean forward, and exhale.

Heart sounds
• S_1: best heard at the apex of the heart; corresponds to closure of the mitral and tricuspid valves
• S_2: best heard at the base of the heart; corresponds to closure of the pulmonic and aortic valves
• S_3: commonly heard in patients with high cardiac output or heart failure (called ventricular gallop); a normal finding in children, young adults, and pregnant patients
• S_4: adventitious sound called atrial gallop; heard in patients who are older adults or in those with hypertension, aortic stenosis, or a history of myocardial infarction

Assessing the vascular system
• Inspect the patient's general appearance, skin, fingernails, and toenails.
• Check carotid artery and jugular vein pulsations.

(Continued)

Cardiovascular system review *(continued)*

• Palpate the patient's skin over the upper and lower extremities for temperature, texture, and turgor.
• Check capillary refill time (should be less than 3 seconds).
• Palpate arterial pulses on each side of the body, moving from head to toe (temporal, carotid, brachial, radial, femoral, popliteal, posterior tibial, and dorsalis pedis arteries, in that order).
• Auscultate over each artery in this same order, listening for hums or bruits.

Abnormal findings
• Chest pain: sensation that varies in severity and presentation depending on the cause
• Palpitations: a conscious awareness of one's heartbeat
• Fatigue: a feeling of excessive tiredness, lack of energy, or exhaustion accompanied by a strong desire to rest or sleep
• Thrill: palpable vibration indicating valvular dysfunction
• Heave: lifting of the chest wall felt during palpation; indicates

ventricular hypertrophy (when felt on the sternal border) or ventricular aneurysm (when felt over the left ventricle)
• Murmur: sound made by turbulent blood flow; may increase in intensity (crescendo) or decrease in intensity (decrescendo) or it may be plateau-shaped (no change in intensity throughout the cardiac cycle)
• Bruit: a murmurlike sound heard over blood vessels

Quick quiz

1. When listening to heart sounds, you can hear S_1 best at the:
    A. base of the heart.
    B. apex of the heart.
    C. second intercostal space to the right of the sternum.
    D. fifth intercostal space to the right of the sternum.

Answer: B. S_1 is best heard at the apex of the heart.

2. You're auscultating for heart sounds in a 3-year-old and hear an S_3. You assess this sound to be a:
    A. normal finding.
    B. probable sign of heart failure.
    C. possible sign of atrial septal defect.
    D. possible sign of patent ductus arteriosus.

Answer: A. S_3 is a normal finding in a child. This sound can indicate heart failure in an adult.

3. Capillary refill time is normally:
    A. 1 to 3 seconds.
    B. 4 to 6 seconds.
    C. 7 to 10 seconds.
    D. 11 to 15 seconds.

Answer: A. Capillary refill time that's longer than 3 seconds is considered delayed and indicates decreased perfusion.

4.   As you auscultate heart sounds in a 53-year-old patient you hear an S_4. This sound may indicate:
    A.   heart failure.
    B.   a normal finding in the last trimester of pregnancy.
    C.   ventricular gallop.
    D.   hypertension.

Answer: D. An S_4 may be heard in older adult patients or in those with hypertension, aortic stenosis, or a history of MI.

5.   You suspect that your patient has a pericardial friction rub but you have trouble hearing it. What should you do?
    A.   Ask the patient to hold their breath.
    B.   Ask the patient to exhale forcefully.
    C.   Ask the patient to lie on their left side.
    D.   Ask the patient to lie flat on their back.

Answer: A. If you suspect a pericardial rub but have trouble hearing one, ask the patient to hold their breath.

Scoring

☆☆☆ If you answered all five questions correctly, take a bow! You're a star of the heart.

☆☆ If you answered four questions correctly, sensational! You're pumped with information.

☆ If you answered fewer than four questions correctly, keep at it! You're just getting into the rhythm.

Just for fun

Match the heart sound in column 1 with its defining characteristics in column 2.

Heart sound

1. S_1 _____

2. S_2 _____

3. S_3 _____

4. S_4 _____

Defining characteristics

A. Low-pitched galloping sound (similar to the y in "Ken-tuck-y") caused by rapid ventricular filling and best heard with patient lying on their left side

B. Low-pitched, dull "lub" sound that's best heard over the mitral area and caused by rising ventricular pressure and closure of the mitral and tricuspid valves at the beginning of systole

C. Adventitious sound called an atrial gallop (similar to the word "Ten-nes-see") that occurs when the atria contract and eject blood into resistant ventricles

D. Short, high-pitched "dub" sound best heard at the base of the heart at the end of systole, when ventricular pressure falls and aortic and pulmonic valves close

Answer: 1. B, 2. D, 3. A, 4. C

Chapter 10

Respiratory system

Just the facts

In this chapter, you'll learn:

♦ anatomy and physiology of the respiratory system

♦ methods for assessing the respiratory system

♦ abnormal respiratory system findings and their causes.

A look at the respiratory system

The respiratory system includes the airways, lungs, bony thorax, respiratory muscles, and central nervous system (CNS). (See *A close look at the respiratory system*, page 232.) They work together to deliver oxygen to the bloodstream and remove excess carbon dioxide from the body.

Anatomy and physiology

Knowing the basic structures and functions of the respiratory system will help you perform a comprehensive respiratory assessment and recognize any abnormalities.

Airways and lungs

The airways are divided into the upper and lower airways. The upper airways include the nasopharynx (nose), oropharynx (mouth), laryngopharynx, and larynx. Their purpose is to warm, filter, and humidify inhaled air. They also help to make sound and send air to the lower airways.

Swallowing safely

The epiglottis is a flap of tissue that closes over the top of the larynx when the patient swallows. The epiglottis protects the patient from aspirating food or fluid into the lower airways.

A close look at the respiratory system

The major structures of the upper and lower airways are illustrated at right. The alveoli, or acini, are shown in the lower illustration.

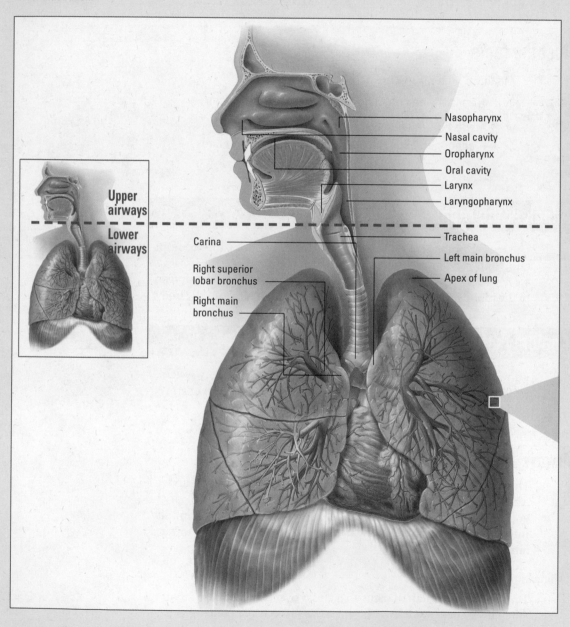

Vocal point

The larynx is located at the top of the trachea and houses the vocal cords. It's the transition point between the upper and lower airways.

Anterior view

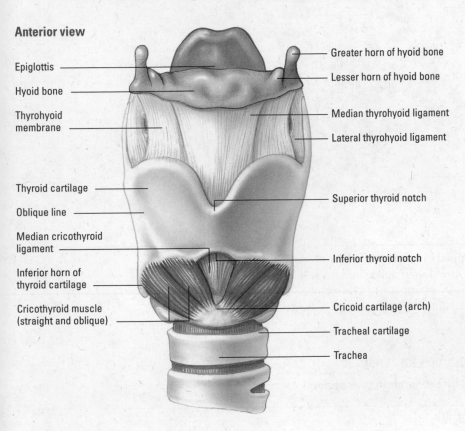

Epiglottis

Hyoid bone

Thyrohyoid membrane

Thyroid cartilage

Oblique line

Median cricothyroid ligament

Inferior horn of thyroid cartilage

Cricothyroid muscle (straight and oblique)

Greater horn of hyoid bone

Lesser horn of hyoid bone

Median thyrohyoid ligament

Lateral thyrohyoid ligament

Superior thyroid notch

Inferior thyroid notch

Cricoid cartilage (arch)

Tracheal cartilage

Trachea

The lowdown on the lower airways

The lower airways begin with the trachea, which then divides into the right and left mainstem bronchi. The mainstem bronchi divide into the lobar bronchi, which are lined with mucus-producing ciliated epithelium, one of the lungs' major defense systems.

The lobar bronchi then divide into secondary bronchi, tertiary bronchi, terminal bronchioles, respiratory bronchioles, alveolar ducts, and, finally, into the alveoli, the gas exchange units of the lungs. An adult's lungs typically contain about 300 million alveoli.

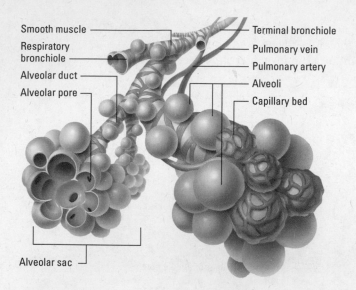

Smooth muscle
Respiratory bronchiole
Alveolar duct
Alveolar pore
Terminal bronchiole
Pulmonary vein
Pulmonary artery
Alveoli
Capillary bed
Alveolar sac

Lungs and lobes

Each lung is wrapped in a lining called the *visceral pleura*. The right lung is larger and has three lobes: upper, middle, and lower. The left lung is smaller and has only an upper and a lower lobe. The space between the lungs is the mediastinum. (See *A close look at the lobes and pleurae*.)

A close look at the lobes and pleurae

The lobes of the lungs and the pleurae are illustrated below.

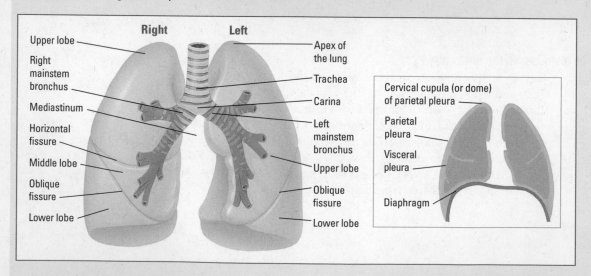

Right   Left

Upper lobe
Right mainstem bronchus
Mediastinum
Horizontal fissure
Middle lobe
Oblique fissure
Lower lobe

Apex of the lung
Trachea
Carina
Left mainstem bronchus
Upper lobe
Oblique fissure
Lower lobe

Cervical cupula (or dome) of parietal pleura
Parietal pleura
Visceral pleura
Diaphragm

Smooth moves

The lungs share space in the thoracic cavity with the heart and great vessels, the trachea, the esophagus, and the bronchi. All areas of the thoracic cavity that come in contact with the lungs are lined with parietal pleura.

A small amount of fluid fills the area between the two layers of the pleura. This pleural fluid allows the layers to slide smoothly over each other as the chest expands and contracts. The parietal pleura also contains nerve endings that transmit pain signals when inflammation occurs.

Thorax

The bony thorax includes the clavicles, sternum, scapulae, 12 sets of ribs, and 12 thoracic vertebrae. You can use specific parts of the thorax, along with some imaginary vertical lines drawn on the chest, to help describe the locations of your findings. (See *Respiratory assessment landmarks*.)

Rack of ribs

Ribs are part of the bony structure that surrounds the chest and provides support and protection to the heart and lungs. All ribs attach to the thoracic vertebrae. The first seven ribs also attach directly to the sternum with cartilage, which allows the chest wall to expand and contract with each breath. The eighth, ninth, and tenth ribs attach to the cartilage of the preceding rib. The eleventh and twelfth ribs are called *floating ribs* because they don't attach to anything in the anterior thorax.

Respiratory muscles

The diaphragm and the external intercostal muscles are the primary muscles used in breathing. They contract when the patient inhales and relax when the patient exhales. (See *Mechanics of breathing*, page 237.)

Message in a nerve

The respiratory center in the brain stem initiates each breath by sending messages to the primary respiratory muscles over the phrenic nerve. Impulses from the phrenic nerve adjust the rate and depth of breathing, depending on the carbon dioxide and pH levels in the cerebrospinal fluid.

Respiratory assessment landmarks

The illustrations below show common landmarks used in respiratory assessment.

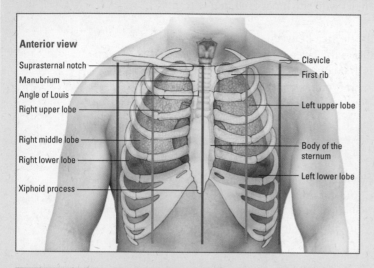

Anterior view

- Suprasternal notch
- Manubrium
- Angle of Louis
- Right upper lobe
- Right middle lobe
- Right lower lobe
- Xiphoid process
- Clavicle
- First rib
- Left upper lobe
- Body of the sternum
- Left lower lobe

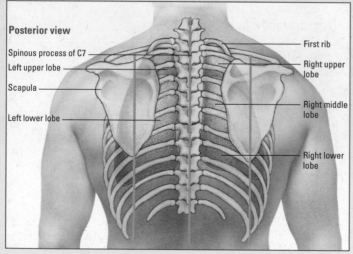

Posterior view

- Spinous process of C7
- Left upper lobe
- Scapula
- Left lower lobe
- First rib
- Right upper lobe
- Right middle lobe
- Right lower lobe

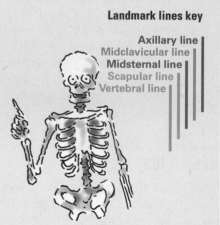

Landmark lines key

- Axillary line
- Midclavicular line
- Midsternal line
- Scapular line
- Vertebral line

Accessory to breathing

Other muscles assist in breathing. Accessory inspiratory muscles include the trapezius, the sternocleidomastoid, and the scalenes, which combine to elevate the scapulae, clavicles, sternum, and upper ribs. That elevation expands the front-to-back diameter of the chest when use of the diaphragm and intercostal muscles isn't effective.

Expiration occurs when the diaphragm and external intercostal muscles relax. If the patient has an airway obstruction, they may also

Mechanics of breathing

Breathing results from differences between atmospheric and intrapulmonary pressures, as described below.

1. Before inspiration, intrapulmonary pressure equals atmospheric pressure, at about 760 mm Hg. Intrapleural pressure equals 756 mm Hg.

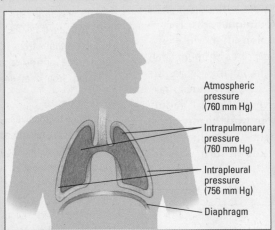

Atmospheric pressure (760 mm Hg)

Intrapulmonary pressure (760 mm Hg)

Intrapleural pressure (756 mm Hg)

Diaphragm

2. During inspiration, the diaphragm and external intercostal muscles contract, enlarging the thorax vertically and horizontally. As the thorax expands, intrapleural pressure decreases and the lungs expand to fill the enlarging thoracic cavity.

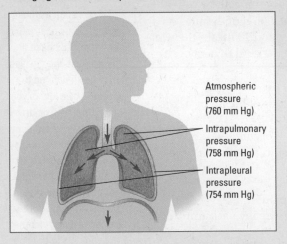

Atmospheric pressure (760 mm Hg)

Intrapulmonary pressure (758 mm Hg)

Intrapleural pressure (754 mm Hg)

3. The intrapulmonary atmospheric pressure gradient pulls air into the lungs until the two pressures are equal.

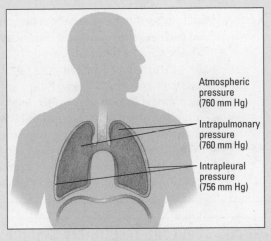

Atmospheric pressure (760 mm Hg)

Intrapulmonary pressure (760 mm Hg)

Intrapleural pressure (756 mm Hg)

4. During normal expiration, the diaphragm slowly relaxes and the lungs and thorax passively return to resting size and position. During deep or forced expiration, contraction of internal intercostal and abdominal muscles reduces thoracic volume. Lung and thorax compression raises intrapulmonary pressure above atmospheric pressure.

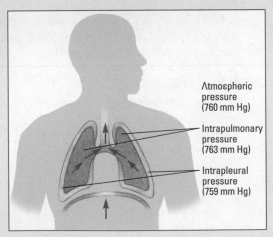

Atmospheric pressure (760 mm Hg)

Intrapulmonary pressure (763 mm Hg)

Intrapleural pressure (759 mm Hg)

use the abdominal muscles and internal intercostal muscles to exhale. Frequent use of accessory muscles may indicate a respiratory problem, particularly when the patient purses the lips, and flares the nostrils when breathing.

Obtaining a health history

When obtaining the health history of a patient with a respiratory disorder, first ask questions pertinent to the respiratory system. Then broaden your assessment to include questions about other health issues.

Questions should be asked about any pulmonary diagnoses they have had such as asthma, chronic obstructive pulmonary disease (COPD), allergies, or frequent respiratory infections. If they use any respiratory medications (prescriptions or herbal) or equipment such as inhalers, nebulizers, CPAP, etc. If they are experiencing any respiratory symptoms: shortness of breath, cough, chest pain with respirations, and circumstances that surround these events. Also ask about smoking history, including vaping. Inquire about work history and chemical exposures as this can provide important clues to lung issues. Be sure to collect information on past immunizations such as pneumonia, COVID-19, and flu vaccines in adults.

Questions about the respiratory system

A patient with a respiratory disorder may report shortness of breath, cough, sputum production, wheezing, and chest pain. (See *Breathtaking facts* and *Listen and learn, then teach*.)

Shortness of breath

You can gain a history of the patient's shortness of breath by using several scales. Ask the patient to rate their usual level of dyspnea on a scale of 0 to 10, in which 0 means no dyspnea and 10 means the worst they have experienced. Then ask them to rate the level that day.

Not to be long-winded, but...

You can learn more about the patient's shortness of breath by asking the following questions:
- When does the shortness of breath seem to occur?
- Is it related to exercise or other activities or to a particular time of day?
- When you cough, do you produce sputum?
- When you breathe in, do you experience pain?
- Do you smoke or vape? How long and how many packs/cartridges a day? Does anyone in the house smoke?
- Have you had recent chest trauma?
- Is it harder to breathe in or breathe out?
- Do you experience any other symptoms such as chest pain at the same time?

Breathtaking facts

Cough it up
Coughing clears unwanted material from the tracheobronchial tree. Sputum from the bronchial tubes traps foreign matter and protects the lungs from damage.

Pain sites
The lungs themselves don't contain pain receptors, but chest pain may be caused by inflammation of the parietal pleura or the costochondral joints at the midclavicular line or at the edge of the sternum.

How much oxygen?
Patients with chronically high partial pressure of arterial carbon dioxide ($PaCO_2$), such as those with chronic obstructive pulmonary disease or a neuromuscular disease, may be stimulated to breathe by a low oxygen level (the hypoxic drive) rather than by a slightly high $PaCO_2$ level, which is normal. For such patients, supplemental oxygen therapy should be provided cautiously because it may depress the stimulus to breathe, further increasing $PaCO_2$.

Listen and learn, then teach

Listening to what your patient says about their respiratory problems will help you know when they need patient education. These typical responses indicate that the patient needs to know more about self-care techniques:

"Whenever I feel short of breath, I use my inhaler." This patient needs to know that continuous and routine use of medications as prescribed decreases exacerbation of symptoms.	**"If I feel all congested, I just smoke a cigarette, and then I can cough up that phlegm!"** This patient needs to know about the dangers of cigarette smoking.	**"None of the other guys wear a mask when we're working."** This patient needs to know the importance of wearing an appropriate safety mask when working around heavy dust and particles in the air, such as sawdust or powders.

- Do you snore or have pauses in your breathing when you sleep?
- Any swelling in your ankles or recent weight gain?
- Do you take any medications to treat your shortness of breath? What medications, and how often do you take them?

Orthopnea

A patient with orthopnea (shortness of breath when lying down) tends to sleep with their upper body elevated.

Need a lift?
Ask the patient how many pillows they use or if they sleep in a recliner. The answer describes the severity of orthopnea. For instance, a patient who uses three pillows can be said to have "three-pillow orthopnea."

Cough

Ask the patient with a cough these questions: Is the cough productive? If the cough is a chronic problem, has it changed recently? If so, how? Is the cough worse in the morning, at night, or the same throughout the day? Does anything make you cough like dust, animals, or movement? What makes the cough better? What makes it worse? Do you take any medication for your cough? If so, what medication and how often? Has it helped?

Sputum

When a patient produces sputum, ask them to estimate the amount produced. Is it clear or thick and cloudy? Is there any blood in the sputum (hemoptysis)?

Now that you've brought it up...

Also ask them these questions: At what time of day do you cough most often? What's the color and consistency of the sputum? If sputum is a chronic problem, has it changed recently? If so, how? Do you cough up blood (hemoptysis)? If so, how much and how often?

Wheezing

If a patient wheezes, ask these questions: When does wheezing occur? What makes you wheeze? Do you get tightness in your chest when you feel like you are wheezing? Do you wheeze loudly enough for others to hear it? What helps stop your wheezing? Have you started any new medications or supplements?

Chest pain

If the patient has chest pain, ask them these questions: Where's the pain located? What does it feel like? Is it sharp, stabbing, burning, or aching? Does it move to another area? How long does it last? What causes it to occur? What makes it better? What makes it worse?

Chest pain associated with a respiratory problem usually results from pneumonia, pulmonary embolism, or pleural inflammation. Coughing or fractures can also cause musculoskeletal chest pain.

Questions about general health

Remember to look at the patient's medical and family history, being particularly watchful for a smoking habit, allergies, previous operations, and respiratory diseases, such as pneumonia and tuberculosis.

Also, ask about environmental exposure to irritants such as asbestos. People who work in mining, farming, construction, or chemical manufacturing are commonly exposed to environmental irritants. People can also be exposed to environmental irritants or respiratory disease where they live.

Assessing the respiratory system

Any patient can develop a respiratory disorder. By using a systematic assessment, you'll be able to detect subtle or obvious respiratory changes. The depth of your assessment will depend on several factors, including the patient's primary health problem and their risk of developing respiratory complications.

A physical examination of the respiratory system follows four steps: inspection, palpation, percussion, and auscultation. Before you begin, make sure the room is well lit and warm.

First impressions

Make a few observations about the patient as soon as you enter the room. Note how the patient is seated, which will most likely be the position in which it's most comfortable for them to breathe. Take note of their level of awareness and general appearance. Do they appear relaxed? Anxious? Uncomfortable? Are they having trouble breathing? You'll include these observations in your final assessment.

Inspecting the chest

Introduce yourself and explain why you're there and what will happen. Help the patient into an upright position. The patient should be undressed from the waist up or clothed in an examination gown that allows you easy access to their chest.

Back, then front

Examine the back of the chest first, using inspection, palpation, percussion, and auscultation. Always compare left side to right (not to be confused with front to back). Then examine the front of the chest using the same sequence. The patient can lie back when you examine the front of the chest if that's more comfortable for them.

Beauty in symmetry

Note masses or scars that indicate trauma or surgery. Look for chest wall symmetry. Both sides of the chest should be equal at

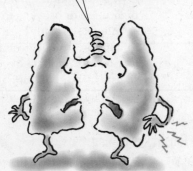

While inspecting the chest, look for characteristics that may put a CRAMP in your patient's respiratory system.

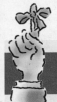

Memory jogger

To help you remember what to check for when inspecting your patient's chest, use the mnemonic **CRAMP**:

- Chest wall asymmetry
- Respiratory rate and pattern (abnormal)
- Accessory muscle use
- Masses or scars
- Paradoxical movement.

rest and expand equally as the patient inhales. The diameter of the chest, from front to back, should be about one-half the width of the chest.

A new angle

Also, look at the angle between the ribs and the sternum at the point immediately above the xiphoid process. This angle—the costal angle—should be less than 90° in an adult. The angle will be larger if the chest wall is chronically expanded because of an enlargement of the intercostal muscles, as can happen with COPD.

Every breath you take

To determine the patient's respiratory rate, count their respirations for a full minute—longer if you note abnormalities. Don't tell them what you're doing or they might alter their natural breathing pattern. One trick is to count respirations while the patient thinks you're taking their pulse or listening to their heart.

Adults normally breathe at a rate of 12 to 20 breaths/min. An infant's breathing rate may reach about 40 breaths/min. The respiratory pattern should be even, coordinated, and regular, with occasional sighs. The ratio of inspiration to expiration (I:E) is about 1:2. Note any periods of apnea, and measure how long they last and how often they occur. (See *Types of breathing*.)

Raising a red flag

Watch for paradoxical, or uneven, movement of the chest wall. Paradoxical movement may appear as an abnormal collapse of part of the chest wall when the patient inhales or an abnormal expansion when the patient exhales. In either case, this uneven movement indicates a loss of normal chest wall function.

Muscles in motion

When the patient inhales, their diaphragm should descend and the intercostal muscles should contract. This dual motion causes the abdomen to push out and the lower ribs to expand laterally. When the patient exhales, their abdomen and ribs return to their resting position. The upper chest shouldn't move much.

Helping more than they should

Accessory muscles may hypertrophy, indicating frequent use. Frequent use of accessory muscles may be normal in some athletes, but for other patients it indicates a respiratory problem, particularly when the patient purses their lips and flares their nostrils when breathing.

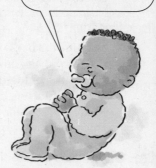

An infant's breathing rate may reach about 40 breaths/minute.

Types of breathing

Male adults, children, and infants usually use abdominal, or diaphragmatic, breathing. Athletes and singers do as well. Most female adults, however, use chest, or intercostal, breathing.

Inspecting related structures

Inspection of the skin, tongue, mouth, fingers, and nail beds also may provide information about respiratory status.

Colorful clues

Skin color varies considerably among patients, but in all cases, patients with a bluish tint to their skin and mucous membranes are considered cyanotic. Cyanosis, which occurs when oxygenation to the tissues is poor, is a late sign of hypoxemia.

Where to look

The most reliable place to check for cyanosis is the tongue and mucous membranes of the mouth. A chilled patient may have cyanotic nail beds, nose, or ears, indicating low blood flow to those areas but not necessarily to major organs.

Join the club

When you check the fingers, look for clubbing, a possible sign of long-term hypoxia. A fingernail normally enters the skin at an angle of less than 180°. When clubbing occurs, the angle is greater than or equal to 180°.

Palpating the chest

Palpation of the chest provides important information about the respiratory system and the processes involved in breathing. (See *Palpating the chest*, page 244.)

Here's what to look for when palpating the chest.

Snap, crackle, pop

The chest wall should feel smooth, warm, and dry. Crepitus indicates subcutaneous air in the chest, an abnormal condition. Crepitus feels like puffed rice cereal crackling under the skin and indicates that air is leaking from the airways or lungs.

If a patient has a chest tube, you may find a small amount of subcutaneous air around the insertion site. If the patient has no chest tube or the area of crepitus is getting larger, alert the doctor immediately.

Tender touch

Gentle palpation shouldn't cause the patient pain. If the patient reports pain during palpation, note the area of the chest wall. Painful costochondral joints are typically located at the midclavicular line or next to the sternum. Rib or vertebral fractures will be quite painful over the fracture, although pain may radiate around the chest as

Peak technique

Palpating the chest

To palpate the chest, place the palm of your hand (or hands) lightly over the thorax, as shown. Palpate for tenderness, alignment, bulging, and retractions of the chest and intercostal spaces. Assess the patient for crepitus. Repeat this procedure on the patient's back.

Next, use the pads of your fingers, as shown, to palpate the front and back of the thorax. Pass your fingers over the ribs and any scars, lumps, lesions, or ulcerations. Note the skin temperature, turgor, and moisture. Also note tenderness and bony or subcutaneous crepitus. The muscles should feel firm and smooth.

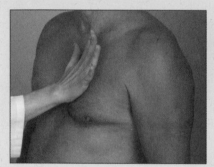

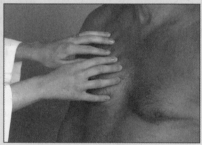

well. Pain may also be caused by sore muscles as a result of protracted coughing. A collapsed lung may also cause pain.

Vibratin' fremitus

Palpate for tactile fremitus, palpable vibrations caused by the transmission of air through the bronchopulmonary system. Fremitus is decreased over areas in which pleural fluid collects, at times when the patient speaks softly, and in those with pneumothorax, atelectasis, or emphysema. Fremitus is increased normally over the large bronchial tubes and abnormally over areas in which alveoli are filled with fluid or exudate, as happens in pneumonia. (See *Checking for tactile fremitus*.)

Equal measure

To evaluate the patient's chest wall symmetry and expansion, place your hands on the front of the chest wall with your thumbs touching each other at the second intercostal space. As the patient inhales deeply, watch your thumbs. They should separate simultaneously and equally to a distance several centimeters away from the sternum.

Repeat the measurement at the fifth intercostal space. The same measurement may be made on the back of the chest near the tenth rib.

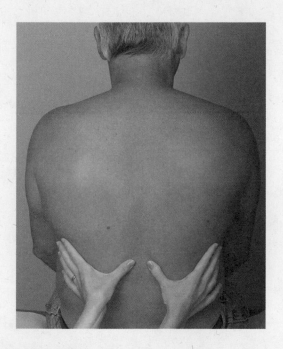

Checking for tactile fremitus

When you check the back of the thorax for tactile fremitus, ask the patient to fold their arms across their chest. This movement shifts the scapulae out of the way.

What to do

Check for tactile fremitus by lightly placing your open palms on both sides of the patient's back, as shown, without touching their back with your fingers. Ask the patient to repeat the phrase "ninety-nine" loud enough to produce palpable vibrations. Then palpate the front of the chest using the same hand positions.

What the results mean

Vibrations that feel more intense on one side than the other indicate tissue consolidation on that side. Less intense vibrations may indicate emphysema, pneumothorax, or pleural effusion. Faint or no vibrations in the upper posterior thorax may indicate bronchial obstruction or a fluid-filled pleural space.

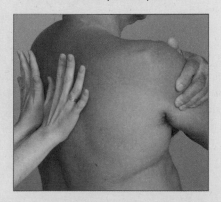

Warning signs

The patient's chest may expand asymmetrically if they have pleural effusion, atelectasis, pneumonia, or pneumothorax. Chest expansion may be decreased at the level of the diaphragm if the patient has emphysema, respiratory depression, diaphragm paralysis, atelectasis, obesity, or ascites.

Percussing the chest

You'll percuss the chest to find the boundaries of the lungs, to determine whether the lungs are filled with air or fluid or solid material, and to evaluate the distance the diaphragm travels between the patient's inhalation and exhalation. (See *Percussing the chest*.)

Different sites, different sounds

Percussion allows you to assess structures as deep as 3″ (7.6 cm). You'll hear different percussion sounds in different areas of the chest. (See *Percussion sounds*.)

Peak technique

Percussing the chest

To percuss the chest, hyperextend the middle finger of your nondominant hand. Place your hand firmly on the patient's chest. Use the tip of the middle finger of your dominant hand to tap on the middle finger of your other hand just below the distal joint (as shown).

The movement should come from the wrist of your dominant hand, not your elbow or upper arm. Keep the fingernail you use for tapping short so you won't hurt yourself. Follow the standard percussion sequence over the front and back chest walls.

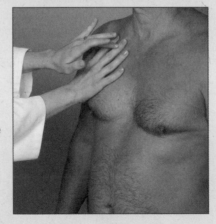

Interpretation station

Percussion sounds

Use this chart to help you become more comfortable with percussion and to interpret percussion sounds quickly. Learn the different percussion sounds by practicing on yourself, your patients, and other people willing to help.

Sound	Sound Description	Clinical significance
Flat	Short, soft, high-pitched, extremely dull, found over the thigh	Consolidation, as in atelectasis and extensive pleural effusion
Dull	Medium in intensity and pitch, moderate length, thudlike, found over the liver	Solid area, as in lobar pneumonia
Resonant	Long, loud, low-pitched, hollow	Normal lung tissue; bronchitis
Hyperresonant	Very loud, low-pitched, found over the stomach	Hyperinflated lung, as in emphysema or pneumothorax
Tympanic	Loud, high-pitched, moderate length, musical, drumlike, found over a puffed-out cheek	Air collection, as in a gastric air bubble, air in the intestines, or a large pneumothorax

Peak technique

Double-check percussion findings

Use other assessment findings to verify the results of respiratory percussion. For example, if you hear low-pitched, loud, booming sounds when you percuss the chest of a patient with chronic obstructive pulmonary disease, an x-ray can be used to confirm emphysema.

Tainted by treatments

You may also hear different sounds after certain treatments. For example, if your patient has atelectasis and you percuss their chest before chest physiotherapy, you'll hear a high-pitched, dull, soft sound. After physiotherapy, you should hear a low-pitched, hollow sound. In all cases, make sure you use other assessment techniques to confirm percussion findings. (See *Double-check percussion findings*.)

Ringing with resonance

You'll hear resonant sounds over normal lung tissue, which you should find over most of the chest. In the left front chest from the third or fourth intercostal space at the sternum to the third or fourth intercostal space at the midclavicular line, you should hear a dull sound. Percussion is dull there because that's the space occupied by the heart. Resonance resumes at the sixth intercostal space. The sequence of sounds in the back is slightly different. (See *Percussion sequences*, page 248.)

Percussion sequences

Follow these percussion sequences to distinguish between normal and abnormal sounds in the patient's lungs. Remember to compare sound variations from one side with the other as you proceed. Carefully describe abnormal sounds you hear and include their locations. You'll follow the same sequences for auscultation.

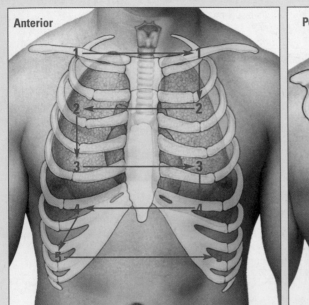

Anterior

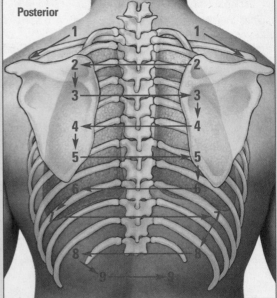

Posterior

Sounds serious

When you hear hyperresonance during percussion, it means you've found an area of increased air in the lung or pleural space. Expect hyperresonance with pneumothorax, acute asthma, bullous emphysema (large holes in the lungs from alveolar destruction), or gastric distention that pushes up on the diaphragm.

When you hear abnormal dullness, it means you've found areas of decreased air in the lungs. Expect abnormal dullness in the presence of pleural fluid, consolidation, atelectasis, or a tumor.

On the move

Percussion also allows you to assess how much the diaphragm moves during inspiration and expiration. The normal diaphragm descends 1¼″ to 2″ (3 to 5 cm) when the patient inhales. The diaphragm doesn't move as far in a patient with emphysema, respiratory depression, diaphragm paralysis, atelectasis, obesity, or ascites. (See *Measuring diaphragm movement*.)

Measuring diaphragm movement

You can measure how much the diaphragm moves by asking the patient to exhale. Percuss the back on one side to locate the upper edge of the diaphragm, the point at which normal lung resonance changes to dullness. Use a pen to mark the spot indicating the position of the diaphragm at full expiration on that side of the back.

Then ask the patient to inhale as deeply as possible. Percuss the back when the patient has breathed in fully until you locate the diaphragm. Use the pen to mark this spot as well. Repeat on the opposite side of the back.

Measure

Use a ruler or tape measure to determine the distance between the marks. The distance, normally 11/4″ to 2″ (3 to 5 cm), should be equal on both the right and left sides.

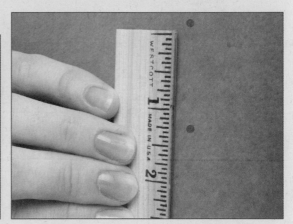

Auscultating the chest

As air moves through the bronchi, it creates sound waves that travel to the chest wall. The sounds produced by breathing change as air moves from larger airways to smaller airways. Sounds also change if they pass through fluid, mucus, or narrowed airways.

Auscultation of these sounds helps you to determine the condition of the alveoli and surrounding pleura. (See *Auscultation sequence.*)

Familiar sites

Auscultation sites are the same as percussion sites. Listen to a full inspiration and a full expiration at each site, using the diaphragm of the stethoscope. Ask the patient to breathe through their mouth; nose breathing alters the pitch of breath sounds. If the patient has abundant chest hair, mat it down with a damp washcloth so the hair doesn't make sounds like crackles.

Auscultation sequence

To distinguish between normal and adventitious breath sounds in the patient's lungs, press the diaphragm of the stethoscope firmly against the skin. Listen to a full inspiration and a full expiration at each site in the sequence shown. Remember to compare sound variations from one side to the other. Document adventitious sounds that you hear and include their locations.

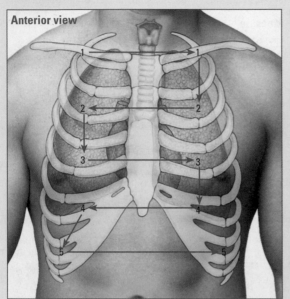

Anterior view

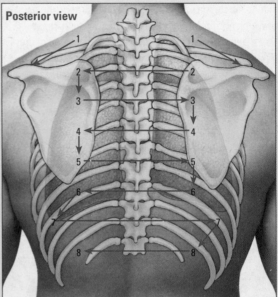

Posterior view

Be firm

To auscultate for breath sounds, you'll press the stethoscope firmly against the skin. Remember that if you listen through clothing or dry chest hair, you may hear unusual and deceptive sounds.

Sounds perfectly normal!

You'll hear four types of breath sounds over normal lungs:
- tracheal (heard when a patient inhales or exhales)
- bronchial (heard loudest when the patient exhales; discontinuous)
- bronchovesicular (heard when the patient inhales or exhales; continuous)
- vesicular (are prolonged during inhalation and shortened during exhalation). (See *Qualities of normal breath sounds.*)

The type of sound you hear depends on where you listen. (See *Locations of normal breath sounds.*)

Qualities of normal breath sounds

Breath sound	Quality	Inspiration expiration (I:E) ratio	Location
Tracheal	Harsh, high-pitched	I = E	Above the supraclavicular notch
Bronchial	Loud, high-pitched	I < E	Just above the clavicles on each side of the sternum, between the scapulae, over the manubrium
Bronchovesicular	Medium in loudness and pitch	I = E	Next to the sternum, between the scapulae
Vesicular	Soft, low-pitched	I > E	Remainder of the lungs

Locations of normal breath sounds

These photographs show the normal locations of different types of breath sounds.

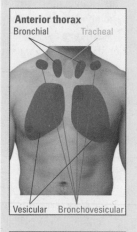

Anterior thorax
Bronchial   Tracheal

Vesicular   Bronchovesicular

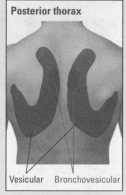

Posterior thorax

Vesicular   Bronchovesicular

In a class by itself

Classify each sound according to its intensity, location, pitch, duration, and characteristic. Note whether the sound occurs when the patient inhales, exhales, or both.

Sounds of silence

If you hear diminished but normal breath sounds in both lungs, the patient may have emphysema, atelectasis, severe bronchospasm, or shallow breathing. If you hear breath sounds in one lung only, the patient may have pleural effusion, pneumothorax, a tumor, or mucus plugs in the airways. In such cases, the doctor may order a chest x-ray and pulmonary function tests (PFTs) to further assess the patient's condition. (See *PFT results.*)

Voicing concerns

Also check the patient for vocal fremitus—voice sounds resulting from chest vibrations that occur as the patient speaks. Abnormal transmission of voice sounds—the most common of which are bronchophony, egophony, and whispered pectoriloquy—may occur over consolidated areas.

Sound check

To test for bronchophony, ask the patient to say "ninety-nine" or "blue moon." Over normal lung tissue, the words sound muffled. Over consolidated areas, the words sound unusually loud. To test for egophony, ask the patient to say "E." Over normal lung tissue, the

PFT result

You may need to interpret results of pulmonary function tests (PFTs) in your assessment of a patient's respiratory status. Use the chart below as a guide to common PFTs.

Restrictive and obstructive

The chart mentions restrictive and obstructive defects. A restrictive defect is one in which a person can't inhale a normal amount of air. It may occur with chest wall deformities, neuromuscular diseases, or acute respiratory tract infections.

An obstructive defect is one in which something obstructs the flow of air into or out of the lungs. It may occur with a disease such as asthma, chronic bronchitis, emphysema, or cystic fibrosis.

Test	Implications
Tidal volume (V_T): amount of air inhaled or exhaled during normal breathing	Decreased V_T may indicate restrictive disease and requires further tests, such as full pulmonary function studies or chest x-rays.
Total lung capacity (TLC): amount of air contained in the lung after maximum inspiration	Decreased TLC may indicate restrictive disease, such as pulmonary fibrosis.
Inspiratory reserve volume (IRV): amount of air inhaled after normal inspiration	Abnormal IRV alone doesn't indicate respiratory dysfunction. IRV decreases during normal exercise.
Expiratory reserve volume (ERV): amount of air that can be exhaled after normal expiration	ERV varies, even in healthy people.
Vital capacity (VC): amount of air that can be exhaled after maximum inspiration	Normal or increased VC with decreased flow rates may indicate reduction in functional pulmonary tissue. Decreased VC with normal or increased flow rates may indicate decreased respiratory effort, decreased thoracic expansion, or limited movement of the diaphragm.
Inspiratory capacity (IC): amount of air that can be inhaled after normal expiration	Decreased IC indicates restrictive disease.
Forced vital capacity (FVC): amount of air that can be exhaled after maximum inspiration	Decreased FVC indicates flow resistance in the respiratory system from obstructive disease, such as chronic bronchitis, emphysema, and asthma.
Forced expiratory volume (FEV): volume of air exhaled in the first second (FEV_1), second second (FEV_2), or third second (FEV_3) of a forced expiratory maneuver	Decreased FEV_1 and increased FEV_2 and FEV_3 may indicate obstructive disease. Decreased or normal FEV_1 may indicate restrictive disease.

sound is muffled. Over consolidated lung tissue, it will sound like the letter *a*. To test for whispered pectoriloquy, ask the patient to whisper "1, 2, 3." Over normal lung tissue, the numbers will be almost indistinguishable. Over consolidated lung tissue, the numbers will be loud and clear. (See *Assessing vocal fremitus*.)

Assessing vocal fremitus

To assess for vocal fremitus, ask the patient to repeat the words below while you listen. Auscultate over an area where you heard abnormally located bronchial breath sounds to check for abnormal voice sounds.

"Ninety-nine" Bronchophony	"E" Egophony	"1, 2, 3" Whispered pectoriloquy
• Ask the patient to say "ninety-nine." • Over normal lung tissue, the words sound muffled. • Over consolidated areas, the words sound unusually loud.	• Ask the patient to say "E." • Over normal lung tissue, the sound is muffled. • Over consolidated lung tissue, it will sound like the letter *A*.	• Ask the patient to whisper "1, 2, 3." • Over normal lung tissue, the numbers will be almost indistinguishable. • Over consolidated lung tissue, the numbers will be loud and clear.

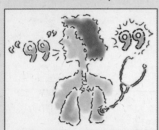 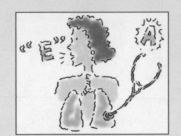 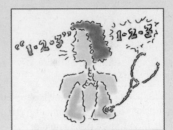

The next step

A patient with abnormal findings during a respiratory assessment may be further evaluated using such diagnostic tests as a chest x-ray, arterial blood gas analysis, and PFTs.

Abnormal findings

Your assessment of the chest may reveal several abnormalities of the chest wall and lungs. In this section, we'll look at chest wall abnormalities, abnormal respiratory patterns, and abnormal breath sounds. (See *Respiratory abnormalities*.)

Chest wall abnormalities

Chest wall abnormalities may be congenital or acquired. As you examine a patient for chest wall abnormalities, keep in mind that a patient with a deformity of the chest wall might have completely normal lungs and that the lungs might be cramped within the chest. The patient might have a smaller-than-normal lung capacity

Interpretation station

Respiratory abnormalities

The chart below shows commonly reported respiratory signs and symptoms, their accompanying signs and symptoms, and their probable causes.

Sign or symptom and findings	Probable cause
Cough	
• Nonproductive cough • Pleuritic chest pain • Dyspnea • Tachypnea • Anxiety • Decreased vocal fremitus • Tracheal deviation toward the affected side	Atelectasis
• Productive cough with small amounts of purulent (or mucopurulent), blood-streaked sputum or large amounts of frothy sputum • Dyspnea • Anorexia • Fatigue • Weight loss • Wheezing • Clubbing	Lung cancer
• Nonproductive cough • Dyspnea • Pleuritic chest pain • Decreased chest motion • Pleural friction rub • Tachypnea • Tachycardia • Flatness on percussion • Egophony	Pleural effusion
Dyspnea	
• Acute dyspnea • Tachypnea • Crackles and rhonchi in both lung fields • Intercostal and suprasternal retractions • Restlessness • Anxiety • Tachycardia	Acute respiratory distress syndrome

Sign or symptom and findings	Probable cause
• Progressive exertional dyspnea • A history of smoking • Barrel chest • Accessory muscle hypertrophy • Diminished breath sounds • Pursed lip breathing • Prolonged expiration • Anorexia • Weight loss	Emphysema
• Acute dyspnea • Tachypnea • Anxiety or restlessness • Pleuritic chest pain • Tachycardia • Decreased breath sounds • Low-grade fever • Dullness on percussion • Cool, clammy skin	Pulmonary embolism
Hemoptysis	
• Sputum ranging in color from pink to dark brown • Productive cough • Dyspnea • Chest pain • Crackles on auscultation • Chills • Fever	Pneumonia
• Frothy, blood-tinged, pink sputum • Severe dyspnea • Orthopnea • Gasping • Diffuse crackles • Cold, clammy skin • Anxiety	Pulmonary edema
• Blood-streaked or blood-tinged sputum • Chronic productive cough	Pulmonary tuberculosis

(Continued)

Respiratory abnormalities *(continued)*

Sign or symptom and findings	Probable cause
Hemoptysis (continued)	
• Fine crackles after coughing • Dyspnea • Dullness on percussion • Increased tactile fremitus	
Wheezing	
• Sudden onset of wheezing • Stridor • Dry, paroxysmal cough • Gagging • Hoarseness • Decreased breath sounds • Dyspnea • Cyanosis	Aspiration of a foreign body
• Audible wheezing on expiration • Prolonged expiration	Asthma

Sign or symptom and findings	Probable cause
Wheezing (continued)	
• Apprehension • Intercostal and supraclavicular retractions • Rhonchi • Nasal flaring • Tachypnea	
• Wheezing • Coarse crackles • Hacking cough that later becomes productive • Dyspnea • Barrel chest • Clubbing • Edema • Weight gain	Chronic bronchitis

and limited exercise tolerance, and they may more easily develop respiratory failure from a respiratory tract infection. (See *Chest deformities*, page 256.)

Paradoxical movement

Paradoxical (uneven) movement of the chest wall is abnormal. It can occur as a result of chest wall injury, such as multiple rib fractures or blunt force trauma to the chest. With spontaneous breathing, paradoxical movement occurs on the injured chest side, which collapses during inspiration and expands during exhalation.

Barrel chest

A barrel chest looks like its name implies: The chest is abnormally round and bulging, with a greater-than-normal front-to-back diameter. Barrel chest may be normal in infants and older adult patients. In other patients, barrel chest occurs as a result of COPD.

Chest deformities

As you inspect the patient's chest, note deviations in size and shape. The illustrations here show a normal adult chest and four common chest deformities.

Normal adult chest	*Barrel chest*	*Funnel chest*	*Pigeon chest*	*Thoracic kyphoscoliosis*

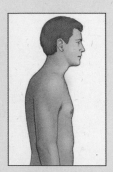 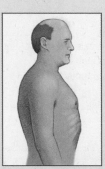 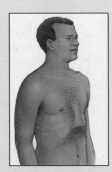 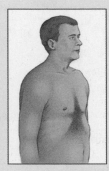 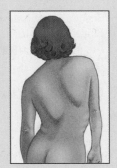

| | Increased anteroposterior diameter | Depressed lower sternum | Anteriorly displaced sternum | Raised shoulder and scapula, thoracic convexity, and flared interspaces |

Calling for backup

In patients with COPD, barrel chest indicates that the lungs have lost their elasticity and that the diaphragm is flattened. You'll note that this patient typically uses accessory muscles when they inhale and easily becomes breathless. You'll also note kyphosis of the thoracic spine, ribs that run horizontally rather than tangentially, and a prominent sternal angle.

Pigeon chest

A patient with pigeon chest, or pectus carinatum, has a chest with a sternum that protrudes beyond the front of the abdomen. The displaced sternum increases the front-to-back diameter of the chest. This congenital defect is commonly associated with scoliosis.

Funnel chest

A patient with funnel chest, or pectus excavatum, has a funnel-shaped depression on all or part of the sternum. The shape of the chest may interfere with respiratory and cardiac function. Compression of the heart and great vessels may cause murmurs.

Thoracic kyphoscoliosis

In thoracic kyphoscoliosis, the patient's spine curves to one side and the vertebrae are rotated. Because the rotation distorts lung tissues, it may be more difficult to assess respiratory status. This is usually a congenital defect.

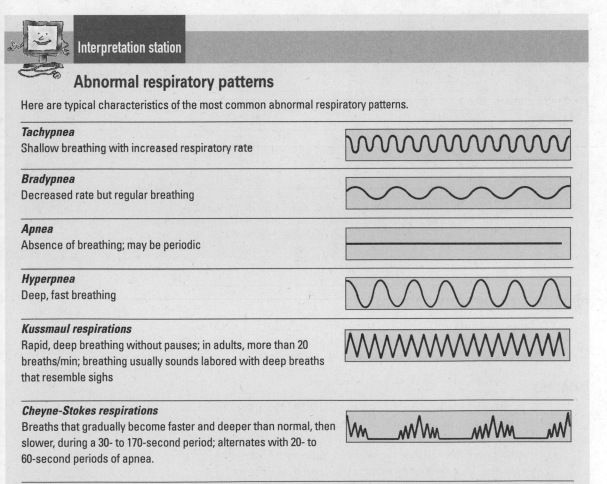

Interpretation station

Abnormal respiratory patterns

Here are typical characteristics of the most common abnormal respiratory patterns.

Tachypnea
Shallow breathing with increased respiratory rate

Bradypnea
Decreased rate but regular breathing

Apnea
Absence of breathing; may be periodic

Hyperpnea
Deep, fast breathing

Kussmaul respirations
Rapid, deep breathing without pauses; in adults, more than 20 breaths/min; breathing usually sounds labored with deep breaths that resemble sighs

Cheyne-Stokes respirations
Breaths that gradually become faster and deeper than normal, then slower, during a 30- to 170-second period; alternates with 20- to 60-second periods of apnea.

Biot respirations
Rapid, deep breathing with abrupt pauses between each breath; equal depth to each breath

Respiratory rate in children and adolescents

Use the table below as a quick reference for lower limit, normal range, and upper limit respiratory rates for patients ages 0 months to 18 years.

Age	Respiratory rate (breaths/minute)		
	Lower limit (1st percentile)	Normal range (10th to 90th percentile)	Upper limit (99th percentile)
0–3 months	25	34–57	66
3 to <6 months	24	33–55	64
6 to <9 months	23	31–52	61
9 to <12 months	22	30–50	58
12 to <18 months	21	28–46	53
18 to <24 months	19	25–40	46
2 to <3 years	18	22–34	38
3 to <4 years	17	21–29	33
4 to <6 years	17	20–27	29
6 to <8 years	16	18–24	27
8 to <12 years	14	16–22	25
12 to <15 years	12	15–21	23
15–18 years	11	13–19	22

Data from Fleming, S., Thompson, M., Stevens, R., Heneghan, C., Pluddemann, A., Maconochie, I., Tarassenko, L., & Mant, D. (2011). Normal ranges of heart rate and respiratory rate in children from birth to 18 years of age: A systematic review of observational studies. *The Lancet, 377*(9770), 1011–1018. https://doi.org/10.1016/S0140-6736(10)62226-X

Abnormal respiratory patterns

Identifying abnormal respiratory patterns can help you assess more completely a patient's respiratory status and their overall condition. (See *Abnormal respiratory patterns*.)

Tachypnea

Tachypnea is a respiratory rate greater than 20 breaths/min with shallow breathing. It's commonly seen in patients with restrictive lung disease, pain, sepsis, obesity, and anxiety. Babies and young children breathe faster than adults, so you need to know normal rates for all age groups. (See *Respiratory rate in children and adolescents*.)

Hot and bothered

Fever may be another cause of tachypnea. The respiratory rate may increase by 4 breaths/minute for every 1° F (0.6° C) rise in body temperature.

Bradypnea

Bradypnea is a respiratory rate below 10 breaths/minute and is typically noted just before a period of apnea or full respiratory arrest.

Feeling depressed
Patients with bradypnea might have CNS depression as a result of excessive sedation, tissue damage, or diabetic coma, which all depress the brain's respiratory control center. (The respiratory rate normally decreases during sleep.)

Apnea

Apnea is the absence of breathing. Periods of apnea may be short and occur sporadically during Cheyne-Stokes respirations, Biot respirations, or other abnormal respiratory patterns. This condition may be life-threatening if periods of apnea are prolonged. (See *Snoring and sleep apnea*.)

Hyperpnea

Characterized by deep, rapid breathing, hyperpnea occurs in patients after strenuous exercise or in those who have anxiety, pain, lung disease such as asthma and COPD, or metabolic acidosis. In a comatose patient, hyperpnea may indicate hypoxia or hypoglycemia.

Kussmaul respirations

Kussmaul respirations are rapid, deep, sighing breaths that occur in patients with metabolic acidosis, especially when associated with diabetic ketoacidosis.

Cheyne–Stokes respirations

Cheyne-Stokes respirations are deep breaths that alternate with short periods of apnea. They have a regular pattern of variations in the rate and depth of breathing. This respiratory pattern occurs in patients with heart failure, kidney failure, or CNS damage. The presence of

Handle with care

Snoring and sleep apnea

If an overweight patient reports a history of snoring, make a note to observe them during sleep. Snoring and obesity are both associated with obstructive sleep apnea, a condition that causes a chronic decrease in oxygen saturation and can eventually affect overall health. It can also affect daytime function. For instance, children who snore and have sleep apnea may feel sleepy during the day and perform poorly in school. More than 50% of the 12 million people affected with sleep apnea are overweight, and most snore heavily.

Cheyne-Stokes respiration can be an indication of worsening and can indicate possible impending death. However, Cheyne-Stokes respirations may be normal during sleep in children and older patients.

Biot respirations

Biot respirations involve rapid, deep breaths that alternate with abrupt periods of apnea. Biot respirations are an ominous sign of severe CNS damage.

Abnormal breath sounds

If you hear a sound in an area other than where you would expect to hear it when auscultating the lungs, consider the sound abnormal. For example, if you hear bronchial or bronchovesicular breath sounds in an area where you would normally hear vesicular breath sounds, then the alveoli and small bronchioles in that area might be filled with fluid or exudate, as occurs in pneumonia and atelectasis. You won't hear vesicular sounds in those areas because no air is moving through the small airways.

Keep in mind that solid tissue transmits sound better than air or fluid. Therefore, breath sounds (as well as spoken or whispered words) will be louder than normal over areas of consolidation.

On the other hand, if pus, fluid, or air fills the pleural space, breath sounds will be quieter than normal. If a foreign body or secretions obstruct a bronchus, breath sounds will be diminished or absent over lung tissue located distal to the obstruction.

Taking advantage of the situation

Other breath sounds, called *adventitious sounds,* are abnormal no matter where you hear them in the lungs. Those sounds include fine and coarse crackles (rales), wheezes, rhonchi, stridor, and pleural friction rub.

Crackles

Crackles are intermittent, nonmusical, brief crackling sounds that are caused by collapsed or fluid-filled alveoli popping open. Heard primarily when the patient inhales, crackles are classified as either fine or coarse and usually don't clear with coughing. If crackles do clear with coughing, secretions most likely caused them. (See *Types of crackles*.)

Wheezes

Wheezes are high-pitched sounds heard first when a patient exhales. (See *When wheezing stops*.) The sounds occur when airflow is blocked. As severity of the block increases, wheezes may also be heard when the patient inhales. The sound of a wheeze doesn't change with coughing. Patients may wheeze as a result of asthma, infection, heart failure, or airway obstruction from a tumor or foreign body. (See *Signs and symptoms of upper airway obstruction*.)

Types of crackles

Here's how to differentiate fine crackles from coarse crackles, a critical distinction when assessing the lungs.

Fine crackles
These characteristics distinguish fine crackles:
- occur when the patient stops inhaling
- are usually heard in lung bases
- sound like a piece of hair being rubbed between the fingers or like Velcro being pulled apart
- are unaffected by coughing
- occur in restrictive diseases, such as pulmonary fibrosis, asbestosis, silicosis, atelectasis, heart failure, and pneumonia.

Coarse crackles
These characteristics distinguish coarse crackles:
- occur when the patient starts to inhale; may be present when the patient exhales
- may be heard through the lungs and even at the mouth
- sound more like bubbling or gurgling, as air moves through secretions in larger airways
- usually clear or diminish after coughing
- in chronic obstructive pulmonary disease, bronchiectasis, and pulmonary edema and in severely ill patients who can't cough; also called the "death rattle."

When wheezing stops

If you no longer hear wheezing in a patient having an acute asthma attack, the attack may be far from over. When bronchospasm and mucosal swelling become severe, little air can move through the airways. As a result, you won't hear wheezing.

If all other assessment criteria—labored breathing, prolonged expiratory time, and accessory muscle use—point to acute bronchial obstruction, act to maintain the patient's airway and give oxygen as ordered. The patient may begin to wheeze again when the airways open.

Signs and symptoms of upper airway obstruction

If a patient can't maintain a patent airway, they may end up in respiratory arrest. Refer to this list of potential signs and symptoms when assessing a patient for partial or complete airway obstruction:
- anxiety
- dyspnea
- stridor
- wheezing
- decreased or absent breath sounds
- use of accessory muscles
- seesaw movement between chest and abdomen
- inability to speak (complete obstruction)
- cyanosis.

Rhonchi

Rhonchi are low-pitched, snoring, rattling sounds that occur primarily during exhalation, although they may also be heard on inhalation. Rhonchi usually change or disappear with coughing. The sounds occur when fluid partially blocks the large airways.

Stridor

Stridor is a loud, high-pitched, turbulent sound that's heard, usually without a stethoscope, during inspiration or exhalation. Stridor, which is caused by an obstruction in the upper airway, requires immediate attention.

Pleural friction rub

Pleural friction rub is a low-pitched, grating, rubbing sound heard when the patient inhales and exhales. Pleural inflammation causes the two layers of pleura to rub together. The patient may report pain in areas where the rub is heard. (See *Discontinuous and continuous adventitious breath sounds* and *Auscultation findings for common disorders*.)

Discontinuous and continuous adventitious breath sounds

The characteristics of some discontinuous and continuous adventitious breath sounds are compared in the chart below. Note the timing of each sound during inspiration and expiration on the corresponding graphs.

Sound		Characteristics
Discontinuous sounds		
Fine crackles	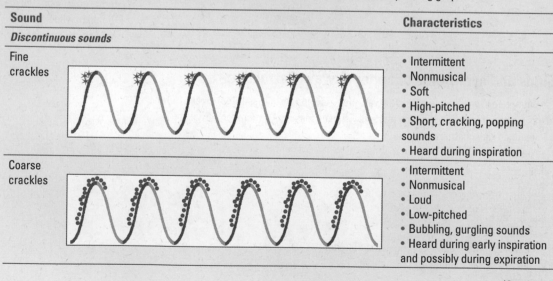	• Intermittent • Nonmusical • Soft • High-pitched • Short, cracking, popping sounds • Heard during inspiration
Coarse crackles		• Intermittent • Nonmusical • Loud • Low-pitched • Bubbling, gurgling sounds • Heard during early inspiration and possibly during expiration

(Continued)

Discontinuous and continuous adventitious breath sounds *(continued)*

Sound	Characteristics
Continuous sounds	
Wheezes 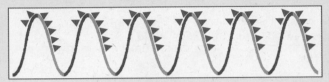	• Musical • High-pitched • Squeaky, whistling sounds • Predominantly heard during expiration but may also occur during inspiration
Rhonchi	• Musical • Low-pitched • Snoring, moaning sounds • Heard during both inspiration and expiration but are more prominent during expiration

Auscultation findings for common disorders

Disorder	Auscultation findings
Asbestosis	• Bronchial breath sounds in both lung bases • High-pitched crackles heard at the end of inspiration • Pleural friction rub
Asthma	• Diminished breath sounds • Musical, high-pitched expiratory polyphonic wheezes • With status asthmaticus, loud and continuous random monophonic wheezes, along with prolonged expiration and possible silent chest if severe
Atelectasis	• High-pitched, hollow, tubular bronchial breath sounds, crackles, and wheezes • Fine, high-pitched, late inspiratory crackles • Bronchophony, egophony, and whispered pectoriloquy when right upper lobe is affected
Bronchiectasis	• Profuse, low-pitched crackles heard during mid inspiration
Chronic obstructive pulmonary disease (COPD)	• Diminished, low-pitched breath sounds • Sonorous or sibilant wheezes • Inaudible bronchophony, egophony, and whispered pectoriloquy • Prolonged expiration • Fine inspiratory crackles
Pleural effusion	• Absent or diminished low-pitched breath sounds • Occasionally loud bronchial breath sounds • Normal breath sounds on contralateral side • Bronchophony, egophony, and whispered pectoriloquy at upper border of pleural effusion

(Continued)

Auscultation findings for common disorders *(continued)*

Disorder	Auscultation findings
Pneumonia	• High-pitched, tubular bronchial breath sounds over affected area during inspiration and expiration • Bronchophony, egophony, and whispered pectoriloquy • Late inspiratory crackles not affected by coughing or position changes
Pneumothorax	• Absent or diminished low-pitched breath sounds • Inaudible bronchophony, egophony, and whispered pectoriloquy • Normal breath sounds on contralateral side
Upper airway obstruction	• Stridor • Decreased or absent breath sounds • Wheezing

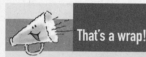

That's a wrap!

Respiratory system review

Anatomy and physiology
Upper airways
• Include the nasopharynx, oropharynx, laryngopharynx, and larynx
• Warm, filter, and humidify inhaled air
• Help to make sound and send air to lower airways

Lower airways
• Trachea—divides into the right and left mainstem bronchi and continues to divide into smaller passages
• Bronchioles—terminate in the alveolar ducts and the alveoli
• Alveoli—gas-exchanging units of the lungs

Thorax
• Includes the clavicles, sternum, scapulae, 12 sets of ribs (which protect the chest and allow it to expand and contract during each breath), and 12 thoracic vertebrae

Respiratory muscles
• Diaphragm and external intercostal muscles (primary breathing muscles)—contract on inhalation and relax on exhalation
• Accessory inspiratory muscles (trapezius, sternocleidomastoid, and scalenes)—combine to elevate the scapulae, clavicles, sternum, and upper ribs when primary breathing muscles aren't effective

Health history
• Ask the patient about shortness of breath, and rate their dyspnea on a scale of 0 to 10.
• Determine if the patient has orthopnea, and ask how many pillows they use to sleep at night.
• Ask if the patient has a cough. If they do, ask them whether it's productive or nonproductive. If it's productive, have them describe the sputum.

• Have the patient describe any chest pain, including its location, how it feels, if it radiates, what brings it on, and what makes it better or worse.
• Ask about the patient's medical history, including smoking, pneumonia, and exposure to irritants.

Assessment
Inspection
• Watch for chest wall symmetry as the patient breathes. Note any paradoxical, or uneven, chest wall movement.
• Count the patient's respiratory rate for a full minute (longer if you note abnormalities) and note periods of apnea; normal respiratory rate for an adult is 12 to 20 breaths/min; for infants, up to 40 breaths/min.
• Observe the patient's respiratory pattern; it should be even, coordinated, and regular with occasional sighs.

(Continued)

Respiratory system review *(continued)*

• Inspect the skin, tongue, mouth, fingers, and nail beds, which can provide more information about the patient's respiratory status.

Palpation

• Gently use your palms to palpate the chest for crepitus, tenderness, alignment, bulging, or retractions. Palpate the front and back of the chest.
• Use the pads of your fingers to palpate the chest, including over the ribs. Note skin temperature, turgor, and moisture as well as the presence of scars, lumps, lesions, or ulcerations.
• Palpate for tactile fremitus.
• Assess chest wall symmetry and expansion by placing your hands on the front of the chest with thumbs touching each other, and ask the patient to inhale deeply.

Percussion

• Resonant sounds are heard over normal lung tissue.
• Hyperresonance is found over areas of increased air in the lung or pleural space (hyperinflated lung, emphysema).
• Dullness is found over areas of decreased air in the lungs (atelectasis, pneumonia).
• Flatness is found over consolidated areas (atelectasis, pleural effusion).
• Tympany is found over areas in which air has collected (large pneumothorax).

Auscultation

• Use the diaphragm of the stethoscope to listen to a full inspiration and a full expiration at each site.
• Ask the patient to breathe through their mouth. (Nose breathing alters the pitch of breath sounds.)
• Wet chest hair to prevent crackles that would be heard if auscultating over dry hair.

Normal Breath Sounds

• Tracheal—harsh, high-pitched, and discontinuous
• Bronchial—loud, high-pitched, and discontinuous
• Bronchovesicular—medium-pitched and continuous
• Vesicular—soft and low-pitched

Vocal Fremitus

• Bronchophony—ask the patient to say "ninety-nine"
• Egophony—ask the patient to say "E"
• Whispered pectoriloquy—ask the patient to whisper "1, 2, 3"

Abnormal findings
Chest wall abnormalities

• Barrel chest—large front-to-back diameter
• Pigeon chest—sternum protrudes beyond front of abdomen; increased front-to-back diameter of chest
• Funnel chest—depression on all or part of the sternum
• Thoracic kyphoscoliosis—curvature of spine; rotation of vertebrae; distortion of lung tissues

Abnormal respiratory patterns

• Tachypnea—respiratory rate greater than 20 breaths/min with shallow breathing
• Bradypnea—respiratory rate below 10 breaths/min
• Apnea—the absence of breathing; may be life-threatening if it's prolonged
• Hyperpnea—deep, rapid breathing
• Kussmaul respirations—rapid, deep, sighing breaths
• Cheyne-Stokes respirations—deep breaths alternating with periods of apnea
• Biot respirations—rapid, deep breaths that alternate with abrupt apneic periods

Abnormal breath sounds

• Crackles—intermittent, nonmusical, crackling sounds heard during inspiration; classified as fine or coarse
• Wheezes—high-pitched sounds caused by blocked airflow; heard on exhalation
• Rhonchi—low-pitched snoring or rattling sound; heard primarily on exhalation
• Stridor—loud, high-pitched sound heard during inspiration
• Pleural friction rub—low-pitched grating sound heard during inspiration and expiration; accompanied by pain

Quick quiz

1. In a patient with COPD, a barrel chest indicates:
    A. loss of lung elasticity.
    B. rotation of the spinal column.
    C. increased elasticity of the intercostal muscles.
    D. accessory muscle use.

Answer: A. Barrel chest in patients with COPD is an indication of the loss of elasticity of the lungs and a flattening of the diaphragm.

2. The percussion sound usually heard over most of the lungs is:
    A. dullness.
    B. resonance.
    C. hyperresonance.
    D. tympany.

Answer: B. The lungs, made up of tissue and air, make a resonant percussion sound. Solid tissue is flat or dull; air-filled spaces are hyperresonant or tympanic.

3. When you auscultate the lower lobes of a healthy patient's lungs, you would expect to hear:
    A. tracheal breath sounds.
    B. bronchial breath sounds.
    C. vesicular breath sounds.
    D. bronchovesicular sounds.

Answer: C. Vesicular breath sounds are soft, low-pitched, and prolonged during inspiration and can be heard over the lower lobes.

4. When you're evaluating a patient's breathing, you should note:
    A. respiratory rate and pattern.
    B. swelling of the feet.
    C. hoarseness.
    D. chest pain.

Answer: A. When evaluating a patient's breathing, you should determine their respiratory rate and the pattern of their breathing, noting slow or rapid breaths, dyspnea, shallow breathing, and periods of apnea. Although swelling of the feet, hoarseness, and chest pain may be linked to a respiratory problem, they should be evaluated during a full assessment.

5. When assessing your patient's lungs for egophony, you ask them to say "E," but it sounds like the letter "A." This finding may indicate which condition?
    A. Normal lung tissue
    B. Fluid in the lung
    C. Lung consolidation
    D. Collapsed lung

Answer: C. When testing for egophony, the spoken letter *E* should sound muffled, indicating normal lung tissue. Over consolidated lung tissue, it will sound like the letter *A*.

Scoring

☆☆☆ If you answered all five questions correctly, excellent! You've left us breathless with your expertise.

☆☆ If you answered four questions correctly, hoorah! You're our resident respiratory guru.

☆ If you answered fewer than four questions correctly, that's okay! Rereading the chapter is sure to expand your knowledge on the subject.

 Just for fun

Take a long, deep breath before tackling this test. Match the pulmonary function test in column 1 with its corresponding definition in column 2.

Pulmonary function test

1. Vital capacity _____

2. Minute volume _____

3. Tidal volume _____

4. Expiratory reserve volume _____

5. Inspiratory reserve volume _____

6. Inspiratory capacity _____

Definitions

A. Amount of air breathed per minute

B. Amount of air that can be inhaled after normal expiration

C. Amount of air inhaled or exhaled during normal breathing

D. Amount of air that can be exhaled after maximum inspiration

E. Amount of air that can be exhaled after normal expiration

F. Amount of air inhaled after normal inspiration

Answer: 1. D, 2. A, 3. C, 4. E, 5. F, 6. B

Chapter 11

Breasts and axillae

Just the facts

In this chapter, you'll learn:

- ◆ structures that make up the breasts
- ◆ breast changes that occur with age, pregnancy, and other conditions
- ◆ the proper way to obtain a patient history about breasts
- ◆ techniques for performing a physical assessment of the breasts and axillae
- ◆ causes of breast and axillae abnormalities and how to recognize them.

*In this chapter: Female = assigned female at birth.
Male = assigned male at birth.

A look at the breasts and axillae

With breast cancer becoming increasingly prominent in the news and on social media, more people are aware of the disease's risk factors, treatments, and diagnostic measures. By staying informed, getting regular mammograms, and performing breast self-examinations, patients can take control of their health and seek medical care when they notice a change in their breasts.

A delicate matter

No matter how informed a person is, they can still feel anxious during breast examinations, even if they haven't noticed a problem. That's because the social and psychological significance of female breasts goes far beyond their biological function. The breast is more than just a delicate structure; it's a delicate subject. Keep this in mind during your assessment. It will let you proceed carefully and professionally, helping your patient feel more at ease.

Anatomy and physiology

The breasts, also called *mammary glands* in female patients, lie on the anterior chest wall. (See *A close look at the female breast.*) They're located vertically between the second or third and the sixth or seventh ribs over the pectoralis major muscle and the serratus anterior muscle, and horizontally between the sternal border and the midaxillary line.

A close look at the female breast

This illustration shows the anatomy of the female breast.

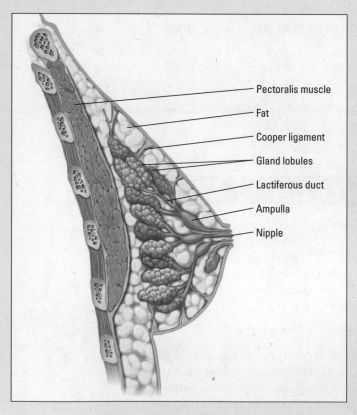

- Pectoralis muscle
- Fat
- Cooper ligament
- Gland lobules
- Lactiferous duct
- Ampulla
- Nipple

Breast structures

Each breast has a centrally located nipple of pigmented erectile tissue ringed by an areola that's darker than the adjacent tissue. (See *Differences in areola pigmentation.*) Montgomery glands (or *tubercles*) are sebaceous glands scattered on the areolar surface, along with hair follicles. These glands secrete a protective lipid material during lactation.

Support structures

Beneath the skin are glandular, fibrous, and fatty tissues that vary with age, weight, sex, heredity, and other factors such as pregnancy. A small triangle of tissue, called the *tail of Spence,* projects into the axilla. Attached to the chest wall musculature are fibrous bands, called *Cooper ligaments,* that support each breast.

Lobes and ducts

In female adults, each breast is surrounded by 12 to 25 glandular lobes containing alveoli that produce milk. The lactiferous ducts from each lobe transport milk to the nipple. In male adults, the breast has a nipple, an areola, and mostly flat tissue bordering the chest wall.

Lymph nodes

The breasts also hold several lymph node chains, each serving different areas. The pectoral lymph nodes drain lymph fluid from most of the breast and anterior chest. The brachial nodes drain most of the arm. The subscapular nodes drain the posterior chest wall and part of the arm. The midaxillary nodes, located near the ribs and the serratus anterior muscle high in the axilla, are the central draining nodes for the pectoral, brachial, and subscapular nodes.

Female focus

In female breasts, the internal mammary nodes drain the mammary lobes. The superficial lymphatic vessels drain the skin.

Cancer connection

In all patients, the lymphatic system is the most common route of spread of cells that cause breast cancer. (See *A close look at the lymph nodes,* page 256.)

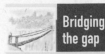

Bridging the gap

Differences in areola pigmentation

The pigment of the nipple and areola varies among people of different skin tones, getting darker as skin tone darkens. People with light skin have light-colored nipples and areolae, usually pink or light beige. People with darker complexions, such as people of African or Asian descent, have medium brown to almost black nipples and areolae.

How the breasts change with age

Female breasts make many transformations throughout the life cycle. Their appearance starts changing at puberty and continues changing

A close look at the lymph nodes

This illustration shows the different lymph nodes in the breast, axilla, and upper arm.

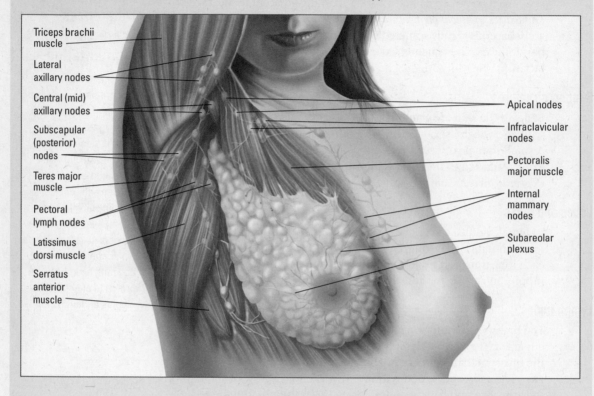

Triceps brachii muscle

Lateral axillary nodes

Central (mid) axillary nodes

Subscapular (posterior) nodes

Teres major muscle

Pectoral lymph nodes

Latissimus dorsi muscle

Serratus anterior muscle

Apical nodes

Infraclavicular nodes

Pectoralis major muscle

Internal mammary nodes

Subareolar plexus

during the reproductive years, pregnancy, and menopause. (See *Breast changes throughout life*.)

Changes during puberty

Breast development is an early sign of puberty in female children. It usually occurs between ages 8 and 13. Menarche, the start of the menstrual cycle, typically occurs about 2 years later. Development of breast tissue in a female child younger than age 10 requires a referral to a healthcare provider.

In the beginning…

Breast development usually starts with the breast and nipple protruding as a single mound of flesh, commonly called the breast

Breast changes throughout life

These illustrations show how female breasts typically change from before puberty through menopause.

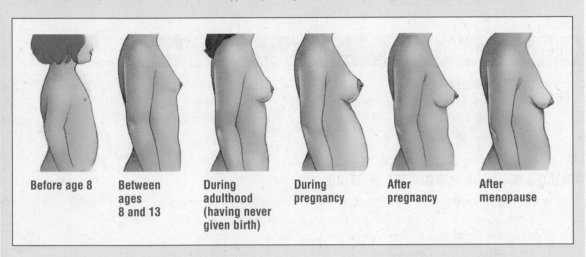

| Before age 8 | Between ages 8 and 13 | During adulthood (having never given birth) | During pregnancy | After pregnancy | After menopause |

bud stage. The shape of the adult female breast is formed gradually. During puberty, breast development is commonly unilateral or asymmetrical.

Changes during the reproductive years

During the reproductive years, female breasts may become full or tender in response to hormonal fluctuations during the menstrual cycle.

Altered state

During pregnancy and lactation, breast changes occur in response to hormones from the corpus luteum, the placenta, and the pituitary gland. The areola becomes deeply pigmented and increases in diameter. The nipple becomes darker, more prominent, and erect. The breasts enlarge because of the proliferation and hypertrophy of the alveolar cells and lactiferous ducts. As veins engorge, a venous pattern may become visible. In addition, striae may appear as a result of stretching, and Montgomery tubercles may become prominent.

Changes after menopause

After menopause, estrogen levels decrease, causing glandular tissue to atrophy and be replaced with fatty deposits. The breasts become less dense and smaller than they were before menopause. As the ligaments relax, the breasts hang loosely from the chest. The nipples flatten, losing some of their erectile quality. The ducts around the nipples may feel like firm strings.

Obtaining a health history

You'll typically begin your health history by asking the patient about their reason for seeking care. You'll then want to ask the patient questions about their personal and family medical history as well as their current health.

Asking about the reason for seeking care

Common presenting problems about the breasts include breast pain, nipple discharge and rash, lumps, masses, and other changes. Signs and symptoms such as these—whether they come from female or male patients—warrant further investigation. (See *Male concerns* and *Evaluating a breast lump*.)

Handle with care

Male concerns

Keep in mind that male patients also need breast examinations and that the incidence of breast cancer in males is rising. Some men with breast disorders may feel uneasy or embarrassed about being examined because they see their condition as being "unmanly." Remember that a male patient needs a gentle, professional hand as much as a female patient does.

Male breast cancer and gynecomastia

Be sure to examine a male patient's breasts thoroughly during a complete physical assessment. Don't overlook palpation of the nipple and areola in male patients; assess for the same changes you would in a female patient. Breast cancer in males usually occurs in the areolar area.

Gynecomastia is abnormal enlargement of the male breast. It may be a benign finding, or it may be caused by medications (especially digoxin and spironolactone), cirrhosis, malnutrition, neoplasms, illicit drug use, alcohol consumption, or a hormonal imbalance.

Breasts in younger and older male patients

Adolescent males may have temporary stimulation of breast tissue caused by the hormone estrogen, which is produced in males and females. Breast enlargement in male children usually stops when they begin producing adequate amounts of the male sex hormone testosterone during puberty. Older males may experience gynecomastia as a result of age-related hormonal alterations or an adverse effect of certain medications.

Evaluating a breast lump

If you find a breast lump during your assessment, note the following characteristics. All breast lumps should be further evaluated with a mammography, ultrasound, fine needle aspiration, or core biopsy.

Characteristics	Benign	Malignant
Appearance	Breast shows no change	Breast is dimpled, scaly, or puckered, with an orange peel appearance or accentuated veins
Consistency	Lump is firm to soft	Lump is firm and hard
Delineation	Lump is well defined	Lump is poorly defined
Mobility	Lump is easy to move	Lump is fixed in breast tissue
Tenderness	Breast is usually nontender but may be tender before menstruation	Breast may be nontender or tender, based on advancement of cancer
Nipple changes	Nipple shows no changes	Nipple may be inverted, retracted, or itchy with bloody, yellow, green, or clear discharge
Number	Single or multiple lumps may be in one or both breasts	Usually a single lump
Location	Lump may occur anywhere in breast	Lump may occur anywhere in breast, but more commonly occurs in upper outer quadrant

Dig deeper

To investigate these signs and symptoms, ask about the onset, duration, and severity. What day of the menstrual cycle do the signs or symptoms appear, if applicable? What relieves or worsens them?

Asking about medical history

Ask the patient if they have ever had breast lumps, a biopsy, or breast surgery, including enlargement or reduction. Also ask if they have a history of breast disease or trauma. If they have had breast cancer, fibroadenoma, or fibrocystic disease, ask for more information, such as whether they underwent surgery, chemotherapy, or radiation treatment.

Periods and pregnancies

Inquire about the patient's menstrual cycle, including what age it started, and record the date of their last menses. If the patient has been pregnant, ask how many pregnancies and live births they have had. How old were they at each pregnancy? Were there complications? Did the patient breastfeed?

All in the family

Ask the patient if any family members have had breast disorders, especially breast cancer. Also ask about the incidence of other types of cancer. Having a close relative with breast cancer greatly increases the patient's risk of having the disease. Teach the patient how to perform breast self-examination and the importance of regular breast examinations and mammograms. (See *Scheduling breast examinations*.)

It is recommended that if a patient is expected to live at least 10 more years, they should continue biennial or annual mammogram screenings.

Asking about current health

Some breast changes are a normal part of aging, so be sure to ask the patient their age. If they have noticed a breast change, ask the patient to describe it in detail. Exactly where on the breast is the change? When did it occur? Do they have pain, tenderness, discharge, or rash? Have they had changes or pain in their underarm area? Does the problem come and go, or is it always present?

Down on the pharm

Ask the patient what drugs they use regularly, such as birth control pills, contraceptive patches, or a vaginal ring with estrogen. Hormonal birth control methods can cause breast swelling and tenderness. Ask about their diet, especially caffeine intake. Caffeine has been linked to fibrocystic disease of the breasts. Ask if the patient is under a lot of

Scheduling breast examinations

The American Cancer Society is now recommending regular mammograms over breast examinations as prevention and detection of breast cancer. The table below gives the guidelines for mammogram testing. With that in mind, it is still important to perform self-examinations and become familiar with the way your breasts feel in order to report any changes in breast shape or feel to your healthcare provider for further investigation.

Depending on their needs, some patients may follow schedules that have been modified by their doctors. Female patients with a family history of or a genetic predisposition for breast cancer—as well as female patients who have a personal history of cancer—may need earlier or more frequent screening tests and examinations. Female patients at high risk for breast cancer should also have an annual magnetic resonance imaging scan.

Age	Breast self-examinations	Mammography
40-44	• Monthly	• Optional to start yearly
45-54	• Monthly	• Yearly
55 and older	• Monthly	• Biennial or maintain annually depending on risk factors

stress, smokes, or drinks alcohol. Discuss the possible link between those factors and breast cancer. Note the patient's weight. If the patient is overweight, explain the link between increased weight and breast cancer development, and refer them to information on weight control. (See *BMI and breast cancer risk*.)

Assessing the breasts and axillae

Having a breast examination can be stressful for your patient. To reduce their anxiety, provide privacy, make them as comfortable as possible, and explain what the examination involves. If possible, perform the examination 7 to 10 days after the onset of menses in a premenopausal patient.

Examining the breasts

Before examining the breasts, make sure the room is well lit. Have the patient disrobe from the waist up and sit with their arms at their sides. Keep both breasts uncovered so you can observe them simultaneously to detect differences.

Inspection

Breast skin should be smooth, undimpled, and the same color as the rest of the skin. Check for edema, which can accompany lymphatic obstruction and may signal cancer. Note breast size and symmetry. Asymmetry may occur normally in some female adults, with the left breast usually larger than the right. Inspect the nipples, noting their size and shape. If a nipple is inverted, dimpled, or creased, ask the patient when they first noticed the abnormality. Lifelong nipple inversion may be normal, but any changes of the nipple call for further evaluation.

Reach for the sky…

Next, inspect the patient's breasts while they hold their arms over their head, and then again while their hands are pressed against their hips. Having the patient assume these positions will help you detect skin or nipple dimpling that might not have been obvious before.

Alternate pose

If the patient has large or pendulous breasts, have them stand with their hands on the back of a chair or the examination table and lean forward. This position helps reveal subtle breast or nipple asymmetry.

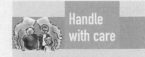

Handle with care

BMI and breast cancer risk

Extra weight can be bad for your patient's health in more ways than one. Female patients who have a body mass index (BMI) of 30 or higher have an increased risk of developing breast cancer, especially after menopause. This is because fat tissue produces small amounts of estrogen, and higher levels of estrogen increase the risk of breast cancer. The outlook is even worse for patients with a BMI greater than 35 who develop breast cancer; they're three times more likely to die of the disease.

Palpation

Before palpating the breasts, ask the patient to lie in a supine position, and place a small pillow under the shoulder on the side you're examining. This causes the breast on that side to protrude. (See *Palpating the breast.*)

Hands behind your head! You're under examination.

Have the patient put their hand behind their head on the side you're examining. This spreads the breast more evenly across the chest and makes finding nodules easier. If the patient's breasts are small, they can leave their arm at their side.

A circuitous route

To perform palpation, place your finger pads flat on the breast and compress the tissues gently against the chest wall, palpating outward from the nipple with a circular, wedged, or vertical strip method. For a patient with pendulous breasts, palpate down or across the breast with the patient sitting upright. (See *Breast palpation methods.*)

Peak technique

Palpating the breast

Use your three middle fingers to palpate the breast systematically. Rotating your fingers gently against the chest wall, move in concentric circles. Make sure you include the tail of Spence and the subareolar area in your examination.

Examining the nipple

If a lump was discovered in the breast, examine the nipple for discharge. Gently squeeze the nipple between your thumb and index finger. Note the color, amount, and consistency of any discharge.

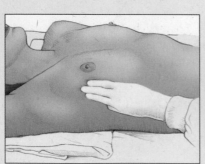

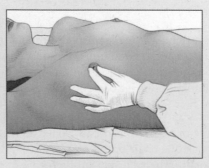

Breast palpation methods

Three methods may be used to palpate the breasts during a clinical examination: circular, wedged, or vertical strip. Whatever method you use, be consistent and palpate the entire breast, including the periphery, tail of Spence, and the areola.

Circular

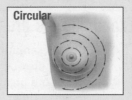

Wedged

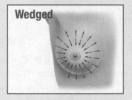

Vertical strip

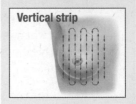

Check the consistency

As you palpate, note the consistency of the breast tissue. Normal consistency varies widely, depending in part on the proportions of fat and glandular tissue. Check for nodules and unusual tenderness. Tenderness may be related to cysts, normal hormonal changes, infection, or, very rarely, cancer. However, nodularity, fullness, and mild tenderness are also premenstrual symptoms. Be sure to ask your patient where they are in their menstrual cycle.

Compare and contrast

A lump or mass that feels different from the rest of the breast tissue may indicate a pathologic change and warrants further investigation by a practitioner. If you find what you think is an abnormality, check the other breast, too. Keep in mind that the inframammary ridge at the lower edge of the breast is normally firm and may be mistaken for a tumor.

Sizing up the situation

If you palpate a mass, record these characteristics:
- number of masses
- size in centimeters
- shape—round, discoid, regular, or irregular
- consistency—soft, firm, or hard
- mobility
- delineation—well defined or not well defined
- degree of tenderness
- location, using the quadrant or clock method (see *Identifying locations of breast lesions,* page 264).

When to get a smear

If the patient complains of a spontaneous nipple discharge (and isn't pregnant or lactating) or has any other abnormal findings on the history or physical examination, perform a thorough examination of the nipple. Compress the nipple and areola to detect discharge. If discharge is present, assess the color, consistency, and quantity of the discharge. If possible, obtain a cytologic smear.

To obtain a smear, put on gloves, place a glass slide over the nipple, and smear the discharge on the slide. Spray the slide with a fixative, label it with the patient's name and the date, and send it to the laboratory, according to your facility's policy.

Memory jogger

To remember what to look for as you assess the nipple, think of the word **DISC:**

Discharge

Inversion

Skin changes

Compare with the other side.

Examining the axillae

To examine the axillae, use the techniques of inspection and palpation. With the patient sitting or standing, inspect the skin of the axillae for rashes, infections, or unusual pigmentation.

Identifying locations of breast lesions

Mentally divide the breast into four quadrants and a fifth segment, the tail of Spence. Describe your findings according to the appropriate quadrant or segment. You can also think of the breast as a clock, with the nipple in the center. Then specify locations according to the time (2 o'clock, for example). Either way, specify the location of a lesion or other findings by the distance in centimeters from the nipple.

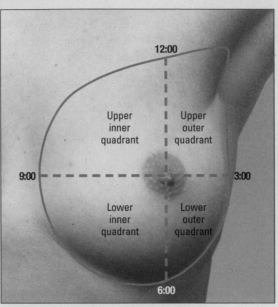

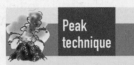

Peak technique

Palpating the axilla

To palpate the axilla, have the patient sit or lie down. Wear gloves if an ulceration or discharge is present. Ask the patient to relax their arm at their side, and support it with your nondominant hand.

Keeping the fingers of your dominant hand together, reach high into the apex of the axilla. Position your fingers so they're directly behind the pectoral muscles, pointing toward the midclavicle. Sweep your fingers downward against the ribs and serratus anterior muscle to palpate the midaxillary or central lymph nodes. Explain to the patient that it's normal for this exam to be mildly uncomfortable.

Prepare to palpate

Before palpating, ask the patient to relax their arm at their side. Support their elbow with one of your hands. Cup the fingers of your other hand, and reach high into the apex of the axilla. Place your fingers directly behind the pectoral muscles, pointing toward the midclavicle. (See *Palpating the axilla*.)

Assessing the axillary nodes

First, try to palpate the central nodes by pressing your fingers downward and in toward the chest wall. You can usually palpate one or more of the nodes, which should be soft, small, and nontender. If you feel a hard, large, or tender lesion, try to palpate the other groups of lymph nodes for comparison.

It's the pits

To palpate the pectoral and anterior nodes, grasp the anterior axillary fold between your thumb and fingers and palpate inside the borders of the pectoral muscles. Palpate the lateral nodes by pressing your fingers along the upper inner arm. Try to compress these nodes against the humerus. To palpate the subscapular or posterior nodes, stand behind the patient and press your fingers to feel the inside of the muscle of the posterior axillary fold.

Assessing the clavicular nodes

If the axillary nodes are abnormal, assess the nodes in the clavicular area. To do this, have the patient relax their neck muscles by flexing their head slightly forward. Stand in front of the patient and hook your fingers over the clavicle beside the sternocleidomastoid muscle. Rotate your fingers deeply into this area to feel the supraclavicular nodes.

Abnormal findings

The menstrual cycle, certain prescription drugs, pregnancy, and other conditions can cause breast changes; therefore, you might have trouble differentiating abnormal changes from those that are normal. To help you, this section describes several common abnormal findings. (See also *Breast abnormalities*.)

Interpretation station

Breast abnormalities

This chart shows some common groups of findings for the chief signs and symptoms of the breasts and axillae, along with their probable causes.

Sign or symptom and findings	Common cause	Sign or symptom and findings	Common cause
Breast dimpling		*Breast nodule*	
• Firm, irregular, nontender lump • Nipple retraction, deviation, inversion, or flattening • Enlarged axillary lymph nodes	Breast cancer	• Single nodule that feels firm, elastic, and round or lobular, with well-defined margins • Extremely mobile, "slippery" feel • No pain or tenderness • Size varies from pinpoint to very large • Grows rapidly • Usually located around the nipple or the lateral side of the upper outer quadrant	Fibroadenoma
• Heat • Erythema • Swelling • Pain and tenderness • Flulike signs and symptoms, such as fever, malaise, fatigue, and aching	Mastitis		

(Continued)

Breast abnormalities *(continued)*

Sign or symptom and findings	Common cause
Breast nodule *(continued)*	
• Hard, poorly delineated nodule • Fixed to the skin or underlying tissue • Breast dimpling • Nipple deviation or retraction • Located in the upper outer quadrant (50% of cases) • Nontender • Serous or bloody nipple discharge • Edema or peau d'orange of the skin overlying the mass • Axillary lymphadenopathy	Breast cancer
• History of trauma to fatty tissue of the breast (patient may not remember such trauma) • Tenderness and erythema • Bruising • Hard, indurated, poorly delineated lump that's fibrotic and fixed to underlying tissue or overlying skin • Nipple retraction	Fat necrosis
• Smooth, round, slightly elastic nodules or generalized "lumpiness" without a discrete mass • Increased size and tenderness just before menstruation • Mobile • Clear, watery (serous), or sticky nipple discharge • Bloating • Irritability • Abdominal cramping	Fibrocystic breast disease

Sign or symptom and findings	Common cause
Breast pain	
• Tender, palpable lymph nodes • Fever • Nipple discharge • Breast pain and enlargement of affected breast • Redness and warmth in the affected breast	Breast cancer abscess
• Unilateral breast pain or tenderness • Serous or bloody nipple discharge, usually only from one duct • Small, soft, poorly delineated mass in the ducts beneath the areola	Intraductal papilloma
• Small, well-delineated nodule • Localized erythema • Induration	Sebaceous cyst (infection)
Nipple retraction	
• Unilateral nipple retraction and inversion • Hard, fixed, nontender breast nodule • Nipple itching, burning, or erosion • Watery or bloody nipple discharge (typically unilateral) • Altered breast contour • Dimpling or peau d'orange • Tenderness, redness, and warmth	Breast cancer
• Unilateral nipple retraction, deviation, cracking, or flattening • Firm, warm, erythematous, tender, swollen area • Possible fatigue, fever, chills, and other flulike symptoms	Mastitis

Breast nodule

A breast nodule, or lump, may be found in any part of the breast, including the axilla. Breast nodules may range in clinical significance from the benign lumps of fibrocystic breast disease to a malignant mass of breast cancer.

Dimpling

Breast dimpling—the puckering or retraction of skin on the breast—results from abnormal attachment of the skin to underlying tissue. It suggests an inflammatory or malignant mass beneath the skin surface and may represent a late sign of breast cancer. (See *Dimpling and peau d'orange*.)

Peau d'orange

Usually another late sign of breast cancer, peau d'orange (orange peel skin) is the edematous thickening and pitting of breast skin. This sign can also occur with breast or axillary lymph node infection of Graves disease. Its striking orange peel appearance stems from lymphatic edema around deepened hair follicles.

Nipple retraction and inversion

Nipple retraction, the inward displacement of the nipple below the level of surrounding breast tissue, may indicate an inflammatory breast lesion or cancer. It results from scar tissue formation within a lesion or large mammary duct. As the scar tissue shortens, it pulls adjacent tissue inward, causing nipple deviation, flattening, and finally retraction.

Nipple inversion is the lack of protrusion of the nipple. It typically occurs in puberty. In a female adult, it may impede breastfeeding and predispose the patient to mastitis and abscess formation.

Nipple discharge

Nipple discharge can occur spontaneously or can be elicited by nipple stimulation. It's characterized as intermittent or constant, unilateral or bilateral, and by color, consistency, and composition. It can be a normal finding; however, nipple discharge can also signal serious underlying disease, particularly when accompanied by other breast changes.

Dimpling and peau d'orange

These illustrations show two common abnormalities in breast tissue: dimpling and peau d'orange.

Dimpling
Dimpling usually suggests an inflammatory or a malignant mass beneath the skin's surface. The illustration shows breast dimpling and nipple retraction caused by a malignant mass above the areola.

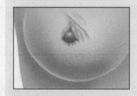

Peau d'orange
Peau d'orange is usually a late sign of breast cancer, but it can also occur with breast or axillary lymph node infection. The skin's orange peel appearance comes from lymphatic edema around deepened hair follicles.

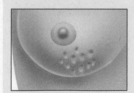

Significant causes include endocrine disorders, cancer, certain drugs, and blocked lactiferous ducts.

Breast pain

Breast pain commonly results from benign breast disease, such as mastitis or fibrocystic breast disease. It may occur during rest or movement and may be aggravated by manipulation or palpation. Breast tenderness refers to pain elicited by physical contact.

Visible veins

Prominent veins in one breast may indicate cancer in some patients; however, they're considered normal in pregnant patients because of engorgement.

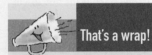

That's a wrap!

Breasts and axillae review

Anatomy and physiology
• Nipple: pigmented erectile tissue located in the center of each breast
• Areola: ringed area that surrounds the nipple; darker in color than adjacent tissue
• Cooper ligaments: fibrous bands that support each breast
• Glandular lobes: contain the alveoli that produce milk
• Lactiferous ducts: transport milk from each lobe to the nipple.

Health history
• Ask the patient about a history of breast lumps, breast surgery, breast cancer, fibrocystic breast disease, or other breast disorders.
• Ask about the patient's menstrual and pregnancy history.
• Ask about a family history of breast disorders, especially breast cancer.

Assessment
• Inspect the breast, noting breast size and symmetry and skin condition.
• Palpate each breast in concentric circles outward from the nipple, including the periphery, tail of Spence, and areola.
• If the patient reports nipple discharge, palpate the nipple and compress to check for discharge.
• Inspect and palpate the axilla.
• Palpate lymph node chains.

Documenting a breast mass
Note these characteristics:
• Diameter
• Shape
• Consistency
• Mobility
• Degree of tenderness
• Location

Abnormal findings
• Breast nodule—breast lump that may be benign or malignant
• Breast dimpling—puckering or retraction of skin on the breast
• Peau d'orange (orange peel skin)—edematous thickening and pitting of breast skin
• Nipple retraction—inward displacement of the nipple below the level of surrounding breast tissue
• Nipple inversion—lack of protrusion of the nipple
• Nipple discharge—may be a normal finding or can signal serious disease
• Breast pain—may occur during rest or movement; may be aggravated by manipulation or palpation
• Visible veins—may indicate cancer but also occur normally in pregnant patients.

Quick quiz

1. Most malignant breast tumors occur in the region of the breast known as the:
    A. lower inner quadrant.
    B. lower outer quadrant.
    C. upper inner quadrant.
    D. upper outer quadrant.

Answer: D. Although a malignancy can occur in any part of the breast, it usually occurs in the upper outer quadrant and appears as a hard, immobile, irregular lump.

2. Normal changes in the breasts of a premenstrual patient include:
    A. a single hard, fixed mass.
    B. nipple inversion and skin dimpling.
    C. tenderness and soft, mobile cysts.
    D. redness and scaling over a portion of the breast.

Answer: C. A week before menses, both breasts are usually tender with soft, benign, mobile, fluid-filled cysts.

3. After obtaining a smear of nipple discharge on a glass slide, you would:
    A. freeze the slide before sending it to the laboratory.
    B. let the smear air-dry before sending it to the laboratory.
    C. spray the slide with a cytologic fixative before sending it to the laboratory.
    D. spread the smear with a cotton swab, apply a coverslip to the slide, and send it to the laboratory.

Answer: C. To obtain a culture of nipple discharge, place a glass slide over the nipple and smear the discharge on the slide. Then spray the slide with a cytologic fixative before sending it to the laboratory.

4. The tail of Spence is located:
    A. above the nipple at the midclavicular line.
    B. in the upper outer quadrant, toward the axilla.
    C. in the upper inner quadrant, near the sternum.
    D. in the lower outer quadrant, close to the ribs.

Answer: B. The tail of Spence is a small triangle of tissue located in the upper outer quadrant of the breast, toward the axilla.

Scoring

★★★ If you answered all four questions correctly, way to go! You're an impeccable inspector and a precision palpator.

★★ If you answered three questions correctly, good job! You've kept abreast of the most important facts in this chapter.

★ If you answered fewer than three questions correctly, that's okay! Feed yourself the information in this chapter again and you're sure to have better results.

 Just for fun

Match the breast finding or disorder in column 1 with the definition or characteristic in column 2.

Breast finding or disorder

1. Peau d'orange _____
2. Gynecomastia _____
3. Mastitis _____
4. Nipple retraction _____
5. Fibrocystic breast disease _____
6. Breast cancer _____
7. Fibroadenoma _____
8. Breast dimpling _____

Definition or characteristic

A. Single nodule that is round with well-defined margins and feels firm, elastic, and "slippery"; usually found around nipple or lateral side of upper outer quadrant

B. Painful, red, hot, swollen area with nipple retraction, deviation, cracking, or flattening; often accompanied by flulike symptoms

C. Abnormal breast enlargement in males; may be hormone related or caused by cirrhosis, leukemia, thyrotoxicosis, or alcohol or illicit/recreational drug use

D. Abnormal puckering of skin, especially around nipple; usually suggests inflammatory or malignant mass beneath skin surface

E. Smooth, round, slightly elastic nodules that increase in size just before menstruation; often associated with bloating, irritability, and abdominal cramping

F. Edematous thickening and pitting of the breast skin that's commonly a late sign of breast cancer; may also be associated with Graves disease

G. Inward displacement of nipple below level of surrounding tissue; may indicate inflammatory breast lesion or cancer

H. Hard, poorly delineated nodule that's fixed to skin or underlying tissue; may be accompanied by nipple retraction, serous or bloody discharge, or other breast changes

Answer: 1. F, 2. C, 3. B, 4. G, 5. E, 6. H, 7. A, 8. D

Chapter 12

Gastrointestinal system

Just the facts

In this chapter, you'll learn:

♦ organs and structures that make up the GI system

♦ questions to ask during a patient history of the GI system

♦ techniques for performing a physical assessment of the GI system

♦ causes and characteristics of GI abnormalities.

A look at the GI system

The GI system's major functions include ingestion and digestion of food and elimination of waste products. When these processes are interrupted, the patient can experience problems ranging from loss of appetite to acid-base imbalances.

Anatomy and physiology

The GI system consists of two major divisions: the GI tract and the accessory organs. (See *A close look at the GI system,* page 288.)

GI tract

The GI tract is a hollow tube that begins at the mouth and ends at the anus. About 25′ (7.5 m) long, the GI tract consists of smooth muscle alternating with blood vessels and nerve tissue. Specialized circular and longitudinal fibers contract, causing peristalsis, which aids in propelling food through the GI tract. The GI tract includes the pharynx, esophagus, stomach, small intestine, and large intestine.

A close look at the GI system

These illustrations show the GI system's major anatomic structures. Knowing these structures will help you conduct an accurate physical assessment.

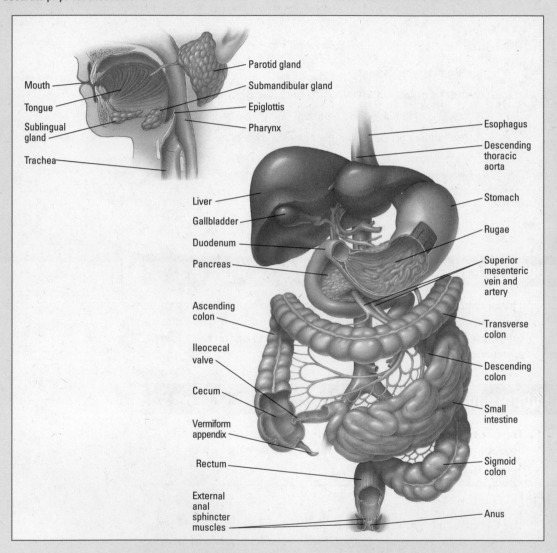

- Mouth
- Tongue
- Sublingual gland
- Trachea
- Parotid gland
- Submandibular gland
- Epiglottis
- Pharynx
- Liver
- Gallbladder
- Duodenum
- Pancreas
- Ascending colon
- Ileocecal valve
- Cecum
- Vermiform appendix
- Rectum
- External anal sphincter muscles
- Esophagus
- Descending thoracic aorta
- Stomach
- Rugae
- Superior mesenteric vein and artery
- Transverse colon
- Descending colon
- Small intestine
- Sigmoid colon
- Anus

Move into the mouth

Digestive processes begin in the mouth with chewing, masticating, salivating, and swallowing. The tongue provides the sense of taste. Saliva is produced by three pairs of salivary glands: the parotid, submandibular, and sublingual.

Proceed to the pharynx

The pharynx, or throat, allows the passage of food from the mouth to the esophagus. The pharynx assists in the swallowing process by secreting mucus that aids in digestion. The epiglottis—a thin, leaf-shaped structure made of fibrocartilage—is directly behind the root of the tongue. When food is swallowed, the epiglottis closes to protect the larynx, and the soft palate lifts to block the nasal cavity. These actions keep food and fluid from being aspirated into the airway.

Enter the esophagus

The esophagus is a muscular, hollow tube about 10″ (25.5 cm) long that moves food from the pharynx to the stomach. When food is swallowed, the upper esophageal sphincter relaxes, and the food moves into the esophagus. Peristalsis then propels the food toward the stomach. The gastroesophageal sphincter at the lower end of the esophagus normally remains closed to prevent reflux of gastric contents. The sphincter opens during swallowing, belching, and vomiting.

Stay awhile in the stomach

The stomach, a reservoir for food, is a dilated, saclike structure that lies obliquely in the left upper abdominal quadrant below the esophagus and diaphragm, to the right of the spleen, and partly under the liver. The stomach contains two important sphincters: the cardiac sphincter, which protects the entrance to the stomach, and the pyloric sphincter, which guards the exit.

The stomach has three major functions. It:

- stores food
- mixes food with gastric juices (hydrochloric acid)
- passes chyme—a watery mixture of partly digested food and digestive juices—into the small intestine for further digestion and absorption.

An average meal can remain in the stomach for 3 to 4 hours. Rugae, accordion-like folds in the stomach lining, allow the stomach to expand when large amounts of food and fluid are ingested.

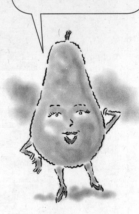

Once food reaches the stomach, it remains there for 3 to 4 hours before moving on to the small intestine.

Slip through the small intestine

The small intestine is about 20′ (6 m) long and is named for its diameter, not its length. It has three sections: the duodenum, the jejunum, and the ileum. As chyme passes into the small intestine, the end products of digestion are absorbed through its thin mucous membrane lining into the bloodstream.

Carbohydrates, fats, and proteins are broken down in the small intestine. Enzymes from the pancreas, bile from the liver, and hormones from glands of the small intestine all aid digestion. These secretions mix with the chyme as it moves through the intestines by peristalsis.

A look at digestion

Digestion is the mechanical, chemical, and enzymatic process by which ingested food is broken down and converted into energy.

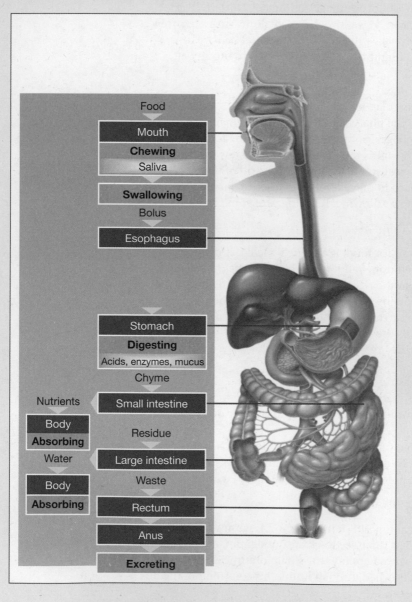

Food

Mouth

Chewing

Saliva

Swallowing

Bolus

Esophagus

Stomach

Digesting

Acids, enzymes, mucus

Chyme

Nutrients

Small intestine

Body

Absorbing

Residue

Water

Large intestine

Body

Waste

Absorbing

Rectum

Anus

Excreting

And leave through the large intestine

The large intestine, or colon, is about 5′ (1.5 m) long. It includes the cecum; the ascending, transverse, descending, and sigmoid colons; the rectum; and the anus—in that order—and is responsible for:
- absorbing water and electrolytes
- storing food residue
- eliminating waste products in the form of feces.

The appendix, a fingerlike projection, is attached to the cecum. Bacteria in the colon produce gas, or flatus.

Accessory organs

Accessory GI organs include the liver, pancreas, gallbladder, and bile ducts. The abdominal aorta and the gastric and splenic veins also aid the GI system.

Look at the liver

The liver is located in the right upper quadrant under the diaphragm. It has two major lobes, divided by the falciform ligament. The liver is the heaviest organ in the body, weighing about 3 lb (1.5 kg) in an adult.

The liver's functions include:
- metabolizing carbohydrates, fats, and proteins
- detoxifying blood
- converting ammonia to urea for excretion
- synthesizing plasma proteins, nonessential amino acids, vitamin A, and essential nutrients, such as iron and vitamins D, K, and B_{12}.

The liver also secretes bile, a greenish fluid that helps break down and digest fats and absorb fatty acids, cholesterol, and other lipids. The absence or presence of bile helps determine the color of stool.

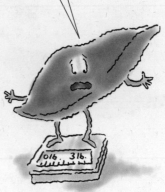

You'd think with all my functions I'd lose a little weight, but I'm the heaviest organ in the body!

Gape at the gallbladder

The gallbladder is a small, pear-shaped organ about 4″ (10 cm) long that lies halfway under the right lobe of the liver. Its main function is to store bile from the liver until the bile is needed by the duodenum. This process occurs when the small intestine initiates chemical impulses that cause the gallbladder to contract, releasing the bile.

Probe the pancreas

The pancreas, which measures 6″ to 8″ (15 to 20.5 cm) in length, lies horizontally in the abdomen, behind the stomach. It consists of a head, tail, and body. The head of the pancreas lies in the lateral aspect of the upper abdominal quadrant, the body of the pancreas is located

A close look at accessory GI organs and vessels

The illustration below shows the position of each of the accessory GI organs and vessels.

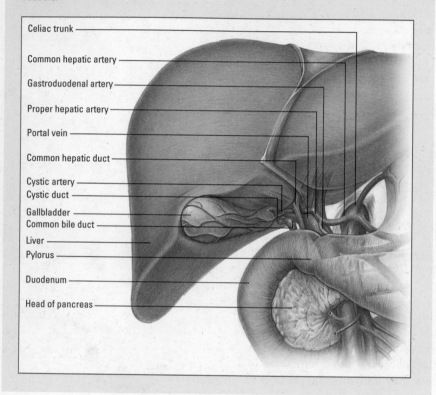

Celiac trunk
Common hepatic artery
Gastroduodenal artery
Proper hepatic artery
Portal vein
Common hepatic duct
Cystic artery
Cystic duct
Gallbladder
Common bile duct
Liver
Pylorus
Duodenum
Head of pancreas

in the right upper quadrant, and the tail is in the left upper quadrant, attached to the duodenum. The tail of the pancreas touches the spleen.

The pancreas releases insulin and glycogen into the bloodstream and produces pancreatic enzymes that are released into the duodenum for digestion.

Behold the bile ducts

The bile ducts provide passageways for bile to travel from the liver to the intestines. Two hepatic ducts drain the liver and the cystic duct drains the gallbladder. These ducts converge into the common bile duct, which empties into the duodenum.

View the vascular structures

The abdominal aorta supplies blood to the GI tract. It enters the abdomen, separates into the common iliac arteries, and then branches into many arteries extending the length of the GI tract.

The gastric and splenic veins drain absorbed nutrients into the portal vein of the liver. After entering the liver, venous blood circulates and then exits the liver through the hepatic vein, emptying into the inferior vena cava.

Obtaining a health history

If your patient has a GI problem, the primary symptom they report will be about abdominal or chest pain, belching, cramping, heartburn, nausea, vomiting, or altered bowel habits. To investigate these and other signs and symptoms, ask your patient about the location, quality, onset, duration, frequency, and severity of each. Also ask your patient what relieves or worsens the symptoms.

Knowing what precipitates and relieves the patient's symptoms will help you perform a more accurate physical assessment and better plan your care.

Asking about past health

To determine if your patient's problem is new or recurring, ask about past GI illnesses, such as an ulcer; liver, pancreas, or gallbladder disease; inflammatory bowel disease; rectal or GI bleeding; hiatal hernia; irritable bowel syndrome; diverticulitis; gastroesophageal reflux disease; or cancer. Also ask if they have had abdominal surgery or trauma.

Asking about current health

Ask the patient about current medications. Several drugs—especially aspirin, nonsteroidal anti-inflammatory drugs, antibiotics, and opioid analgesics—can cause nausea, vomiting, diarrhea, constipation, and other GI signs and symptoms.

Be sure to ask about laxative use; habitual use may cause constipation. Also, ask about enema or suppository use. Don't forget to ask if the patient is allergic to medications or foods. Such allergies commonly cause GI symptoms.

Gnawing problems

In addition, ask the patient about changes in appetite, difficulty chewing or swallowing, and changes in bowel habits. Does the patient have excessive belching or passing of gas? Has there been a change in the color, amount, frequency, and appearance of the stool? Has there been blood in the stool?

Travel plans

If the patient's reason for seeking care is diarrhea, find out if there has been recent travel abroad and where that travel was. Diarrhea, hepatitis, and parasitic infections can result from ingesting contaminated food or water.

Asking about family health

Because some GI disorders are hereditary, ask the patient whether anyone in the family has had a GI disorder. (See *Culture and the GI history*, page 294.)

Disorders with a familial link include:
- ulcerative colitis
- colorectal cancer
- peptic ulcers
- gastric cancer
- alcohol use disorder
- Crohn disease.

Asking about psychosocial health

Inquire about your patient's occupation, home life, financial situation, stress level, and recent life changes. Be sure to ask about alcohol, caffeine, and tobacco use as well as food and fluid consumption, exercise habits, and oral hygiene. Also ask about sleep patterns: How many hours is the patient sleeping and does the patient feel it is enough sleep?

Assessing the GI system

A physical assessment of the GI system should include a thorough examination of the mouth, abdomen, and rectum. To perform an abdominal assessment, use this sequence: inspection, auscultation, percussion, and palpation. Palpating or percussing the abdomen before you auscultate can change the character of the patient's bowel sounds and lead to an inaccurate assessment.

Bridging the gap

Culture and the GI history

When taking a health history, consider your patient's ethnic background. For example, patients from Japan, Iceland, Chile, and Austria are at higher risk for death from gastric cancer than patients from other countries. Also, Crohn disease is more common in patients who are Jewish.

Before beginning your examination, explain the techniques you'll be using and warn the patient that some procedures might be uncomfortable. Perform the examination in a private, quiet, warm, and well-lighted room.

Examining the mouth

Use inspection and palpation to assess the mouth. Be sure to put on gloves before examining the patient.

Open wide

First, inspect the patient's mouth and jaw for color, asymmetry, and swelling. Check their bite, noting malocclusion from an overbite or underbite. Inspect the inner and outer lips, teeth, gums, and oral mucosa with a penlight. Note bleeding; ulcerations; caries; loose, missing, or broken teeth; and color changes, including rashes. If the patient wears partial or complete dentures, assess their color, condition, and fit. Palpate the gums, inner lips, and cheeks for tenderness, lumps, and lesions.

Assess the tongue, checking for coating, tremors, swelling, and ulcerations. Note unusual breath odors. Finally, examine the pharynx by pressing a tongue blade firmly down on the middle of the tongue and asking the patient to say "Ahh." Look for color changes, uvular deviation, tonsillar abnormalities, lesions, plaques, and exudate.

Examining the abdomen

Use inspection, auscultation, percussion, and palpation to examine the abdomen. To ensure an accurate assessment, take these actions before the examination:

- Ask the patient to empty their bladder.
- Drape the genitalia and, if the patient is female, the breasts.
- Place a small pillow under the patient's knees to help relax the abdominal muscles.
- Ask the patient to keep their arms at their sides.
- Keep the room warm. Chilling can cause abdominal muscles to become tense.
- Warm your hands and the stethoscope head.
- Speak softly and encourage the patient to perform breathing exercises or use imagery during uncomfortable procedures.
- Ask the patient to point to any areas of pain.
- Assess painful areas last to help prevent the patient from tensing their abdominal muscles.

Inspection

Begin by mentally dividing the abdomen into four quadrants and then imagining the organs in each quadrant. (See *Abdominal quadrants*, page 296.)

It's all in the terms

You can more accurately pinpoint your physical findings by knowing these three terms:

- epigastric—above the umbilicus and between the costal margins
- umbilical—around the navel
- suprapubic—above the symphysis pubis.

Abdominal quadrants

To perform a systematic GI assessment, try to visualize the abdominal structures by dividing the abdomen into four quadrants, as shown here.

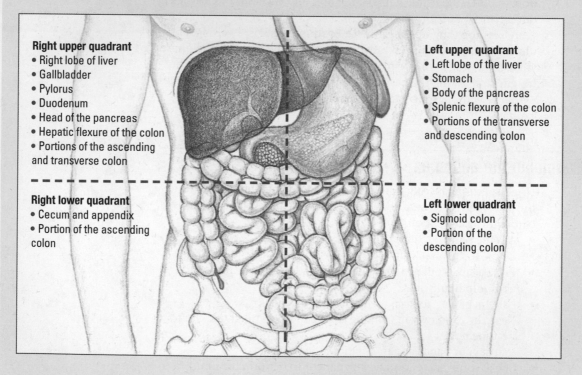

Right upper quadrant
- Right lobe of liver
- Gallbladder
- Pylorus
- Duodenum
- Head of the pancreas
- Hepatic flexure of the colon
- Portions of the ascending and transverse colon

Left upper quadrant
- Left lobe of the liver
- Stomach
- Body of the pancreas
- Splenic flexure of the colon
- Portions of the transverse and descending colon

Right lower quadrant
- Cecum and appendix
- Portion of the ascending colon

Left lower quadrant
- Sigmoid colon
- Portion of the descending colon

Battle of the bulge

Observe the abdomen for color and symmetry, checking for bumps, bulges, lesions, scars, rashes, or masses. A bulge may indicate bladder distention or hernia.

Also note the patient's abdominal shape and contour. The abdomen should be flat to rounded in people of average weight. A protruding abdomen may be caused by obesity, pregnancy, ascites, or abdominal distention. A slender person may have a slightly concave abdomen.

Innie or outie?

Assess the umbilicus, which should be inverted and located midline in the abdomen. Conditions such as pregnancy, ascites, or an underlying mass can cause the umbilicus to protrude. Have the patient raise their head and shoulders. If their umbilicus protrudes, they may have an umbilical hernia.

Stretched to the limit

The skin of the abdomen should be smooth and uniform in color. Striae, or stretch marks, can be caused by pregnancy, excessive weight gain, or ascites. New striae are pink or blue; old striae are silvery white (in patients with darker skin, striae may be dark brown). Note dilated veins. Record the length, location, and condition of any surgical scars on the abdomen.

Riding the peristaltic wave

Note abdominal movements and pulsations. Usually, waves of peristalsis can't be seen; if they're visible, they should look like slight, wavelike motions. Visible, rippling waves may indicate bowel obstruction and should be reported immediately. In thin patients, pulsation of the aorta is visible in the epigastric area. Marked pulsations may occur with hypertension, aortic insufficiency, aortic aneurysm, and other conditions that cause widening pulse pressure.

Auscultation

Lightly place the stethoscope diaphragm in the right lower quadrant, slightly below and to the right of the umbilicus. Auscultate in a clockwise fashion in each of the four quadrants. Note the character and quality of bowel sounds in each quadrant. In some cases, you may need to auscultate for up to 5 minutes before you hear sounds. Be sure to allow enough time to listen in each quadrant before you decide that bowel sounds are abnormal or absent.

Silence the suction

Before auscultating the abdomen of a patient with a nasogastric tube or another abdominal tube connected to suction, clamp the tube or turn off the suction. Suction noises can obscure or mimic actual bowel sounds.

Pardon my borborygmus

Normal bowel sounds are high-pitched, gurgling noises caused by air mixing with fluid during peristalsis. The noises vary in frequency, pitch, and intensity and occur irregularly from 5 to 34 times per minute. They're loudest before mealtimes. Borborygmus, or stomach growling, is the loud, gurgling, splashing bowel sound heard over the large intestine as gas passes through it.

Too much activity or not enough?

Bowel sounds are classified as normal, hypoactive, or hyperactive. Hyperactive bowel sounds—loud, high-pitched, tinkling sounds that occur frequently—may be caused by diarrhea, constipation, laxative use, or certain GI disorders, such as Crohn disease or ulcerative colitis.

Hypoactive bowel sounds are heard infrequently. They're associated with ileus, bowel obstruction, or peritonitis and indicate diminished peristalsis. Paralytic ileus, torsion of the bowel, or the use of opioid analgesics and other medications can decrease peristalsis.

Voice of the vessels

Auscultate for vascular sounds with the bell of the stethoscope. (See *Auscultating vascular sounds*.) Using firm pressure, listen over the aorta and renal, iliac, and femoral arteries for bruits, venous hums, and friction rubs.

Percussion

Direct or indirect percussion is used to detect the size and location of abdominal organs and to detect air or fluid in the abdomen, stomach, or bowel.

In direct percussion, strike your hand or finger directly against the patient's abdomen. With indirect percussion, use the middle finger of your dominant hand or a percussion hammer to strike a finger resting on the patient's abdomen. Begin percussion in the right lower quadrant and proceed clockwise, covering all four quadrants.

Don't percuss the abdomen of a patient with an abdominal aortic aneurysm or a transplanted abdominal organ. Doing so can precipitate a rupture or organ rejection.

Peak technique

Auscultating vascular sounds

Use the bell of your stethoscope to auscultate for vascular sounds at the sites shown in the illustration.

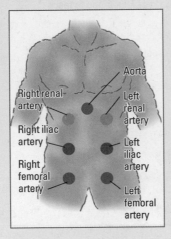

Hollow or dull?

You normally hear two sounds during percussion of the abdomen: tympany and dullness. When you percuss over hollow organs, such as an empty stomach or bowel, you hear a clear, hollow sound like a drum beating. This sound, tympany, predominates because air is normally present in the stomach and bowel. The degree of tympany depends on the amount of air and gastric dilation.

When you percuss over solid organs, such as the liver, kidney, or feces-filled intestines, the sound changes to dullness. Note where percussed sounds change from tympany to dullness. (See *Sites of tympany and dullness*, page 299.)

How large is the liver?

Percussion of the liver can help you estimate its size. (See *Percussing and measuring the liver*.) Hepatomegaly is commonly associated with hepatitis and other liver diseases. Liver borders may be obscured and difficult to assess.

Sites of tympany and dullness

Expect to percuss tympany and dullness in the areas shown here.

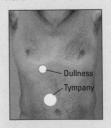

Percussing and measuring the liver

To percuss and measure the liver, follow these steps:
• Identify the upper border of liver dullness. Start in the right midclavicular line in an area of lung resonance, and percuss downward toward the liver. Use a pen to mark the spot where the sound changes to dullness.
• Start in the right midclavicular line at a level below the umbilicus, and lightly percuss upward toward the liver, as shown here. Mark the spot where the sound changes from tympany to dullness.
• Use a ruler to measure the vertical span between the two marked spots. In an adult, a normal liver span ranges from 2½° to 4¾° (6.5 to 12 cm).

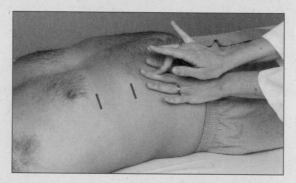

Splenic dullard

The spleen is located at about the level of the 10th rib, in the left midaxillary line. Percussion may produce a small area of dullness, generally 7″ (17.8 cm) or less in adults. However, the spleen usually can't be percussed because tympany from the colon masks the dullness of the spleen. It's also difficult to distinguish between the dullness of the posterior flank and the dullness of the spleen.

Growing problem

Conditions that cause splenomegaly include mononucleosis, trauma, and illnesses that destroy red blood cells, such as sickle cell anemia and some cancers. (See *Spleen or kidney enlargement?* page 301) To assess a patient for splenic enlargement, ask them to breathe deeply. Then percuss along the 6th to 10th intercostal spaces on the left midaxillary line, listening for a change from tympany to dullness. Measure the area of dullness. This is called a *positive splenic percussion sign*.

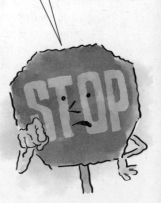

Don't percuss if the patient has an abdominal aortic aneurysm or a transplanted abdominal organ. Doing so can precipitate a rupture or organ rejection.

Palpation

Abdominal palpation includes light and deep touch to help determine the size, shape, position, and tenderness of major abdominal organs and to detect masses and fluid accumulation. Palpate all four quadrants, leaving painful and tender areas for last.

Light touch

Light palpation helps identify muscle resistance and tenderness as well as the location of some superficial organs. To palpate, put the fingers of one hand close together, depress the skin about ½″ (1.5 cm) with your fingertips, and make gentle, rotating movements. Avoid short, quick jabs.

Getting in touch with what you're feeling

The abdomen should be soft and nontender. As you palpate the four quadrants, note organs, masses, and areas of tenderness or increased resistance. Determine whether resistance is due to the patient being cold, tense, or ticklish, or if it's due to involuntary guarding or rigidity from muscle spasms or peritoneal inflammation.

Help the patient relax by putting their hand over yours as you palpate. If the patient complains of abdominal tenderness even before you touch the area, palpate by placing your stethoscope lightly on the abdomen.

Pressing the issue

To perform deep palpation, push the abdomen down 2″ to 3″ (5 to 7.5 cm). In a patient who is obese, put one hand on top of the other and push. Palpate the entire abdomen in a clockwise direction, checking for tenderness, pulsations, organ enlargement, and masses.

Hands off!

If the patient's abdomen is rigid, don't palpate it. The patient could have peritoneal inflammation, and palpation could cause pain or could rupture an inflamed organ.

Palpation precaution

Palpate the patient's liver to check for enlargement and tenderness. (See *Palpating the liver*, page 302.) Unless the spleen is enlarged, it isn't palpable. If you do feel the spleen, stop palpating immediately because compression can cause rupture. (See *Palpating the spleen*, page 302.)

Spleen or kidney enlargement?

To differentiate between spleen and kidney enlargement, ask your patient to take a deep breath. Then percuss along the 9th to 11th intercostal spaces on the left midaxillary line. You should hear tympany produced by colonic or gastric air. If you hear dullness instead, the patient's spleen may be enlarged. If you hear resonance, their left kidney may be enlarged.

Peak technique

Palpating the liver

Method 1: Standard palpation

• Place the patient in the supine position. Standing at the right side, place your left hand under the patient's back at the approximate location of the liver.

• Place your right hand slightly below the mark you made earlier at the liver's upper border. Point the fingers of your right hand toward the patient's head just under the right costal margin.

• As the patient inhales deeply through their mouth, gently press in and up on the abdomen until the liver brushes under your right hand. The edge should be smooth, firm, and somewhat round. Note any tenderness.

Method 2: Hooking the liver

• Hooking is an alternate way of palpating the liver. To hook the liver, stand next to the patient's right shoulder, facing the feet. Place your hands side by side, and hook your fingertips over the right costal margin, below the lower mark of dullness.

• Ask the patient to take a deep breath through the mouth as you push your fingertips in and up. If the liver is palpable, you may feel its edge as it slides down in the abdomen as the patient inhales.

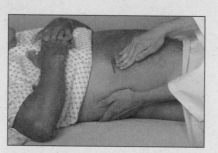

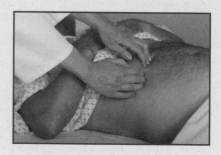

Peak technique

Palpating the spleen

Although a normal spleen isn't palpable, an enlarged spleen is. To palpate the spleen, stand on the patient's right side. Use your left hand to support the posterior left lower rib cage. Ask patient to take a deep breath. Then, with your right hand on their abdomen, press up and in toward the spleen. If you are able to feel the spleen, stop palpating immediately.

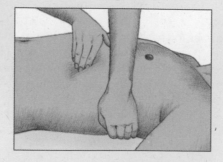

Special assessment procedures

To check for rebound tenderness or ascites, follow these guidelines.

On the rebound

Perform the test for rebound tenderness when you suspect peritoneal inflammation. Check for rebound at the end of your examination.

Choosing a site away from any painful area, position your hand at a 90° angle to the abdomen. Push down slowly and deeply into the abdomen; then withdraw your hand quickly. Rapid withdrawal causes the underlying structures to rebound suddenly and results in a sharp, stabbing pain on the inflamed side. Don't repeat this maneuver because you may rupture an inflamed appendix. (See *Eliciting rebound tenderness in children*, page 303.)

Waterlogged

Ascites, a large accumulation of fluid in the peritoneal cavity, can be caused by advanced liver disease, heart failure, pancreatitis, or cancer.

If ascites is present, use a tape measure to measure the fullest part of the abdomen. Mark this point on the patient's abdomen with indelible ink so you'll be sure to measure it consistently. This measurement is important, especially if fluid removal or paracentesis is performed. (See *Checking for ascites*, page 304.)

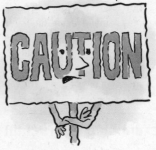

To minimize the risk of rupturing an inflamed appendix, don't repeat the maneuver for assessing rebound tenderness.

Handle with care

Eliciting rebound tenderness in children

Eliciting rebound tenderness in young children who can't verbalize how they feel may be difficult. Be alert for such clues as an anguished facial expression, a grimace, or intensified crying.

When attempting to assess this symptom, use techniques that elicit minimal tenderness. For example, have the child hop or jump to allow tissue to rebound gently while you watch closely for signs of pain. With this technique, the child won't associate the exacerbation of the pain with your actions and you may gain the child's cooperation.

Peak technique

Checking for ascites

To check for ascites, have an assistant place the ulnar edge of their hand firmly on the patient's abdomen at its midline. Then, as you stand facing the patient's head, place the palm of your right hand against the patient's left flank, as shown below. Give the right abdomen a firm tap with your left hand. If ascites is present, you may see and feel a "fluid wave" ripple across the abdomen.

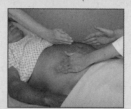

Examining the rectum and anus

If your patient is age 40 or older, perform a rectal examination as part of your GI assessment. Be sure to explain the procedure to the patient.

An outside point of view

First, inspect the perianal area. Put on gloves and spread the buttocks to expose the anus and surrounding tissue, checking for fissures, lesions, scars, inflammation, discharge, rectal prolapse, and external hemorrhoids. Ask the patient to strain as if having a bowel movement; this may reveal internal hemorrhoids, polyps, or fissures. The skin in the perianal area is normally somewhat darker than that of the surrounding area.

The inside story

Next palpate the rectum. Apply a water-soluble lubricant to your gloved index finger. Tell the patient to relax and warn the patient that they will feel some pressure. Ask the patient to bear down. As the sphincter opens, gently insert your finger into the rectum, toward the umbilicus. To palpate as much of the rectal wall as possible, rotate your finger clockwise and then counterclockwise. The rectal walls should feel soft and smooth, without masses, fecal impaction, or tenderness.

Remove your finger from the rectum, and inspect the glove for stool, blood, and mucus. Test fecal matter adhering to the glove for occult blood using a guaiac test.

Patients age 40 and older should undergo a rectal examination.

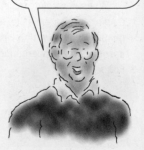

Abnormal findings

GI disorders can affect a patient's ingestion, digestion, and elimination. This section describes common abnormalities you might uncover during a GI assessment. (See *GI abnormalities* and *Abdominal distension*.)

Abdominal distention

Distention may result from gas, a tumor, or a colon filled with feces. It may also be caused by an incisional hernia, which may protrude when the patient lifts the head and shoulders.

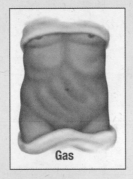

Gas

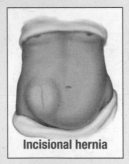

Incisional hernia

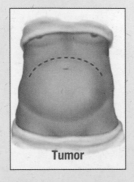

Tumor

GI abnormalities

This chart shows some common groups of findings for signs and symptoms of the GI system, along with their probable causes.

Sign or symptom and findings	Probable cause
Diarrhea	
• Soft, unformed stools or watery diarrhea that may be foul-smelling or grossly bloody • Abdominal pain, cramping, and tenderness • Fever	Clostridium difficile infection
• Diarrhea occurs within several hours of ingesting milk or milk products • Abdominal pain, cramping, and bloating • Borborygmi • Flatus	Lactose intolerance
• Recurrent bloody diarrhea with pus or mucus • Hyperactive bowel sounds • Occasional nausea and vomiting	Ulcerative colitis
Rectal bleeding	
• Moderate to severe rectal bleeding • Epistaxis • Purpura	Coagulation disorders
• Bright-red rectal bleeding with or without pain • Diarrhea or ribbon-shaped stools • Stools may be grossly bloody • Weakness and fatigue • Abdominal aching and dull cramps	Colon cancer
• Chronic bleeding with defecation • Painful defecation	Hemorrhoids
Nausea and vomiting	
• Nausea and vomiting follow or accompany abdominal pain • Pain progresses rapidly to severe, stabbing pain in the right lower quadrant (McBurney sign) • Abdominal rigidity and tenderness • Constipation or diarrhea • Tachycardia	Appendicitis
• Nausea and vomiting of undigested food • Diarrhea • Abdominal cramping • Hyperactive bowel sounds • Fever	Gastroenteritis

GI abnormalities *(continued)*

Sign or symptom and findings	Probable cause
• Nausea and vomiting • Headache with severe, constant, throbbing pain • Fatigue • Photophobia • Light flashes • Increased noise sensitivity	Migraine headache

Nausea and vomiting

Usually occurring together, nausea and vomiting can be caused by existing illnesses, such as myocardial infarction, gastric and peritoneal irritation, appendicitis, bowel obstruction, cholecystitis, acute pancreatitis, food poisoning and neurologic disturbances, or by some medications.

Dysphagia

Dysphagia, or difficulty swallowing, may be accompanied by weight loss. It can be caused by an obstruction, achalasia of the lower esophagogastric junction, or a neurologic disease, such as stroke or Parkinson disease. Dysphagia can lead to aspiration and pneumonia.

Skin color changes

A bluish umbilicus, called *Cullen sign*, indicates intra-abdominal hemorrhage. Areas of abdominal redness may indicate inflammation. Bruising on the flank, or Turner sign, indicates retroperitoneal hemorrhage. Dilated, tortuous, visible abdominal veins may indicate inferior vena cava obstruction. Cutaneous angiomas may signal liver disease.

Constipation

Constipation can be caused by dietary habits, dehydration, substance misuse, immobility, a sedentary lifestyle, or medications. The patient may report a dull ache in the abdomen, a full feeling, and hyperactive bowel sounds, which may be caused by irritable bowel syndrome. A patient with complete intestinal obstruction won't pass flatus or stool and won't have bowel sounds below the obstruction. Constipation occurs more commonly in older patients.

Diarrhea

Diarrhea may be caused by toxins, medications, food intolerance, food poisoning, or a GI condition such as Crohn disease. Cramping, abdominal tenderness, anorexia, and hyperactive bowel sounds may accompany diarrhea. If fever occurs, the diarrhea may be caused by a toxin.

Distention

Distention may occur with gas, a tumor, or a colon filled with feces. It may also be caused by an incisional hernia, which may protrude when the patient lifts their head and shoulders.

Abnormal bowel sounds

Hyperactive bowel sounds indicate increased intestinal motility and have many causes, including laxative use or misuse, gastroenteritis, and life-threatening intestinal obstruction. Hypoactive bowel sounds can be caused by recent bowel surgery, a full colon, or paralytic ileus. (See *Abnormal abdominal sounds*, page 308.)

Interpretation station

Abnormal abdominal sounds

The chart below lists abnormal abdominal sounds that you may encounter. The characteristics and location of a sound can help you determine its possible cause.

Sound and description	Location	Possible cause
Abnormal bowel sounds		
Hyperactive sounds (unrelated to hunger)	Any quadrant	Diarrhea, laxative use, or early intestinal obstruction
Hypoactive, then absent sounds	Any quadrant	Paralytic ileus or peritonitis

Abnormal abdominal sounds *(continued)*

Sound and description	Location	Possible cause
High-pitched tinkling sounds	Any quadrant	Intestinal fluid and air under tension in a dilated bowel
High-pitched rushing sounds coinciding with abdominal cramps	Any quadrant	Intestinal obstruction
Systolic bruits		
Vascular blowing sounds resembling cardiac murmurs	Over abdominal aorta	Partial arterial obstruction or turbulent blood flow
	Over renal artery	Renal artery stenosis
	Over iliac artery	Hepatomegaly
	Over femoral artery	Arterial insufficiency in the legs
Venous hum (rare)		
Continuous, medium-pitched tone created by blood flow in a large engorged vascular organ such as the liver	Epigastric and umbilical regions	Increased collateral circulation between portal and systemic venous systems, as in cirrhosis
Friction rub (rare)		
Harsh, grating sound like two pieces of sandpaper rubbing together	Over liver and spleen	Inflammation of the peritoneal surface of the liver (as from a tumor) or of the spleen (as from an infarct)

Friction rubs and abdominal bruits

Friction rubs over the liver and spleen in the epigastric region may indicate splenic infarction or hepatic tumor. Abdominal bruits may be caused by aortic aneurysms or partial arterial obstruction.

Abdominal pain

Abdominal pain may result from abdominal trauma, ulcers, intestinal obstruction, appendicitis, cholecystitis, peritonitis, or other inflammatory disorders. A duodenal ulcer can cause gnawing abdominal pain in the midepigastrium 1½ to 3 hours after the patient has eaten. The pain may awaken the patient and be relieved by antacids or food. (See *Types of abdominal pain* and *Abdominal pain origins*, page 310.)

Tender situation

Rebound tenderness can be caused by peritonitis or appendicitis. Appendicitis may be accompanied by increased abdominal wall resistance and guarding. Not all patients have the classic right lower

Types of abdominal pain

If your patient reports abdominal pain, ask them to describe the pain and ask how and when it started. This table will help you assess the pain and determine possible causes.

Type of pain	Possible cause
Burning	Peptic ulcer, gastroesophageal reflux disease
Cramping	Biliary colic, irritable bowel syndrome, diarrhea, constipation, flatulence
Severe cramping	Appendicitis, Crohn disease, diverticulitis
Stabbing	Pancreatitis, cholecystitis

Abdominal pain origins

What can you do to figure out which organ is affected if your patient has abdominal pain? Assess the location of the pain, and then look at this chart to get a quick idea of the most likely source of the pain.

Affected organ	Visceral pain	Parietal pain	Referred pain
Stomach	Midepigastrium	Midepigastrium and left upper quadrant	Shoulders
Small intestine	Periumbilical area	Over affected site	Midback (rare)
Appendix	Periumbilical area	Right lower quadrant	Right lower quadrant
Proximal colon	Periumbilical area and right flank for ascending colon	Over affected site	Right lower quadrant and back (rare)
Distal colon	Hypogastrium and left flank for descending colon	Over affected site	Left lower quadrant and back (rare)
Gallbladder	Midepigastrium	Right upper quadrant	Right subscapular area
Kidneys	Costovertebral angle	Over affected site	Groin; scrotum or labia
Pancreas	Midepigastrium and left upper quadrant	Midepigastrium and left upper quadrant	Back and left shoulder
Ovaries, fallopian tubes, and uterus	Hypogastrium and groin	Over affected site	Inner thighs

quadrant pain. Some older adults with appendicitis have less abdominal rigidity than younger patients.

Bloody stools

The passage of bloody stools, also known as *hematochezia,* usually indicates—and may be the first sign of—GI bleeding. It may also result from rectal trauma, colorectal cancer, colitis, Crohn disease, or an anal fissure or hemorrhoids.

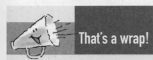

That's a wrap!

Gastrointestinal system review

Anatomy and physiology
- Ingestion and digestion of food
- Elimination of waste products

GI tract
- Mouth—responsible for chewing, salivation, and swallowing
- Pharynx—allows passage of food from the mouth to the esophagus
- Epiglottis—closes to protect the larynx when food is swallowed, preventing aspiration into the airway
- Esophagus—moves food from the pharynx to the stomach
- Stomach—serves as a reservoir for food and secretes gastric juices that aid in digestion
- Small intestine—consists of the duodenum, the jejunum, and the ileum; absorbs end products of digestion into the bloodstream and digests carbohydrates, fats, and proteins
- Large intestine—consists of the cecum; the ascending, transverse, descending, and sigmoid colons; the rectum; and the anus; responsible for

absorbing excess water and electrolytes, storing food residue, and eliminating waste products

Accessory organs
- Liver—metabolizes carbohydrates, fats, and proteins; detoxifies the blood; converts ammonia to urea; and synthesizes proteins and essential nutrients
- Gallbladder—stores bile from the liver until it's needed by the duodenum
- Pancreas—releases insulin and glycogen into the bloodstream; secretes pancreatic enzymes that aid digestion
- Bile ducts—serve as passageways for bile from the liver to the intestines
- Abdominal aorta—supplies blood to the GI tract

Health history
Ask the patient about:
- past GI illnesses, surgery, and trauma
- medications, including laxative, enema, and suppository use

- current GI signs or symptoms
- family medical history, especially history of ulcerative colitis, colorectal cancer, peptic ulcers, and gastric cancer
- diet, exercise patterns, and alcohol, caffeine, and tobacco use.

Assessment
Mouth
- Inspect the mouth and jaw as well as the inner and outer lips, teeth, gums, and oral mucosa.
- Inspect the tongue.
- Palpate for areas of tenderness or lesions.

Abdomen
- Inspect the abdomen for color, symmetry, shape, and contour.
- Note abdominal movements and pulsations.
- Auscultate in each of the four abdominal quadrants to assess bowel sounds and over the abdominal arteries to check for bruits, venous hums, and friction rubs.

(Continued)

Gastrointestinal system review *(continued)*

• Percuss the abdomen, listening for tympany over hollow organs (such as an empty stomach or intestine) and for dullness over solid organs (such as the liver) or feces-filled intestines.
• Palpate in all four quadrants of the abdomen, leaving painful areas for last.
• Check for rebound tenderness if you suspect peritoneal inflammation; also check for ascites, a large accumulation of fluid in the peritoneal cavity.

Rectum and anus
• Inspect the perianal area.
• Palpate the rectum using a water-soluble lubricant on your gloved index finger.

Abnormal findings
• Nausea and vomiting—may be caused by existing illness or by certain medications
• Dysphagia—difficulty swallowing; has various causes; may lead to aspiration and pneumonia
• Cullen sign—a bluish umbilicus; indicates intra-abdominal hemorrhage
• Turner sign—bruising on the flank; indicates retroperitoneal hemorrhage
• Constipation—may cause a dull abdominal ache, a full feeling, and hyperactive bowel sounds
• Diarrhea—may cause cramping, abdominal tenderness, anorexia, and hyperactive bowel sounds

• Abdominal distention—may occur with gas, a tumor, or a colon filled with feces
• Abnormal bowel sounds—may be hyperactive (indicating increased intestinal motility), hypoactive, or absent
• Friction rubs—may indicate splenic infarction or hepatic tumor
• Abdominal pain—may result from abdominal trauma, ulcers, intestinal obstruction, appendicitis, cholecystitis, peritonitis, or other inflammatory disorders

Quick quiz

1. The nurse is performing an abdominal assessment and inspects the skin of the abdomen. The nurse performs which assessment technique next?
    A. Palpates the abdomen for size
    B. Palpates the liver at the right rib margin
    C. Listens to bowel sounds in all four quadrants
    D. Percusses the right lower abdominal quadrant

Answer: C. After visual examination, and prior to any palpation or percussion, bowel sounds should be assessed.

2. What is the name of the action the GI tract uses to propel food?
    A. Digestion
    B. Peristalsis
    C. Swallowing
    D. Metabolizing

Answer: B. Peristalsis is the wavelike movements of the muscles of the GI tract as it moves food for digestion.

3. A patient reports a gnawing, burning pain in the midepigastric area that is aggravated by bending over or lying down. Which additional question does the nurse ask as part of a symptom analysis?
    A. "Do you have a family history of this type of pain?"
    B. "How long ago did you eat?"
    C. "Is the pain worse after eating or when your stomach is empty?"
    D. "Have you noticed any yellow coloring in your eyes or on your skin?"

Answer: C. Burning can indicate gastroesophageal reflux.

4. During visual assessment of the abdomen, the nurse notices a bluish tinge around the patient's umbilicus. This indicates what?
    A. Intra-abdominal hemorrhage
    B. Hypothermia
    C. Ascites
    D. Constipation

Answer: A. A bluish umbilicus, also known as Cullen sign, means a patient is bleeding in the abdomen.

Scoring

★★★ If you answered all four questions correctly, congratulations! You effectively digested an abundance of facts concerning GI assessments.

★★ If you answered three questions correctly, super! Your ability to chew up the information in this chapter is truly impressive!

★ If you answered fewer than three questions correctly, that's okay! All the information on GI assessments may have been a lot to swallow in one sitting. Why not go over it again?

Just for Fun

Label structures found in each quadrant using word bank below.

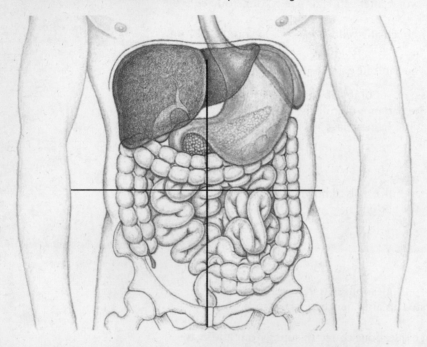

Word bank: portion of descending colon, right lobe of liver, left lobe of liver, gallbladder, duodenum, head of pancreas, hepatic flexure of the colon, portions of ascending and transverse colon, cecum, appendix, stomach, splenic flexure of colon, portions of descending and transverse colon, sigmoid colon, portion of ascending colon

Answers:
RLQ—cecum, appendix, portion of ascending colon
LLQ—sigmoid colon, portion of descending colon
RUQ—right lobe of liver, gallbladder, pylorus, duodenum, head of pancreas, hepatic flexure of colon, portions of ascending and transverse colon
LUQ—left lobe of liver, stomach, body of pancreas, splenic flexure of colon, portions of transverse and descending colon

Chapter 13

Female genitourinary system

Just the facts

In this chapter, you'll learn:

♦ organs and structures that make up the female genitourinary (GU) system

♦ questions to ask during a patient history of the female GU system

♦ techniques for performing a physical assessment of the female GU system

♦ causes and characteristics of female GU system abnormalities.

♦ pregnancy anatomy and assessment during prepartum, intrapartum, and postpartum

♦ abnormal pregnancy findings.

**In this chapter: Female = People assigned female at birth. Male = People assigned male at birth.

A look at the female GU system

The female genitourinary (GU) system encompasses the urinary tract and the reproductive organs and structures. Disorders of this system can have wide-ranging effects on other body systems. For example, ovarian dysfunction can alter hormonal balance. Kidney dysfunction can alter blood pressure, disrupt serum electrolytes, and affect production of the hormone erythropoietin, which regulates the production of red blood cells.

Subtle signs and symptoms

Assessing the female GU system can be a challenging task. Many patients with urinary disorders don't realize they're ill because they have only mild signs and symptoms or no symptoms at all. It's easy to overlook underlying problems.

It's complicated...

More female patients seek health care for reproductive disorders than for anything else. Assessing those problems can be difficult because the reproductive system is complex and its functions have far-reaching psychosocial implications.

Anatomy and physiology

To perform an accurate assessment, you'll need to have a firm grasp of the anatomy and physiology of the GU system. This section reviews the urinary system and the reproductive system.

Urinary system

The urinary system consists of the kidneys, ureters, bladder, and urethra. (See *A close look at the urinary system.*)

Kidneys

The essential functions of the urinary system—such as forming urine and maintaining the proper balance of fluids, minerals, and organic substances for homeostasis—take place in the highly vascular kidneys. Each kidney is approximately 4″ (10 cm) long, 2″ to 2½″ (5 to 6 cm) wide, and 1″ to 1½″ (2.5 to 4 cm) thick. Located retroperitoneally on either side of the lumbar vertebrae, the kidneys lie behind the abdominal organs and in front of the muscles attached to the vertebral column. The peritoneal fat layer protects them.

Two's a crowd
The right kidney is slightly lower than the left; it's displaced downward by the overlying liver. Each kidney contains roughly one million nephrons. Urine gathers in the collecting tubules and ducts of the nephrons and eventually drains into the ureters, down into the bladder and, when urination occurs, out through the urethra.

Ureters

The ureters are 10″ to 12″ (25.5 to 30.5 cm) long. The left ureter is slightly longer than the right because of the left kidney's higher position. The diameter of each ureter varies from ⅛″ to ¼″ (3 to 6.5 mm), with the narrowest part at the ureteropelvic junction.

The rhythm of the flow
Located along the posterior abdominal wall, the ureters enter the bladder anteromedially. They carry urine from the kidneys to the bladder by peristaltic contractions that occur one to five times per minute.

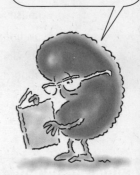

Says here I'm shaped like a kidney bean. So that's why they call them kidney beans…

A close look at the urinary system

This illustration shows the main structures of the urinary system.

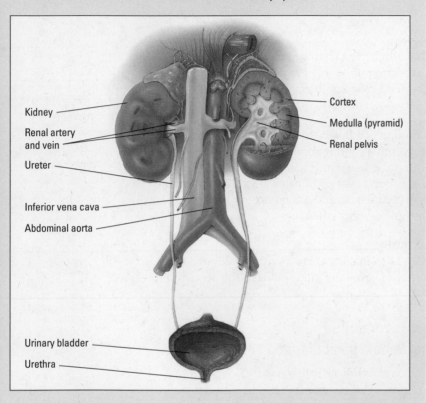

Kidney

Renal artery and vein

Ureter

Inferior vena cava

Abdominal aorta

Cortex

Medulla (pyramid)

Renal pelvis

Urinary bladder

Urethra

Bladder

Located in the pelvis, the bladder is a hollow, muscular organ that serves as a container for urine collection. The bladder lies directly behind the symphysis, the connecting point for pelvic bone structures. Bladder capacity ranges from 500 to 1,000 mL in healthy adults. The bladders of children and older people have a lower capacity.

Urethra

The urethra is a small duct that carries urine from the bladder to the outside of the body. The female urethra is only 1″ to 1½″ (2.5 to 4 cm) long and anterior to the vaginal opening.

Reproductive system

The female reproductive system consists of external and internal genitalia. Let's start with external genitalia.

External genitalia

The external genitalia, collectively called the *vulva*, consist of the mons pubis, labia majora, labia minora, clitoris, vagina, urethra, and Skene and Bartholin glands. (See *A close look at external female genitalia*.)

Mons pubis

The mons pubis is a mound of adipose tissue overlying the symphysis pubis. It protects the symphysis during coitus (sexual intercourse). In adults, it's covered with pubic hair. Pubic hair usually first appears at age 10½. It may become sparse after menopause because of hormonal changes. People of Native American and Asian ancestry usually have less pubic hair than people of other ethnicities.

Labia majora and minora

The outer vulval lips, or labia majora, are two vertical folds of adipose tissue that extend posteriorly from the mons pubis to the perineum.

A close look at external female genitalia

This illustration shows the main parts of the external female genitalia.

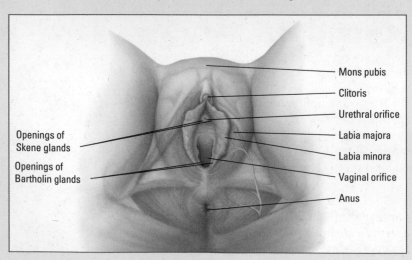

- Mons pubis
- Clitoris
- Urethral orifice
- Labia majora
- Labia minora
- Vaginal orifice
- Anus
- Openings of Skene glands
- Openings of Bartholin glands

The labia majora surround two thinner vertical folds of reddish epithelium called the labia minora.

The anterior labia minora form the prepuce and the frenulum (a fold connecting the under surface of the clitoris with the labia minora).

Clitoris, vestibule, and urethral opening

The clitoris is a small, cylindrical organ composed of erectile tissue and lies between the labia minora at the top of the vestibule, which contains the urethral and vaginal openings. The urethral orifice is a small opening below the clitoris.

Vaginal opening and perineum

The vaginal opening, or introitus, is posterior to the urethral orifice. This opening is narrow and vertical in people who have intact hymens (the thin fold of mucous membrane that partially covers the vaginal opening). The opening is larger with irregular edges in those whose hymens have been perforated. In some female patients, the hymen is absent.

The perineum is the area bordered anteriorly by the top of the labial fold and posteriorly by the anus.

Skene and Bartholin glands

Two kinds of glands have ducts that open into the vulva. Skene glands are tiny structures just below the urethra, each containing 6 to 31 ducts. Bartholin glands are found posterior to the vaginal opening. Neither of these glands can be seen, but they can be palpated if enlarged.

Fluid generators

Skene and Bartholin glands produce lubricating fluids important for the reproductive process. They can become infected, usually with organisms known to cause sexually transmitted infections (STIs).

Internal genitalia

The internal genitalia include the vagina, uterus, ovaries, and fallopian tubes. (See *A close look at internal female genitalia*, page 320.)

Vagina

A pink, hollow, collapsed tube, the vagina is located between the urethra and the rectum, extending up and back from the vulva to the uterus. It's the route of passage for childbirth and menstruation.

A close look at internal female genitalia

These illustrations show the main internal structures of the female reproductive system.

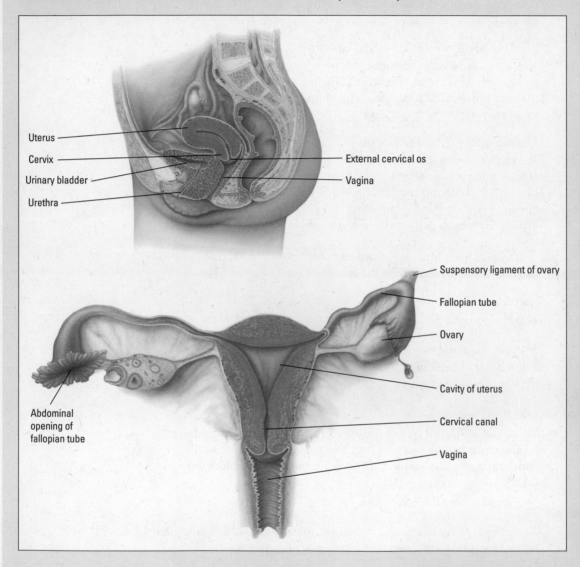

Uterus

Cervix

Urinary bladder

Urethra

External cervical os

Vagina

Suspensory ligament of ovary

Fallopian tube

Ovary

Cavity of uterus

Abdominal opening of fallopian tube

Cervical canal

Vagina

Uterus

The uterus is a hollow, pear-shaped, muscular organ that lies between the rectum and the bladder. It's divided into the fundus (the upper portion of the uterus) and the cervix, which protrudes into the vagina. The cervix contains mucus-secreting glands that help in reproduction and protect the uterus from pathogens. The function of the uterus is to nurture the fetus during pregnancy and then expel the fetus during labor.

Locations may vary

The position of the uterus in the pelvic cavity may vary, depending on bladder fullness. The uterus may also tilt in different directions.

Ovaries

A pair of oval glands about 1¼″ (3 cm) long, the ovaries are usually found in the lower abdominal cavity, one on each side of the uterus. They produce ova (eggs) and release the hormones estrogen and progesterone. The ovaries become fully developed after puberty and shrink after menopause.

Fallopian tubes

Each approximately 4″ (10 cm) long, the two fallopian tubes extend from the ovaries into the upper portion of the uterus. Their funnel-shaped ends curve toward the ovaries and, during ovulation, help guide the ova to the uterus after expulsion from the ovaries. The fallopian tube is also the usual site of fertilization of the ova by the sperm.

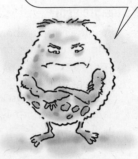

The cervix's mucus-secreting glands protect the uterus from pathogens. I'm not happy about that.

Obtaining a health history

Because the urinary and reproductive systems are located so close together in female patients, you and your patient may have trouble differentiating signs and symptoms. Even if the patient's reported symptom seems minor, investigate it. Ask about its onset, duration, and severity and ask about measures taken to treat it. The information you gain will help you formulate a more appropriate care plan.

Asking about the urinary system

The most common complaints of the urinary system include output changes, such as polyuria, oliguria, and anuria; voiding pattern changes, such as hesitancy, frequency, urgency, nocturia, and incontinence; urine color changes; and pain that may occur in the abdomen, in the flank, or while urinating.

Dredging up the past

Past illnesses and pre-existing conditions can affect a patient's urinary tract health. For example, has the patient ever had a urinary tract infection (UTI), kidney trauma, or kidney stones? Kidney stones or trauma can alter the structure and function of the kidneys and bladder. Also ask about any surgery involving the urinary tract.

What's the problem?

Ask the patient about current problems and medications, as patients taking immunosuppressing medications can be at an increased risk for frequent UTIs. Does the patient have diabetes, cardiovascular disease, or hypertension? Patients with diabetes have an increased risk of UTIs. Cardiovascular disease can alter kidney perfusion. Hypertension can contribute to kidney failure and nephropathy.

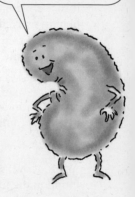

Remember, kidney stones affect female patients, too!

The urination situation

Has the patient noticed a change in the amount, color, or odor of their urine? Is there pain or burning during urination? Do they have problems with incontinence or urinary frequency? Are there any allergies to foods or medications? Allergic reactions can cause tubular damage. A severe anaphylactic reaction can cause temporary renal failure and permanent tubular necrosis.

Discuss drugs

Make a list of all the prescribed medications, herbal preparations, and over-the-counter drugs the patient takes. Some drugs can affect the appearance of urine; nephrotoxic drugs can alter urinary function.

Familial factors

Also ask about the patient's family history to get information about their risk of developing kidney failure or kidney disease.

Asking about the reproductive system

The most common reproductive system symptoms patients report are abdominal pain, vaginal discharge, abnormal uterine bleeding, vaginal pruritus, and infertility. To obtain the most complete data about these problems, focus on the patient's current complaints, and then explore their reproductive, sexual-social, and family history. Ask them to describe the symptoms in their own words, encouraging open communication about the symptoms.

Ease into it

Many patients feel uncomfortable answering questions about their sexual health or reproductive system. Start with the less personal questions to help establish a rapport.

Go with the flow

Start by asking the patient about their menstrual cycle. How old were they when they began to menstruate? How long does their menses usually last? How often does it occur? The typical cycle for menstruation is one menses every 21 to 35 days. The typical duration is 2 to 8 days.

Does the patient have cramps, spotting, or an unusually heavy or light blood flow? Spotting between menses, or metrorrhagia, may be normal in patients taking low-dose hormonal contraceptives or progesterone; otherwise, spotting may indicate infection, cancer, or other abnormality.

Menses generally starts by age 12½ and could occur as early as age 8. If it hasn't and if no secondary sex characteristics have developed, the patient should be evaluated by a doctor.

The sexual side

When the patient seems comfortable, ask about their sexual practices, the number of sexual partners they currently have, whether they experience pain with intercourse, if they have ever had an STI, and their human immunodeficiency virus (HIV) status. If the patient is sexually active, ask about the type of birth control they use, when their last Papanicolaou (Pap) test was performed, and what the results were. Finally, ask if they have questions or concerns about sexual development or practices. If the patient is sexually active, talk about the importance of safe sex and the prevention of STIs.

Past, present, and possible pregnancy

Ask if the patient has ever been pregnant or had problems with infertility. Ask how many times they have been pregnant and how many times they have given birth. Have they had any miscarriages or therapeutic abortions? Did they have a vaginal or cesarean delivery? Did they experience any complications before or after delivery?

Pause to reflect

If your patient is postmenopausal, ask for the date of their last normal menses. To find out more about their menopausal symptoms, ask if they are having hot flashes, night sweats, mood swings, flushing, vaginal dryness or itching, or changing sleep patterns.

Assessing the female GU system

To perform a physical assessment of the GU system, you'll use the techniques of inspection, percussion, and palpation.

Examining the urinary system

Before assessing specific structures of the urinary system, evaluate your patient's vital signs, weight, and mental status. These observations can provide clues about renal dysfunction.

For example, a patient's vital signs might reveal hypertension, which can either cause renal dysfunction if it's uncontrolled or actually stem from renal dysfunction. Be sure to check the blood pressure in each arm. Weighing the patient can provide information about fluid status and is important for patients with urinary disorders or renal failure, especially those receiving dialysis. If your patient has known or suspected renal dysfunction, you may also want to ask if they have noticed any extremity swelling or increased shortness of breath. This could warrant some further investigation into their renal function.

Catch the clues

Observing the patient's behavior can give you clues about their mental status. Do they have trouble concentrating, have memory loss, or seem disoriented? Kidney dysfunction can cause those symptoms. Progressive, chronic kidney failure can cause lethargy, confusion, disorientation, stupor, seizures, and coma.

Inspection

First, observe the color and shape of the area around the kidneys and bladder. The skin should be free from lesions, discolorations, inflammation, and swelling.

Percussion

Kidney percussion checks for costovertebral angle tenderness that occurs with inflammation. To percuss over the kidneys, have the patient sit up. Place the ball of your nondominant hand on her back at the costovertebral angle of the 12th rib. Strike the ball of that hand with the ulnar surface of your other hand. Use just enough force to cause a painless but perceptible thud. (See *A close look at percussing the kidneys*.)

A close look at percussing the kidneys

The image below illustrates the proper technique to percuss a patient's kidneys.

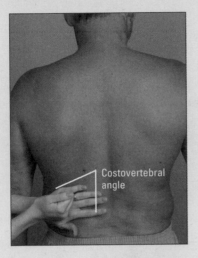

Costovertebral angle

The bladder matters

To percuss the bladder, first ask the patient to empty it. Then have the patient lie in the supine position. Start at the symphysis pubis and percuss upward toward the bladder and over it. You should hear tympany. A dull sound signals retained urine.

Palpation

Because the kidneys lie behind other organs and are protected by muscle, they normally aren't palpable unless they're enlarged. However, in very thin patients, you may be able to feel the lower end of the right kidney as a smooth round mass that drops on inspiration. (See *Palpating the kidneys*.)

In older patients, you may be able to palpate both kidneys because of decreased muscle tone and elasticity. If the kidneys feel enlarged, the patient may have hydronephrosis, cysts, or tumors.

If the bladder is full, you'll feel it

You won't be able to palpate the bladder unless it's distended. With the patient in a supine position, use the fingers of one hand to palpate the lower abdomen in a light dipping motion. A distended bladder will feel firm and relatively smooth, extending above the symphysis pubis. If the patient is 12 or more weeks pregnant, you might actually be feeling the fundus of the uterus, palpable just above the symphysis pubis.

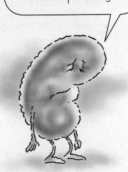

Enlarged kidneys may indicate hydronephrosis, cysts, or tumors. How depressing.

Palpating the kidneys

To palpate the kidneys, first have the patient lie in a supine position. To palpate the right kidney, stand on their right side. Place your left hand under their back and your right hand on their abdomen.

Instruct the patient to inhale deeply, so their kidney moves downward. As they inhale, press up with your left hand and down with your right, as shown at right.

To palpate the left kidney, reach across the patient's abdomen, placing your left hand behind their left flank. Place your right hand over the area of the left kidney. Ask the patient to inhale deeply again. As they do so, pull up with your left hand and press down with your right.

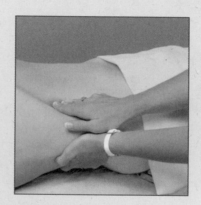

Handle with care

Examining the reproductive system

Before the examination, ask the patient to void to prevent discomfort and inaccurate findings during palpation. Have them disrobe and put on an examination gown. Help the patient into the dorsal lithotomy position, and drape all areas not being examined. Make sure you explain the procedure before the examination.

You'll begin by examining the external genitalia, followed by the internal genitalia.

Inspecting the external genitalia

First, put on a pair of gloves. Spread the labia and locate the urethral meatus. It should be a pink, irregular, small opening at the midline, just above the vagina. Note the presence of discharge (a sign of urethral infection) or ulcerations (a sign of an STI). Inspect the external genitalia and pubic hair to assess sexual maturity. (See *Pubic hair development*.)

Pubic hair development

Pubic hair changes in density, color, and texture throughout a female patient's life. Before adolescence, the pubic area is covered only with body hair. In adolescence, this body hair grows thicker, darker, coarser, and curlier. In full maturity, it spreads over the symphysis pubis and inner thighs. In later years, the hair grows thin, gray, and brittle.

A look at the labia

Using your index finger and thumb, gently spread the labia majora and minora. They should be moist and free from lesions. You may detect a normal discharge that varies from clear and stretchy before ovulation to white and opaque after ovulation. The discharge should be odorless and nonirritating to the mucosa. Atypical appearance and odor may indicate vaginitis. (See *Vaginitis and abnormal discharge.*)

Vaginitis and abnormal discharge

Vaginitis usually results from an overgrowth of infectious organisms. It causes redness, itching, dyspareunia (painful intercourse), dysuria, and a malodorous discharge. Vaginitis occurs with bacterial vaginosis, *Candida albicans* infection (a fungal infection), trichomoniasis, and mucopurulent cervicitis.

Bacterial vaginosis
• Produces thin, grayish white discharge with fishy odor

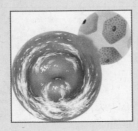

Mucopurulent cervicitis
• Produces purulent yellow discharge from the cervical os
• Occurs with chlamydia and gonorrhea

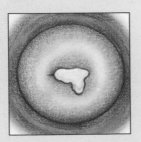

C. albicans infection
• Produces thick, white, curdlike discharge with a yeast-like odor
• Appears in patches on the cervix and vaginal walls

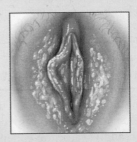

Trichomoniasis
• May produce a malodorous yellow or green, frothy or watery, foul-smelling discharge
• May also involve red papules on the cervix and vaginal walls, giving the tissue a "strawberry" appearance

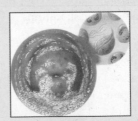

View the vestibule

Examine the vestibule, especially the area around the Bartholin and Skene glands. Check for swelling, redness, lesions, discharge, and unusual odor. If you detect any of these conditions, notify the doctor and obtain a specimen for culture. Finally, inspect the vaginal opening, noting whether the hymen is intact or perforated.

Palpating the external genitalia

Spread the labia with one hand and palpate with the other. The labia should feel soft and the patient shouldn't feel any pain. Note swelling, hardness, or tenderness. If you detect a mass or lesion, palpate it to determine its size, shape, and consistency.

A gentle touch

If you find swelling or tenderness, see if you can palpate Bartholin glands, which normally aren't palpable. (See *Palpating Bartholin glands*.)

Under fire

If the urethra is inflamed, milk it and the area of Skene glands. First, moisten your gloved index finger with water. Then separate the labia with your other hand, and insert your index finger about 1¼″ (3 cm) into the anterior vagina. With the pad of your finger, gently press and pull outward. Continue palpating down to the introitus. This procedure shouldn't cause the patient discomfort. Culture the discharge.

Inspecting the internal genitalia

Nurses don't routinely inspect internal genitalia unless they're in advanced practice. However, you may be asked to assist with this examination. To start, select an appropriate speculum for your patient. (See *Speculum types*.) If your patient is young or is small, you may need a pediatric speculum.

Warm welcome

Hold the speculum under warm, running water to lubricate and warm the blades. Don't use other lubricants; many of them are bacteriostatic and can alter Pap test results.

Talk about it

Sit or stand at the foot of the examination table. Tell the patient they'll feel internal pressure and possibly some slight, transient discomfort as you insert and open the speculum.

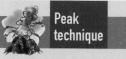

Peak technique

Palpating Bartholin glands

To palpate Bartholin glands, insert your gloved index finger carefully into the patient's posterior introitus, as shown. Then place your thumb along the lateral edge of the swollen or tender labium and gently squeeze the labium. If discharge from the duct results, culture it.

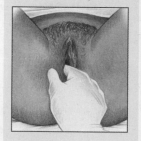

Speculum types

Specula come in various shapes and sizes. Choose an appropriate one for your patient. A Graves speculum is usually used. However, if the patient has an intact hymen, has never given birth through the vaginal canal, or has a contracted introitus from menopause, use a Pederson speculum, which has narrower blades. The illustrations here show the parts of a typical speculum and three types of specula available.

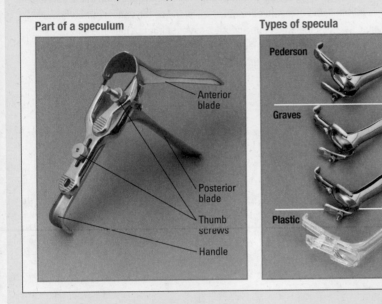

Part of a speculum

- Anterior blade
- Posterior blade
- Thumb screws
- Handle

Types of specula

- Pederson
- Graves
- Plastic

Just relax

Using your dominant hand, hold the speculum by the base with the blades anchored between your index and middle fingers. This causes less discomfort and keeps the blades from accidentally opening during insertion. Encourage the patient to take slow, deep breaths during insertion to relax the abdominal muscles. (See *Inserting a speculum.*)

A look inside

After inserting the speculum, observe the color, texture, and integrity of the vaginal lining. A thin, white, odorless discharge on the vaginal walls is normal. Using the thumb of the hand holding the speculum, press the lower lever to open the blades. Lock them in the open position by tightening the thumb screw above the lever.

Inserting a speculum

Initial insertion
Place the index and middle fingers of your nondominant hand about 1" (2.5 cm) into the vagina and spread the fingers to exert pressure on the posterior vagina. Hold the speculum in your dominant hand, and insert the blades between your fingers, as shown below.

Deeper insertion
Ask the patient to bear down to open the introitus and relax the perineal muscles. Point the speculum slightly downward, and insert the blades until the base of the speculum touches your fingers, inside the vagina.

Rotate and open
Rotate the speculum in the same plane as the vagina, and withdraw your fingers. Open the blades as far as possible and lock them. You should now be able to view the cervix clearly.

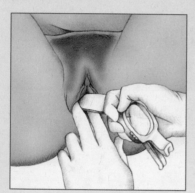
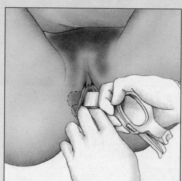
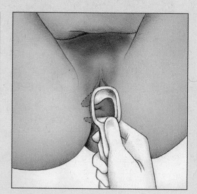

The typical view
Examine the cervix for color, shape, and dilation of the os; erosions; nodules; masses; discharge; and bleeding. It should be smooth and round. The central cervical opening, or cervical os, is circular in a patient who hasn't given birth vaginally and a horizontal slit in a patient who has. Expect to see a clear, watery cervical discharge during ovulation and a slightly bloody discharge just before menstruation. (See *The normal os*.)

Obtain a specimen for a Pap test if needed. Then, unlock and close the blades and withdraw the speculum.

Palpating the internal genitalia
To palpate the internal genitalia, lubricate the index and middle fingers of your gloved dominant hand. Stand at the foot of the

examination table and position the hand for insertion into the vagina by extending your thumb and index and middle fingers and curling your ring and little finger toward your palm.

Use the thumb and index finger of your other hand to spread the labia majora. Insert your two lubricated fingers into the vagina, exerting pressure posteriorly to avoid irritating the anterior wall and urethra.

Probing the issue

When your fingers are fully inserted, note tenderness or nodularity in the vaginal wall. Ask the patient to bear down so you can assess the support of the vaginal outlet. Bulging of the vaginal wall may indicate a cystocele or a rectocele.

Making a clean sweep

To palpate the cervix, lubricate the index and middle fingers of your gloved dominant hand, and then sweep your fingers from side to side across the cervix and around the os. The cervix should be smooth and firm and protrude ¼″ to 1¼″ (0.5 to 3 cm) into the vagina. If you palpate nodules or irregularities, the patient may have cysts, tumors, or other lesions.

Moving right along

Next, place your fingers into the recessed area around the cervix. The cervix should move in all directions. If the patient reports pain during this part of the examination, they may have inflammation of the uterus or adnexa (ovaries, fallopian tubes, and ligaments of the uterus).

Two hands are better than one

A bimanual examination allows you to palpate the uterus and ovaries. Usually, only nurses in advanced practice perform bimanual palpation. (See *Performing a bimanual examination.*)

The last step

Rectovaginal palpation, the last step in a genital assessment, examines the posterior part of the uterus and the pelvic cavity. Warn the patient that this procedure may be uncomfortable. (See *Performing a rectovaginal examination*, page 332.)

To begin, put on a new pair of gloves and apply water-soluble lubricant to the index and middle fingers of your dominant hand. Instruct the patient to bear down with her vaginal and rectal muscles; then insert your index finger a short way into her vagina and your middle finger into her rectum.

The normal os

These illustrations show the difference between the os of a patient who has never given birth vaginally (is nulliparous) and the os of a patient who has (is parous).

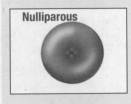

Nulliparous

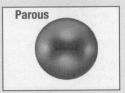

Parous

Performing a bimanual examination

During a bimanual examination, palpate the uterus and ovaries from the inside and the outside simultaneously. The illustrations here show how to perform such an examination.

1. Proper position

After putting on gloves, place the index and middle fingers of your dominant hand in the patient's vagina and move them up to the cervix. Place the fingers of your other hand on the patient's abdomen between the umbilicus and the symphysis pubis, as shown at right.

Elevate the cervix and uterus by pressing upward with the two fingers inside the vagina. At the same time, press down and in with the hand on the abdomen. Try to grasp the uterus between your hands.

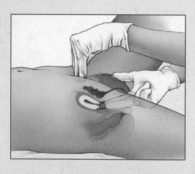

2. Note the position

Next, move your fingers into the posterior fornix, pressing upward and forward to bring the anterior uterine wall up to your nondominant hand. Use your dominant hand to palpate the lower portion of the uterine wall, as shown at right. Note the position of the uterus.

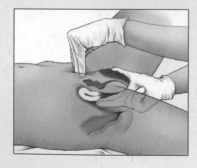

3. Palpate the walls

Slide your fingers farther into the anterior section of the fornix, the space between the uterus and cervix. You should feel part of the posterior uterine wall with this hand. You should feel part of the anterior uterine wall with the fingertips of your nondominant hand. Note the size, shape, surface characteristics, consistency, and mobility of the uterus as well as tenderness.

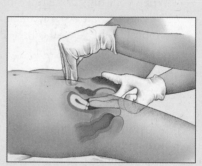

4. Palpate the ovaries

After palpating the anterior and posterior walls of the uterus, move your nondominant hand toward the right lower quadrant of the abdomen. Slip the fingers of your dominant hand into the right fornix and palpate the right ovary. Then palpate the left ovary. Note the size, shape, and contour of each ovary. The ovaries may not be palpable in patients who aren't relaxed or who are obese. They shouldn't be palpable in postmenopausal patients. Remove your hand from the patient's abdomen and your fingers from the vagina.

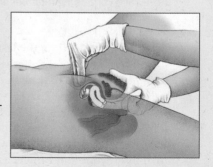

Peak technique

Performing a rectovaginal examination

To perform a rectovaginal examination, begin by putting on a pair of gloves and applying water-soluble lubricant to the index and middle fingers of your dominant hand. Then instruct the patient to bear down with the vaginal and rectal muscles and insert your index finger a short way into the vagina and your middle finger into the rectum. Use your middle finger to assess rectal muscle and sphincter tone.

Next, insert your middle finger deeper into the rectum and palpate the rectal wall. Sweep the rectum with your finger, assessing for masses or nodules, and palpate the posterior wall of the uterus through the anterior wall of the rectum, evaluating the uterus for size, shape, tenderness, and masses. The rectovaginal septum (the wall between the rectum and vagina) should feel smooth and springy.

Place your nondominant hand on the patient's abdomen at the symphysis pubis. With your index finger in the vagina, palpate deeply to feel the posterior edge of the cervix and the lower posterior wall of the uterus. If stool testing for occult blood is ordered, put on a new glove and apply water-soluble lubricant to your gloved index finger. Slide

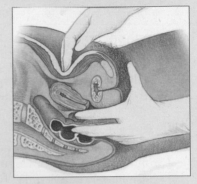

your index finger into the patient's anus to obtain a small stool sample. Withdraw your finger and test the stool for occult blood using a guaiac test. When you're finished, discard the gloves and wash your hands.

Testing the tone

Use your middle finger to assess rectal muscle and sphincter tone. Insert your finger deeper into the rectum, and palpate the rectal wall with your middle finger. Sweep the rectum with your finger, assessing for masses or nodules.

Palpate the posterior wall of the uterus through the anterior wall of the rectum, evaluating the uterus for size, shape, tenderness, and masses. The rectovaginal septum, the wall between the rectum and the vagina, should feel smooth and springy.

On the edge of discovery

Place your nondominant hand on the patient's abdomen at the symphysis pubis. With your index finger in the vagina, palpate deeply to feel the posterior edge of the cervix and the lower posterior wall of the uterus.

When you're finished, discard the gloves and wash your hands. Help the patient to a sitting position, and provide privacy for dressing and personal hygiene.

Abnormal findings

This section discusses common abnormalities of the GU system. (See *Female GU abnormalities*.)

Urinary abnormalities

Common abnormal findings in the female urinary system include polyuria; hematuria; urinary frequency, urgency, and hesitancy; nocturia; urinary incontinence; and dysuria.

Polyuria

A fairly common finding, polyuria is the production and excretion of more than 3,000 mL of urine daily. It usually results from diabetes insipidus, hypercalcemia, diabetes mellitus, or diuretic use.

Plenty of polyuria causes

Other causes of polyuria include psychological, neurologic, or renal disorders. Urologic disorders, such as pyelonephritis and obstructive uropathy, can also cause polyuria. Patients with polyuria are at risk for developing hypovolemia.

Hematuria

Hematuria, the presence of blood in the urine, causes dark brownish gold or bright red urine. The timing of hematuria suggests the location of the underlying problem. Bleeding at the start of urination is caused by a disorder of the urethra; bleeding at the end of urination signifies a disorder of the bladder neck.

Above or below the neck

Bleeding that occurs throughout urination indicates a disorder located above the bladder neck. Hematuria can also be caused by GI, vaginal, or certain coagulation disorders.

Urinary frequency, urgency, and hesitancy

Urinary frequency, abnormally frequent urination, commonly results from decreased bladder capacity and is a classic symptom of a UTI. Frequency also occurs with urethral stricture, neurologic disorders, pregnancy, and uterine tumors.

It's a pain

In many cases, the sudden urge to urinate, or urinary urgency, is accompanied by bladder pain and is another symptom of a UTI. Even small amounts of urine in the bladder can cause pain because inflammation

Interpretation station

Female GU abnormalities

This chart shows some common groups of findings for disorders of the female genitourinary (GU) system, along with their probable causes.

Sign or symptom and findings	Probable cause
Dysmenorrhea	
• Steady, aching pain that begins before menses and peaks at the height of menstrual flow; may occur between menses • Pain may radiate to the perineum or rectum • Premenstrual spotting • Dyspareunia • Infertility • Nausea and vomiting • Tender, fixed adnexal mass palpable on bimanual examination	Endometriosis
• Severe abdominal pain • Fever • Malaise • Foul-smelling, purulent vaginal discharge • Menorrhagia • Cervical motion tenderness and bilateral adnexal tenderness on pelvic examination	Pelvic inflammatory disease
• Cramping pain that begins with menstrual flow and diminishes with decreasing flow • Abdominal bloating • Breast tenderness • Depression • Irritability • Headache • Diarrhea	Premenstrual syndrome

Sign or symptom and findings	Probable cause
Dysuria	
• Urinary frequency • Nocturia • Straining to void • Hematuria • Perineal or low-back pain • Fatigue • Low-grade fever	Cystitis
• Dysuria throughout voiding • Bladder distention • Diminished urinary stream • Urinary frequency and urgency • Sensation of bloating or fullness in the lower abdomen or groin	Urinary system obstruction
• Urinary urgency • Hematuria • Bladder spasms • Feeling of warmth or burning during urination	Urinary tract infection
Urinary incontinence	
• Urge or overflow incontinence • Hematuria • Dysuria • Nocturia • Urinary frequency • Suprapubic pain from bladder spasms • Palpable mass on bimanual examination	Bladder cancer

(Continued)

Female GU abnormalities *(continued)*

Sign or symptom and findings	Probable cause	Sign or symptom and findings	Probable cause
• Overflow incontinence • Painless bladder distention • Episodic diarrhea or constipation • Orthostatic hypotension • Syncope • Dysphagia	Diabetic neuropathy	• Yellow, mucopurulent, odorless, or acrid discharge • Dysuria • Dyspareunia • Vaginal bleeding after douching or coitus	Chlamydia infection
• Urinary urgency and frequency • Visual problems • Sensory impairment • Constipation • Muscle weakness • Emotional lability	Multiple sclerosis	• Yellow or green, foul-smelling discharge that can be expressed from the Bartholin or Skene ducts • Dysuria • Urinary frequency and incontinence • Vaginal redness and swelling	Gonorrhea
Vaginal discharge			
• Profuse, white, curdlike discharge with a yeasty, sweet odor • Exudate may be lightly attached to the labia and vaginal walls • Vulvar redness and edema • Intense labial itching and burning • External dysuria	Candidiasis		

decreases bladder capacity. Urgency without pain may be a symptom of an upper motor neuron lesion that affects bladder control.

Trouble starting up

Difficulty starting a urine stream, or urinary hesitancy, can occur with a UTI, a partial obstruction of the lower urinary tract, neuromuscular disorders, or the use of certain drugs.

Nocturia

Excessive urination at night, or nocturia, is a common sign of kidney or lower urinary tract disorders. It can result from a disruption of normal urination patterns or from overstimulation of the nerves and muscles that control urination. It may also be caused by perimenopause or by cardiovascular, endocrine, or metabolic disorders and is a common adverse effect of diuretics.

Urinary incontinence

Urinary incontinence is a commonly reported symptom that may be transient or permanent. The amount of urine released may be small or large. Possible physiologic causes include obesity, chronic lung disease, smoking, pelvic floor injury, and surgery. Other causes include stress incontinence, tumor, bladder cancer and calculi, and neurologic disorders such as Guillain-Barré syndrome, multiple sclerosis, and spinal cord injury.

Dysuria

Dysuria, or pain during urination, signals a lower UTI. The onset of pain suggests the cause of dysuria. For example, pain just before urination indicates bladder irritation or distention. Pain at the start of urination usually signals a bladder outlet obstruction. Pain at the end of urination can be a sign of bladder spasm, and pain throughout urination may indicate pyelonephrosis, especially when fever, chills, hematuria, and flank pain are also present.

Genital abnormalities

Common female genital abnormalities include genital lesions, vaginal inflammation and discharge, cervical lesions and polyps, vaginal and uterine prolapse, and rectocele.

Genital lesions

A syphilitic chancre, which appears in the early stage of syphilis, is a red, painless erosion or papule that ulcerates superficially and has a raised, indurated border. The lesion usually appears inside the vagina but may also appear on the external genitalia.

Watch those warts

Genital warts, an STI caused by human papillomavirus, produce painless warts on the vulva, vagina, cervix, or anus. Warts start as tiny red or pink swellings that grow and develop stemlike structures. Multiple swellings with a cauliflower appearance are common.

Herpes breakdown

Genital herpes produces multiple, shallow vesicles, lesions, or crusts inside the vagina, on the external genitalia, on the buttocks, and, sometimes, on the thighs. Dysuria, regional lymph node inflammation, pain, edema, and fever may be present. A Pap test reveals multinucleated giant cells with intranuclear inclusion bodies.

Vaginal inflammation and discharge

Vaginitis usually results from an overgrowth of infectious organisms. It causes redness, itching, dyspareunia (painful intercourse), dysuria, and a malodorous discharge. Bacterial vaginosis causes a fishy odor and a thin, grayish white discharge. Candidiasis, a fungal infection, caused by *Candida albicans* produces pruritus and a thick, white, curdlike discharge that appears in patches on the cervix and vaginal walls. The discharge has a yeast like odor.

Strawberry signs

Trichomoniasis may cause an abundant malodorous discharge that's either yellow or green and frothy or watery. In addition to redness, you may note red papules on the cervix and vaginal walls, giving the tissue a "strawberry" appearance.

STI with subtlety

Chlamydia, a common but in many cases subtle STI caused by *Chlamydia trachomatis*, produces a mucopurulent cervical discharge and cystitis. However, 75% of female patients with chlamydia are asymptomatic.

Getting to know gonorrhea

Gonorrhea commonly produces no symptoms, but it may cause a purulent green-yellow discharge and cystitis.

Cervical lesions and polyps

During a speculum examination, you may detect late-stage cervical cancer as hard, granular, friable lesions; in the early stages, the cervix looks normal. Cervical polyps are bright red, soft, and fragile. They're usually benign, but they may bleed. They usually arise from the endocervical canal.

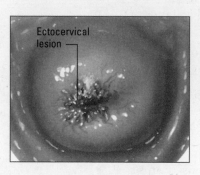

Ectocervical lesion

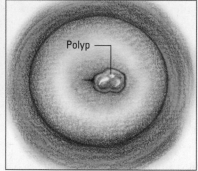

Polyp

Cervical cyanosis

Cervical cyanosis may accompany any disorder that causes systemic hypoxia or venous congestion in the cervix. It's also common during pregnancy and may be observed in women using hormonal contraceptives.

Vaginal and uterine prolapse

Also called *cystocele*, vaginal prolapse occurs when the anterior vaginal wall and bladder prolapse into the vagina. During speculum examination, you'll see a pouch or bulging on the anterior wall as the patient bears down. The uterus may also prolapse into the vagina and even be visible outside the body.

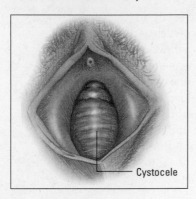

Cystocele

Rectocele

Rectocele is the herniation of the rectum through the posterior vaginal wall. On examination, you'll see a pouch or bulging on the posterior wall as the patient bears down.

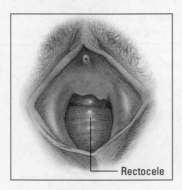

Rectocele

Menstrual abnormalities

Common menstrual abnormalities include dysmenorrhea and amenorrhea.

Dysmenorrhea

Dysmenorrhea—painful menstruation—affects more than 50% of menstruating people; in fact, it's the leading cause of lost time from school and work among female adults of childbearing age. It's usually characterized by mild to severe cramping or colicky pain in the pelvis or lower abdomen that may radiate to the thighs and lower sacrum. The pain gradually subsides as bleeding tapers off.

Amenorrhea

The absence of menstrual flow, amenorrhea, can be classified as primary or secondary. With primary amenorrhea, menarche fails to begin before age 17. The cause may be a congenital defect (such as an imperforate hymen), cervical stenosis, or intrauterine adhesions. With secondary amenorrhea, menarche typically begins at an appropriate age but later ceases for three or more months; in some cases, it is marked by an absence of vaginal fluid for 12 months along with a history of irregular bleeding. Causes of secondary amenorrhea include normal pregnancy, frequent vigorous exercise (such as in athletes), or an emotional disorder, such as depression, anorexia, or bulimia. Secondary amenorrhea may also result from drug or hormonal treatments. Weight can also be a factor. (See *Menstrual disturbances and obesity*.)

Pregnancy

The body undergoes many changes during pregnancy. For example, as a result of hormonal activity (estrogen and progesterone changes), the breasts may double in size and become more nodular. When assessing a pregnant patient, remember that although the pregnant person and fetus have separate and distinct needs, they have an interdependent relationship; factors that influence the pregnant patient's health can also affect the fetus. Changes that occur in fetal well-being can also have an influence on the pregnant person's physical and emotional health.

Handle with care

Menstrual disturbances and obesity

Menstrual disturbances—such as cycle interruption, abnormal flow, amenorrhea, and increased pain during the menstrual cycle—occur three times more frequently in patients who are obese than in those who aren't obese. Obesity also increases the risk of such reproductive disorders as polycystic ovary syndrome. However, a weight loss of just 10% can improve menstrual regularity, ovulation, and pregnancy capability.

Anatomy and assessment of the pregnant patient

The first prenatal visit includes a baseline assessment of vital signs that includes a blood pressure, height, and weight. It is also important to determine the patient's due date at this initial exam using a tool called Naegele rule.

Estimated date of birth

How to use the Naegele rule to calculate the estimated date of birth (EDB).
- Ask the patient the first day of their last menstrual period (LMP).
- Subtract 3 months from the first day.
- Add 7 days to find the EDB.

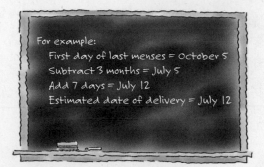

For example:
First day of last menses = October 5
Subtract 3 months = July 5
Add 7 days = July 12
Estimated date of delivery = July 12

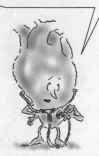

Listen closely! Measuring the patient's blood pressure at each prenatal visit is important because a sudden increase in blood pressure is a danger sign of hypertension in pregnancy.

Breasts

Examine the breasts. In pregnancy, superficial veins appear more prominent and the areolae around the nipples become a darker color. Many patients may also develop striae, which are red color stretch marks that change to silver after the pregnancy. Montgomery tubercles may be visible on the areolae and may begin to express colostrum during the last trimester. Also palpate the breasts to detect abnormalities.

Breast palpation

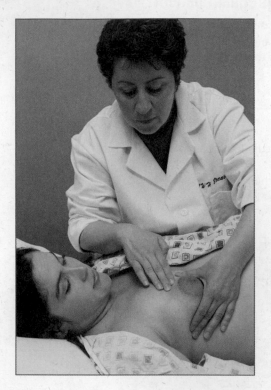

Heart and lungs

Palpate the apical pulse. As the pregnancy advances, the apical pulse may be found slightly higher than the fourth intercostal space because uterine displacement of the diaphragm causes transverse and leftward rotation of the heart.

Abdomen

Observe for a linea nigra, purple-red striae, and scars from previous cesarean births. Palpate the abdomen for the shape and size of the fetus. The abdomen may be flat to round depending on the gestation of the pregnancy. Fetal movement may be felt by a health care provider after the 18th week of gestation.

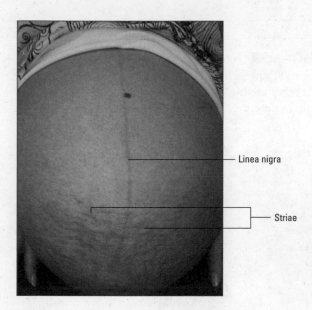

— Linea nigra

— Striae

Fundal height

At about 12 to 14 weeks' gestation, the uterus is palpable over the symphysis pubis as a firm, globular sphere. It reaches the umbilicus at 20 to 22 weeks, reaches the xiphoid at 36 weeks, and then, in many cases, returns to about 4 cm below the xiphoid process at 40 weeks due to lightening. Lightening is caused by the fetus descending into the pelvis. Sometimes this can cause the fetus to press on the nerves in the low abdomen, creating mild pain for the patient. Luckily, this pain should only last for a few seconds at a time.

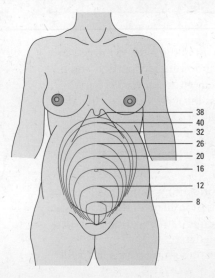

Fetal heart rate

The most common way that fetal heart rate is measured is through fetal doppler. A fetal heart tone (FHT) can be heard between 10 and 12 weeks using fetal Doppler. Another method that can be used is called a fetoscope, which is useful to detect FHT around 18 to 20 weeks.

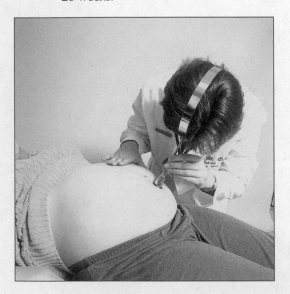
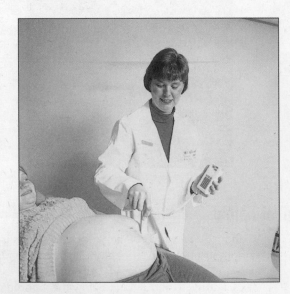

Intrapartum assessment

Fetal presentation

Fetal presentation refers to the relationship of the fetus to the cervix. Assessed through vaginal examination, abdominal inspection and palpation, sonography, or auscultation of fetal heart tones (FHTs), it indicates which part of the fetus will pass through the cervix first during birth. (See *A close look at fetal presentation.*)

Fetal position

Fetal position is the relationship of the presenting part of the fetus to a specific quadrant of the mother's pelvis. It influences the progression of labor and helps determine whether surgical intervention is needed.

Fetal position is defined using three letters:
- The first letter designates whether the presenting part is facing the mother's right (R) or left (L) side.

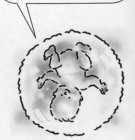

Vertex presentation is considered the most common!

Performing Leopold maneuvers

Use Leopold maneuvers to determine fetal position, presentation, and attitude.

First maneuver

- Place your hands over the patient's abdomen and curl your fingers around the fundus.
- When the fetus is in the vertex position (head first), the buttocks should feel irregularly shaped and firm.
- When the fetus is in the breech position (feet first), the head should feel hard, round, and completely moveable.

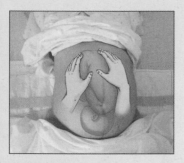

Second maneuver

- Move your hands down the side of the abdomen, applying gentle pressure.
- If the fetus is in the vertex position, you'll feel a smooth, hard surface on one side—the fetal back.
- Opposite, you'll feel lumps and knobs—the knees, hands, feet, and elbows.
- If the fetus is in the breech position, you may not feel the back at all.

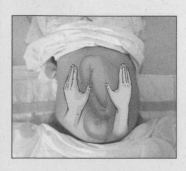

Third maneuver

- Spread your thumb and fingers of one hand, place them just above the patient's symphysis pubis, and then bring your fingers together.
- If the fetus is in the vertex position and hasn't descended, you'll feel the head.
- If the fetus is in the vertex position and has descended, you'll feel a less distinct mass.
- If the fetus is in the breech position, you'll feel a less distinct mass, which could be the feet or knees.

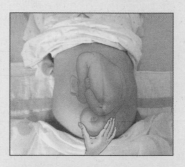

Fourth maneuver

- Use the fourth maneuver to determine flexion or extension of the fetal head and neck.
- Place your hands on both sides of the lower abdomen.
- Gently apply pressure with your fingers as you slide downward toward the symphysis pubis.
- If the head is the presenting part, one of your hands will be stopped by the cephalic prominence.
- If the fetus is in the vertex position, you'll feel the cephalic prominence on the same side as the back.

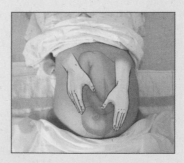

A close look at fetal presentation

The images below depict what the fetus looks like in various presentations.

Cephalic

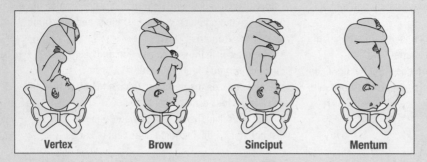

| Vertex | Brow | Sinciput | Mentum |

Breech

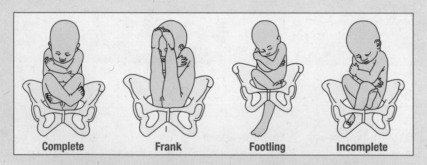

| Complete | Frank | Footling | Incomplete |

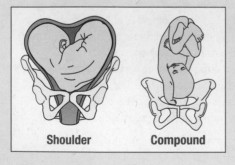

| Shoulder | Compound |

- The second letter or letters refer to the presenting part of the fetus: the occiput (O), mentum (M), sacrum (Sa), or scapula or acromion process (A).
- The third letter designates whether the presenting part is pointing to the anterior (A), posterior (P), or transverse (T) section of the mother's pelvis.

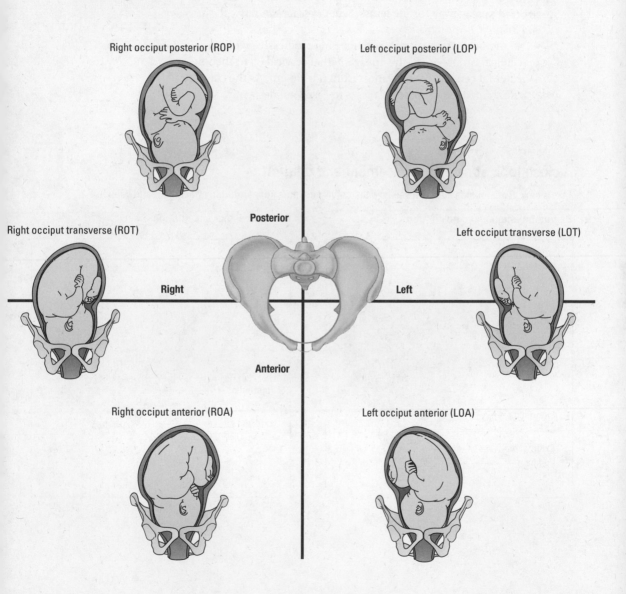

Right occiput posterior (ROP)

Left occiput posterior (LOP)

Posterior

Right occiput transverse (ROT)

Left occiput transverse (LOT)

Right

Left

Anterior

Right occiput anterior (ROA)

Left occiput anterior (LOA)

Cervical effacement and dilation

During effacement, the cervix shortens and its walls become thin, progressing from 0% effacement (palpable and thick) to 100% effacement (fully indistinct or effaced and paper-thin). Full effacement obliterates the constrictive uterine neck to create a smooth, unobstructed passageway for the fetus. (See *A close look at cervical effacement and dilation*.)

- At the same time, dilation occurs. This progressive widening of the cervical canal—from the upper internal cervical os to the lower external cervical os—advances from 0 to 10 cm. As the cervical canal opens, resistance decreases to ease fetal descent.

A close look at cervical effacement and dilation

Take a look at the images below to see how the cervix and fetus appear during effacement and dilation.

Beginning effacement; no dilation

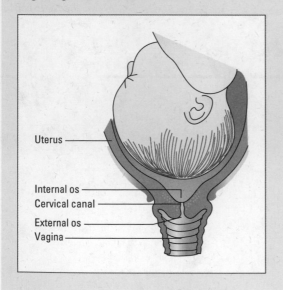

Uterus

Internal os
Cervical canal

External os
Vagina

Full effacement and dilation

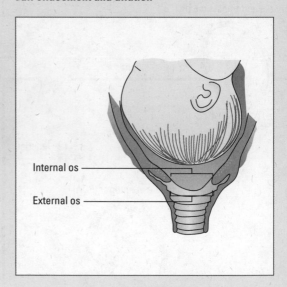

Internal os

External os

Fetal engagement and station

Assess for fetal engagement (the point at which the fetal presenting part advances into the pelvis) during cervical examination. After you have determined fetal engagement, palpate the presenting part and grade the fetal station (where the presenting part lies in relation to the ischial spines of the maternal pelvis).

> You can't assess fetal station unless the presenting part is fully engaged.

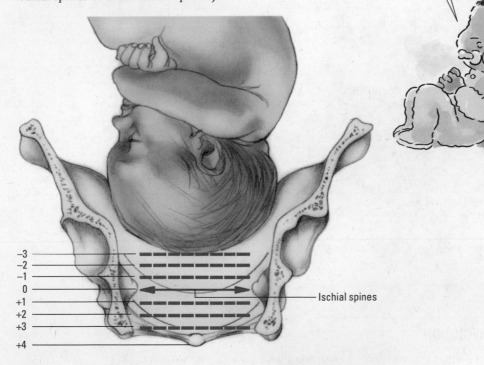

Ischial spines

Postpartum assessment

Breasts

Inspect and palpate the breasts, noting their size, shape, and color. At first, the breasts should feel soft and secrete thin, yellow fluid called colostrum. As they fill with milk—usually around the third postpartum day—they should begin to feel firm and warm.

Fundal assessment

Pregnancy stretches the ligaments that support the uterus, placing it at risk for inversion during palpation. To guard against this:
- Place one hand against the abdomen at the symphysis pubis level to steady the fundus and prevent downward displacement.

- Place the opposite hand at the top of the fundus, cupping it.
- When assessing the uterine fundus, also assess for bladder distention, which can impede downward descent of the uterus by pushing it upward and, possibly, to the right side.

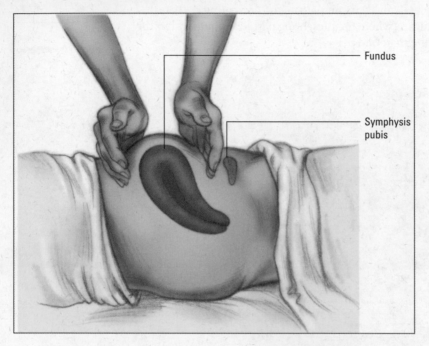

Fundus

Symphysis pubis

Uterine involution

After birth, the uterus begins its descent back into the pelvic cavity. After delivery is complete, the top of the fundus lies midline and halfway in between the symphysis pubis and the umbilicus. Assessment of the fundus 6 to 12 hours later should locate the top of the fundus approximately at the umbilicus level. The uterus continues to descend 1 cm/d until it isn't palpable above the symphysis pubis, at about 9 days after birth.

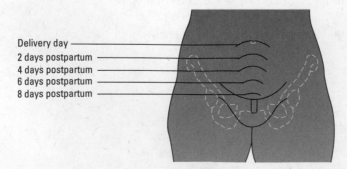

Delivery day
2 days postpartum
4 days postpartum
6 days postpartum
8 days postpartum

Lochia

After birth, the outermost layer of the uterus becomes necrotic and is expelled. This vaginal discharge—called lochia—is similar to menstrual flow and consists of blood, fragments of the decidua, white blood cells, mucus, and some bacteria.

- Assess lochia flow for amount, color, odor, and consistency. A foul or offensive odor may indicate infection. Evidence of large or numerous clots indicates poor uterine contraction and requires further assessment.

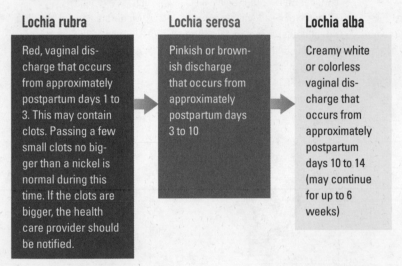

Lochia rubra

Red, vaginal discharge that occurs from approximately postpartum days 1 to 3. This may contain clots. Passing a few small clots no bigger than a nickel is normal during this time. If the clots are bigger, the health care provider should be notified.

Lochia serosa

Pinkish or brownish discharge that occurs from approximately postpartum days 3 to 10

Lochia alba

Creamy white or colorless vaginal discharge that occurs from approximately postpartum days 10 to 14 (may continue for up to 6 weeks)

Perineum and rectum

Assess the perineum and rectum when you assess the lochia. Observe for intactness of skin, positioning of the episiotomy (if one was performed), and appearance of sutures (from episiotomy or laceration repair) and the surrounding rectal area. Note ecchymosis, hematoma, erythema, edema, drainage, or bleeding from sutures; a foul odor; or signs of infection. Also observe for hemorrhoids.

Abnormal findings

Abruptio placenta

Abruptio placenta is premature separation of a normally implanted placenta from the uterine wall. (See *Types of abruptio placentae.*)

Types of abruptio placentae

Mild separation

Begins with small areas of separation and internal bleeding (concealed hemorrhage) between the placenta and uterine wall.

Signs and symptoms
- Gradual onset
- Mild to moderate bleeding
- Vague lower abdominal discomfort
- Mild to moderate abdominal tenderness and uterine irritability
- Strong, regular fetal heart tones (FHTs)

Moderate separation

May develop abruptly or progress from mild to extensive separation with external hemorrhage

Signs and symptoms
- Gradual or abrupt onset
- Moderate, dark red vaginal bleeding
- Continuous abdominal pain
- Tender uterus that remains firm between contractions
- Barely audible or irregular and bradycardic FHTs
- Possible signs of shock

Severe separation

External hemorrhage occurs, along with shock and possible fetal cardiac distress

Signs and symptoms
- Abrupt onset of agonizing, unremitting uterine pain
- Moderate vaginal bleeding
- Boardlike, tender uterus
- Absence of FHTs
- Rapidly progressive shock

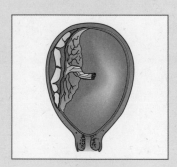 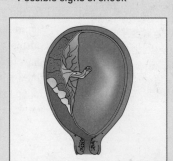 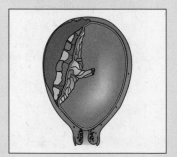

Cephalopelvic disproportion

Narrowing of the birth canal at the inlet, midpelvis, or outlet causes a disproportion between the size of the fetal head and the pelvic diameters, or cephalopelvic disproportion (CPD). CPD results in failure of labor to progress.

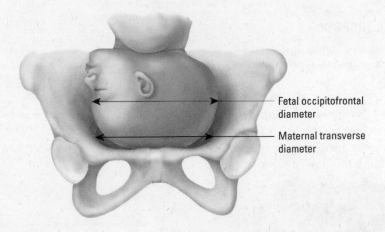

Fetal occipitofrontal diameter

Maternal transverse diameter

Ectopic pregnancy

Ectopic pregnancy occurs when a fertilized ovum implants outside the uterine cavity, most commonly in a fallopian tube. Mild abdominal pain may occur. Typically, the patient reports amenorrhea or abnormal menses (fallopian tube implantation), followed by slight vaginal bleeding and unilateral pelvic pain over the mass. The uterus feels boggy and is tender. The patient may report extreme pain when the cervix is moved.

Sites of ectopic pregnancy

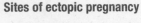

Sites of ectopic pregnancy

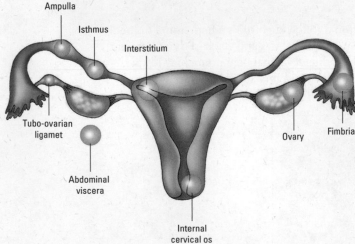

Ampulla

Isthmus

Interstitium

Tubo-ovarian ligamet

Abdominal viscera

Ovary

Fimbria

Internal cervical os

Gestational trophoblastic disease

Gestational trophoblastic disease, or molar pregnancy, is the rapid deterioration of trophoblastic villi cells. As a result of this cell abnormality, the embryo fails to develop.

- Signs and symptoms include mild vaginal bleeding, ranging from brownish red spotting to bright red hemorrhaging. The patient may report passing tissue that resembles grape clusters. The patient's history may also include hyperemesis, lower abdominal cramps, and signs and symptoms of preeclampsia.

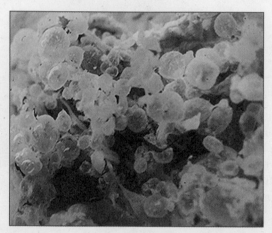

Hematoma

The most common hematoma following birth is a hematoma of the vulva, which results from ruptured arteries and veins in the superficial fascia that seep into nearby tissue. A vaginal hematoma may result after trauma to the soft tissue of the vagina after birth. It can obstruct the urethra, making urination difficult.

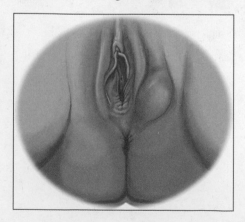

Hypertension in pregnancy

Hypertension in pregnancy is defined as a blood pressure greater than 140 mm Hg systolic and greater than 90 mm Hg diastolic on two occasions at least 4 hours apart after 20 weeks gestation.

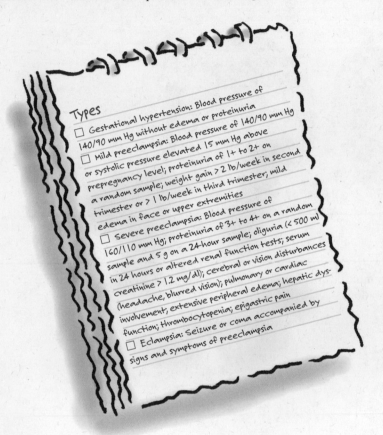

Types

☐ Gestational hypertension: Blood pressure of 140/90 mm Hg without edema or proteinuria

☐ Mild preeclampsia: Blood pressure of 140/90 mm Hg or systolic pressure elevated 15 mm Hg above prepregnancy level; proteinuria of 1+ to 2+ on a random sample; weight gain > 2 lb/week in second trimester or > 1 lb/week in third trimester; mild edema in face or upper extremities

☐ Severe preeclampsia: Blood pressure of 160/110 mm Hg; proteinuria of 3+ to 4+ on a random sample and 5 g on a 24-hour sample; oliguria (< 500 ml in 24 hours or altered renal function tests; serum creatinine > 1.2 mg/dl); cerebral or vision disturbances (headache, blurred vision); pulmonary or cardiac involvement; extensive peripheral edema; hepatic dysfunction; thrombocytopenia; epigastric pain

☐ Eclampsia: Seizure or coma accompanied by signs and symptoms of preeclampsia

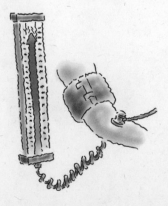

Multiple pregnancy

Multiple pregnancy, or multiple gestation, refers to a pregnancy involving more than one fetus. It's considered a complication of pregnancy because the patient's body must adjust to the effects of carrying multiple fetuses.

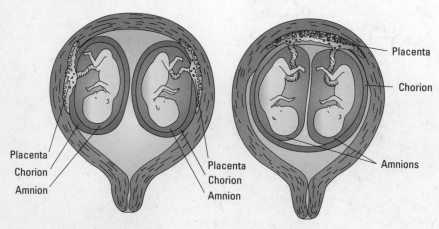

Twin pregnancy presentations

With a twin or other multiple pregnancy, the fetuses can be in several presentation combinations.

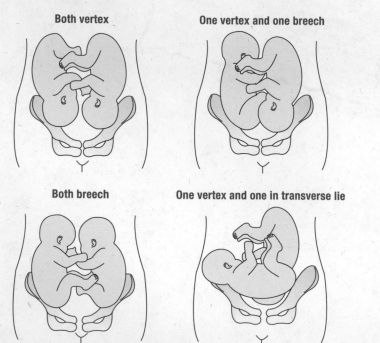

Both vertex

One vertex and one breech

Both breech

One vertex and one in transverse lie

Placenta previa

Placenta previa occurs when the placenta implants in the lower uterine segment, where it encroaches on the internal cervical os. It causes painless, bright red, usually episodic vaginal bleeding after the 20th week of pregnancy. Malpresentation is possible because the placenta's abnormal location interferes with descent of the fetal head. (See *Types of placenta previa.*)

Postpartum hemorrhage

Postpartum hemorrhage is any blood loss from the uterus that exceeds 500 mL during a 24-hour period. It's a major cause of maternal mortality. If your patient starts hemorrhaging postpartum, uterine massage is the first intervention that needs to take place. Other interventions may be necessary such as surgical repair or medication administration. Assess the patient's vital signs and notify the physician immediately if this occurs.

Types of placenta previa

Low implantation

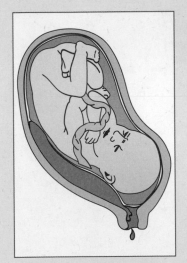

The placenta implants in the lower uterine segment.

Partial placenta previa

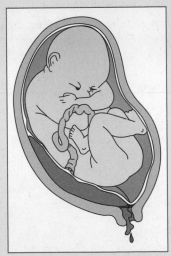

The placenta partially occludes the cervical os.

Total placenta previa

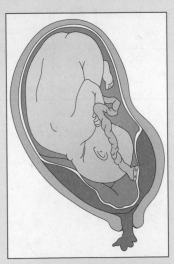

The placenta totally occludes the cervical os.

Causes of postpartum hemorrhage

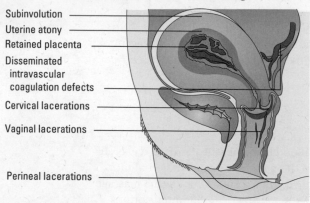

Causes of postpartum hemorrhage

- Subinvolution
- Uterine atony
- Retained placenta
- Disseminated intravascular coagulation defects
- Cervical lacerations
- Vaginal lacerations
- Perineal lacerations

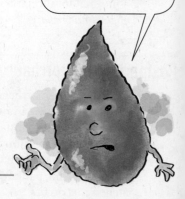

The danger of postpartum hemorrhage from uterine atony is greatest during the first hour after birth.

Spontaneous abortion

Spontaneous abortions occur without medical intervention and in various ways. (See *Types of spontaneous abortion.*)

Umbilical cord prolapse

In umbilical cord prolapse, a loop of the umbilical cord slips in front of the fetal presenting part. It can occur at any time after the membranes rupture, especially if the presenting part isn't firmly engaged in the cervix.

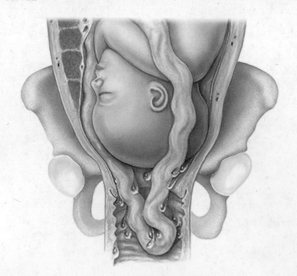

Types of spontaneous abortion

Complete abortion
The uterus passes all products of conception. Minimal bleeding usually accompanies complete abortion because the uterus contracts and compresses the maternal blood vessels that feed the placenta.

Recurrent pregnancy loss
Spontaneous loss of three or more consecutive pregnancies in order.

Incomplete abortion
The uterus retains part of or the entire placenta. Before 10 weeks' gestation, the fetus and placenta are usually expelled together; after the 10th week, they're expelled separately. Because part of the placenta may adhere to the uterine wall, bleeding continues. Hemorrhage is possible because the uterus doesn't contract and seal the large vessels that feed the placenta.

Inevitable abortion
Membranes rupture, and the cervix dilates. As labor continues, the uterus expels the products of conception.

Missed abortion
The uterus retains the products of conception for 2 months or more after the fetus has died. Uterine growth ceases; uterine size may even seem to decrease. Prolonged retention of the dead products of conception causes coagulation defects such as disseminated intravascular coagulation.

Septic abortion
Infection accompanies abortion. This may occur with spontaneous abortion but usually results from a lapse in sterile technique during threatened abortion.

Threatened abortion
Bloody vaginal discharge occurs during the first half of pregnancy. About 20% of pregnant patients have vaginal spotting or actual bleeding early in pregnancy. Of these, about 50% abort.

Other abnormal findings

Bleeding

Vaginal bleeding at any time during a pregnancy is a potential danger sign that requires further investigation. It can range from slight spotting to frank bleeding and may or may not be accompanied by pain.

Premature cervical dilation

In premature cervical dilation, the cervix dilates prematurely and can't hold the fetus until term. Often the first sign is a pink-stained vaginal discharge or increased pelvic pressure, which may be followed by rupture of the amniotic fluid membranes.

Premature rupture of membranes

A sudden gush of clear vaginal fluid suggests rupture of the membranes and onset of labor, which typically occurs at term. Before term (before 37 weeks), it's called preterm premature rupture of membranes (PPROM) and predisposes the mother and fetus to infection. Additionally, PROM can lead to inadequate nutritional supply to the fetus and possible prolapse of the umbilical cord.

Preterm labor

Preterm labor is the onset of rhythmic contractions that produce cervical changes after fetal viability but before fetal maturity. It usually occurs between 20 and 37 weeks' gestation.

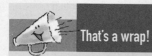

That's a wrap!

Female genitourinary system review

Anatomy and physiology of the urinary system
- Kidneys—form urine; maintain homeostasis; contain nephrons
- Ureters—carry urine from the kidneys to the bladder
- Bladder—container for urine collection
- Urethra—carries urine from the bladder to outside of the body

Anatomy and physiology of external genitalia
- Mons pubis—mound of adipose tissue over symphysis pubis
- Labia majora and minora—vulval lips
- Clitoris—erectile tissue between the labia minora and vestibule
- Vaginal opening—also called the introitus
- Perineum—area between the labial fold and anus

- Skene and Bartholin glands—produce lubricating fluids that are important to reproduction

Anatomy and physiology of the internal genitalia
- Vagina—route of passage for childbirth and menstruation
- Uterus—nurtures and then expels the fetus during pregnancy; divided into the fundus and cervix
- Ovaries—produce ova and release the hormones estrogen and progesterone
- Fallopian tubes—the usual site of fertilization of the ova by the sperm; help to guide the ova to the uterus after expulsion from the ovaries

Health history
Ask about:
- urinary tract infections, kidney disease or kidney stones, and past medical history

- menstruation and sexual practices
- pregnancy and birth control
- menopause.

Assessment
Urinary system
- Inspect the areas over the kidneys and bladder.
- Percuss the kidneys (to check for costovertebral angle tenderness) and bladder.
- Attempt to palpate the kidneys and bladder, although they aren't normally palpable unless the kidneys are enlarged or the bladder is distended.

Reproductive system
- Inspect the external genitalia; note the appearance of pubic hair to determine sexual maturity.
- Palpate the external genitalia—this should be pain-free for the patient.

(Continued)

Female genitourinary system review *(continued)*

- Inspect internal genitalia using a speculum lubricated with warm water.
- Examine the vaginal wall for color, texture, and integrity, and the cervix for color, position, size, shape, mucosal integrity, and discharge.
- Palpate the internal genitalia, including bimanual palpation and rectovaginal palpation.

Abnormal findings
Urinary system
- Polyuria—overproduction of urine
- Hematuria—blood in the urine, causing urine to turn dark brownish or gold
- Urinary frequency—abnormally frequent urination
- Urinary urgency—sudden urge to urinate
- Urinary hesitancy—difficulty starting urine stream
- Nocturia—excessive urination at night
- Urinary incontinence—involuntary release of urine
- Dysuria—painful urination

Reproductive system
- Genital lesions—may result from syphilis (red, painless, eroding lesion with a raised, indurated border); genital warts (painless tiny red or pink swellings that develop stem-like structures); or genital herpes (multiple, shallow vesicles, lesions, or crusts)
- Vaginal discharge—may result from bacterial vaginosis (thin, grayish white discharge); candidiasis (thick, white, curdlike discharge); trichomoniasis (malodorous, yellow or green, and watery or frothy discharge); chlamydia (mucopurulent discharge); or gonorrhea (purulent green-yellow discharge)
- Cervical polyps—bright red, soft, and fragile lesions
- Vaginal and uterine prolapse—anterior vaginal wall and bladder prolapse into the vagina
- Rectocele—herniation of the rectum through the posterior vaginal wall
- Dysmenorrhea—painful menstruation
- Amenorrhea—the absence of menstrual flow

Pregnancy
Anatomy and assessment of the pregnant patient
- Vital signs—blood pressure, height, weight
- Estimated date of birth—use Naegele rule at initial exam to calculate estimated date of birth
- Breasts—breast changes during pregnancy include darkened areolae, more prominent superficial veins, striae (stretch marks), and Montgomery tubercles; palpate breasts to detect abnormalities.
- Heart and lungs—apical pulse may be slightly higher than the fourth intercostal space as pregnancy advances because of the transverse and leftward rotation of the heart caused by uterine displacement of the diaphragm.
- Abdomen—observe for a linea nigra, purple-red striae, and scars from previous cesarean births. Palpate the abdomen for the shape and size of the fetus. Fetal movement may be felt by a health care provider after the 18th week of gestation.
- Fundal height—uterus feels like a firm sphere over symphysis pubis at about 12 to 14 weeks' gestation; reaches umbilicus at 20 to 22 weeks, reaches xiphoid at 36 weeks, and often returns to 4 cm below xiphoid at 40 weeks due to lightening.
- Fetal heart rate—most commonly measured using fetal Doppler at 10 to 12 weeks; fetoscope is also used at 18 to 20 weeks.

Intrapartum assessment
- Fetal presentation—relationship of the fetus to cervix that indicates which part of fetus will pass through cervix first during birth; assessed via vaginal examination, abdominal inspection and palpation, sonography, or auscultation of fetal heart tones
- Fetal position—relationship of presenting part of fetus to specific quadrant of mother's pelvis; influences progression of labor and determines whether surgical intervention is needed
- Cervical effacement and dilation—cervix shortens and its walls thin during effacement to create passageway for fetus; during dilation, cervical canal widens and opens to ease fetal descent
- Fetal engagement and station—fetal engagement is the point at which fetal presenting part advances into pelvis; fetal station is where presenting part lies in relation to the ischial spines of maternal pelvis

(Continued)

Female genitourinary system review *(continued)*

Postpartum assessment

- Breasts—inspect and palpate for size, shape, and color; breasts should feel soft at first and secrete colostrum, then feel firm and warm as they fill with milk
- Fundal assessment—decrease risk of uterine inversion during palpation by placing one hand against abdomen at symphysis pubis level to steady fundus and prevent downward displacement, then place opposite hand at the top of the fundus and cup it; also assess for bladder distension
- Uterine involution—uterus begins to descend back into pelvic cavity after birth, and top of fundus should be located at approximately umbilicus level 6 to 12 hours after birth, continuing to descend 1 cm/d until about 9 days after birth, when it is no longer palpable above the symphysis pubis
- Lochia—vaginal discharge after birth that contains blood, fragments of decidua, white blood cells, mucus, and some bacteria; assess lochia flow for amount, color, and consistency
- Perineum and rectum—assess for intactness of skin, positioning of episiotomy if performed, appearance of sutures, and surrounding rectal area, noting ecchymosis, hematoma, erythema, edema, drainage, or bleeding from sutures; a foul odor; or signs of infection; observe for hemorrhoids

Abnormal findings

- Abruptio placenta—premature separation of normally implanted placenta from the uterine wall; can be mild, moderate, or severe
- Cephalopelvic disproportion—disproportion between size of fetal head and pelvic diameters caused by narrowing of birth canal at inlet, midpelvis, or outlet; results in failure of labor to progress
- Ectopic pregnancy—occurs when fertilized ovum implants outside uterine cavity, usually in a fallopian tube; can cause mild abdominal pain, amenorrhea or abnormal menses, slight vaginal bleeding, unilateral pelvic pain over the mass, tender and "boggy" feel to uterus
- Gestational trophoblastic disease (molar pregnancy)—rapid deterioration of trophoblastic villi cells, which causes embryo to fail to develop; signs and symptoms include vaginal bleeding (spotting to hemorrhaging) and passing tissue resembling grape clusters
- Hematoma—most common post-birth hematoma is hematoma of vulva, caused by ruptured arteries and veins seeping from superficial fascia to nearby tissue; vaginal hematoma may result after trauma to soft tissue of vagina after birth and can obstruct urethra
- Hypertension in pregnancy—blood pressure greater than 140 mm Hg systolic and greater than 90 mm Hg diastolic on two occasions at least 4 hours apart after 20 weeks gestation
- Multiple pregnancy (multiple gestation)—considered complication because of the effects on patient's body from carrying multiple fetuses
- Placenta previa—occurs when the placenta implants in the lower uterine segment, where it encroaches on the internal cervical os; causes painless, bright red, usually episodic vaginal bleeding after the 20th week of pregnancy and possible malpresentation because the placenta's abnormal location interferes with descent of the fetal head
- Postpartum hemorrhage—any blood loss from the uterus that exceeds 500 mL during a 24-hour period
- Spontaneous abortion—occurs without medical intervention and in various ways; types include complete abortion, recurrent pregnancy loss, incomplete abortion, inevitable abortion, missed abortion, septic abortion, and threatened abortion
- Umbilical cord prolapse—when loop of umbilical cord slips in front of the fetal presenting part; can occur at any time after membranes rupture

Other abnormal findings

- Vaginal bleeding
- Premature cervical dilation
- Premature rupture of membranes
- Preterm labor

Quick quiz

1. Using commercial lubricants on speculum blades before inserting them into the vagina should be avoided because:
    A. lubricants can alter test results.
    B. additional lubrication is unnecessary.
    C. many patients are hypersensitive to lubricants.
    D. lubricants can discolor the vaginal tissue.

Answer: A. Most commercial lubricants are bacteriostatic and can alter test and culture results. Hold the speculum blades under warm running water to lubricate them.

2. Your patient reports lower abdominal pressure, and you note a firm mass extending above the symphysis pubis. You suspect:
    A. a distended bladder.
    B. an enlarged kidney.
    C. a UTI.
    D. an inflamed ovary.

Answer: A. The bladder is usually nonpalpable unless it's distended. The feeling of pressure is usually relieved with urination.

3. The ducts of Skene glands open into the:
    A. perianal area.
    B. clitoris.
    C. urethra.
    D. vulva.

Answer: D. Skene glands are multiple, tiny structures located just below the urethra, each containing 6 to 31 ducts that empty into the vulva.

4. Your patient reports a 32-day menstrual cycle. You know this cycle is probably:
    A. a normal variation.
    B. a sign of metrorrhagia.
    C. a precursor to uterine cancer.
    D. a precursor to menopause.

Answer: A. The menstrual cycle varies from patient to patient. If a patient's pattern changes, they should be evaluated further.

5. Your patient reports a thick, white vaginal discharge and vaginal itch. You suspect:
    A. gonorrhea.
    B. candidiasis.
    C. bacterial vaginosis.
    D. trichomoniasis.

Answer: B. Candidiasis, or yeast infection, causes pruritus and a thick, white, curdlike discharge with a yeastlike odor that appears in patches on the labia and vaginal walls.

6. Your patient reports a perineal sore. You suspect:
   A. gonorrhea.
   B. chlamydia.
   C. genital herpes.
   D. cervical polyps.

Answer: C. Genital herpes causes multiple shallow vesicles, lesions, or crusts inside the vagina, on the external genitalia, on the buttocks, and sometimes on the thighs.

Scoring

 If you answered all six questions correctly, fantastic! Your ability to flow through this information is most impressive.

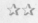 If you answered four or five questions correctly, excellent! Your study of this chapter has "reproduced" wonderful results.

☆ If you answered fewer than four questions correctly, don't despair. Why not cycle through the chapter again?

 Just for fun

Match the disorder in column 1 with the genitourinary findings in column 2.

Disorder

1. Early syphilis _____

2. Diabetic nephropathy _____

3. Urinary system obstruction _____

4. Gonorrhea _____

5. Bladder cancer _____

Genitourinary findings

A. Overflow incontinence and painless bladder distention

B. Dysuria throughout voiding, bladder distention, diminished urinary stream, urinary frequency and urgency, and sensation of bloating or fullness in lower abdomen or groin

C. Urge or overflow incontinence, hematuria, dysuria, nocturia, urinary frequency, suprapubic pain from bladder spasms, and palpable mass on bimanual examination

D. Chancrous red, painless, eroding lesion with a raised, indurated border that usually appears inside the vagina

E. Yellow or green, foul-smelling discharge that can be expressed from Bartholin or Skene ducts; dysuria; urinary frequency and incontinence; vaginal redness and swelling

Answer: 1. D, 2. A, 3. B, 4. E, 5. C

Identify the anatomic structures of pregnancy indicated on this illustration.

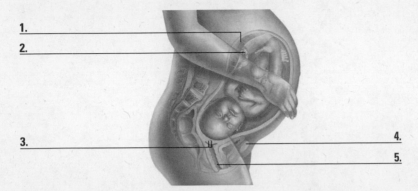

1. _____
2. _____

3. _____   4. _____

5. _____

Answer: 1. Placenta, 2. Umbilical cord, 3. Cervix, 4. Symphysis pubis, 5. Vagina

Matchmaker

Match the abnormal pregnancy findings shown with their correct names.

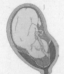

A. Umbilical cord prolapse
B. Abruptio placentae
C. Placenta previa
D. Gestational trophoblastic disease

1. _____

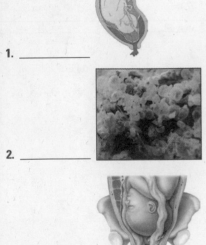

2. _____

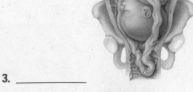

3. _____

4. _____

Answer: 1. C, 2. D, 3. A, 4. B.

Chapter 14

Male genitourinary system

Just the facts

In this chapter, you'll learn:

- ◆ characteristics of the organs and structures of the male genitourinary (GU) system
- ◆ questions to ask during a patient history about the male GU system
- ◆ techniques to conduct a physical assessment of the male GU system
- ◆ causes and characteristics of male GU system abnormalities.

*In this chapter, male = assigned male at birth; female = assigned female at birth.

A look at the male GU system

A disorder of the male urinary or reproductive system can have far-reaching consequences. In addition to affecting the system itself, such a disorder can trigger problems in other body systems. It can also affect the patient's quality of life, self-esteem, and sense of well-being.

Despite these consequences, many patients are reluctant to discuss their problems with nurses of another sex or have intimate areas of their bodies examined. Your challenge, then, is to perform an assessment that's both skilled and sensitive. To do so, you must be aware of your own feelings about sexuality. If you appear comfortable discussing the patient's problem, the patient will be encouraged to talk openly too.

Anatomy and physiology

To thoroughly and accurately assess your patient's GU system, you'll need to know the organs and structures of the urinary and reproductive systems and how they work.

Urinary system

The urinary system helps maintain homeostasis by regulating fluid and electrolyte balance. It consists of the kidneys, ureters, bladder, and urethra. The essential functions of the system, such as forming urine and maintaining homeostasis, occur in the highly vascular kidneys. Each kidney contains roughly one million nephrons. The kidneys maintain acid-base, fluid, and electrolyte balance, as well as assist in blood pressure control. They also form urine to remove waste from the body.

Although the male and female urinary systems function in the same way, the male urethra is approximately 8″ (20 cm) long and the female urethra is approximately 1½″ (4 cm) long. That's because the male urethra must pass through the erectile tissue of the penis.

Reproductive system

In males, the urethra is also part of the reproductive system because it carries semen as well as urine. The male reproductive system also

A close look at the male reproductive system

This illustration shows the important structures of the male reproductive system.

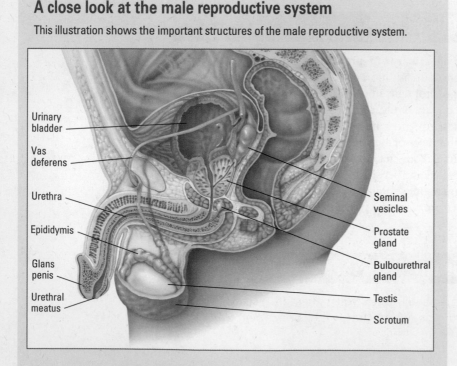

Urinary bladder

Vas deferens

Urethra

Epididymis

Glans penis

Urethral meatus

Seminal vesicles

Prostate gland

Bulbourethral gland

Testis

Scrotum

includes the penis, scrotum, testicles, epididymis, vas deferens, seminal vesicles, and prostate gland. (See *A close look at the male reproductive system.*)

Penis

The penis consists of the shaft, glans, urethral meatus, corona, and prepuce. The skin of the penis is hairless, movable, and usually darker than the skin on other parts of the body.

The shaft contains three columns of vascular erectile tissue. The glans is located at the end of the penis. The urethral meatus is a narrow opening located ventrally at the tip of the glans. The corona is formed by the junction of the glans and the shaft. The prepuce (or foreskin), the loose skin covering the glans, is commonly removed shortly after birth in a surgical procedure called *circumcision.* (See *Circumcision as a religious practice.*)

When the penile tissues are engorged with blood, the erect penis can discharge sperm. During sexual activity, sperm and semen are forcefully ejaculated from the urethral meatus.

Scrotum

A loose, wrinkled, deeply pigmented sac that consists of a muscle layer covered by skin, the scrotum is located at the base of the penis. Each of its two compartments contains a testicle, an epididymis, and portions of the spermatic cord. The left side of the scrotum is usually lower than the right because the left spermatic cord is longer.

Testicles

The testicles are oval, rubbery structures suspended vertically and slightly forward in the scrotum. They produce testosterone and sperm.

Where it all begins

Testosterone stimulates the changes that occur during puberty, which starts between ages 9½ and 13½. The testicles enlarge (the first sign of pubertal changes), pubic hair grows, and penis size increases. Secondary sex characteristics appear, such as axillary, pubic, and facial hair; maturation of reproductive organs; deepening of the voice; and the development of muscle and bone mass.

Epididymis

The epididymis is a reservoir for maturing sperm. It curves over the posterolateral surface of each testicle, creating a visible bulge on the surface. In a small number of males, the epididymis is located anteriorly.

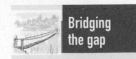

Bridging the gap

Circumcision as a religious practice

In some religions, circumcision is a religious practice. In Judaism, circumcision signifies a covenant between God and the Jewish people. All Jewish males are circumcised when they're 8 days old during a ritual called a *brit milah*, or *bris.* The circumcision may be performed by a mohel (a Jewish person with special training) or by the neonate's father.

In the Islamic religion, circumcision is considered a rule of cleanliness. Islamic boys may be circumcised from the time they're 7 days old until they reach 7 years old. The age varies, depending on family, region, and country.

Vas deferens

The vas deferens—a storage site and the pathway for sperm—begins at the lower end of the epididymis, climbs the spermatic cord, travels through the inguinal canal into the pelvic cavity, and loops over the urinary bladder.

Seminal vesicles

The seminal vesicles are paired structures that lie at the base of the bladder and produce 60% of the volume of semen.

Prostate gland

About 2½″ (6.5 cm) long, the prostate surrounds the neck of the bladder and urethra. It produces a thin, milky, alkaline fluid that mixes with seminal fluid during ejaculation to enhance sperm activity.

Obtaining a health history

Common symptoms patients report about the urinary system include pain during urination and changes in voiding pattern and urine color and output. The most commonly reported symptoms about the reproductive system are penile discharge, erectile dysfunction, infertility, and scrotal or inguinal masses, pain, and tenderness. As you obtain a history, remember that the patient may feel uncomfortable discussing urinary or reproductive problems. (See *Putting your patient at ease*.)

Putting your patient at ease

Here are some tips for helping your patient feel more comfortable during the health history:
• Make sure that the room is private and that you won't be interrupted.
• Tell the patient that their answers will remain confidential, and phrase your questions tactfully.
• Start with less sensitive areas and work up to more sensitive areas such as sexual function.
• Don't rush or omit important facts because the patient seems embarrassed.
• Be especially tactful with older patients, who may see a normal decrease in sexual prowess as a sign of declining health and may be less willing to talk about sexual problems than younger patients are.
• When asking questions, keep in mind that many men view sexual problems as a sign of diminished masculinity. Phrase your questions carefully, and offer reassurance as needed.
• Consider the patient's use of language when reporting information. If the patient uses slang or euphemisms to talk about sexual organs or function, make sure you're both talking about the same thing.

Asking about past health and family health

Ask the patient about their medical history, especially the presence of diabetes or hypertension. Has the patient ever had a kidney or bladder infection or an infection of the reproductive system? Also ask about kidney or bladder trauma, kidney stones, and surgery. Has the patient ever been catheterized? (See *Assessing urine appearance*.)

Factoring in the family

Inquire about the health of the patient's family to get information on the patient's risk of developing renal failure or kidney disease.

Asking about current health

Ask if the patient has been circumcised. If not, ask if the patient can retract and replace the prepuce (foreskin) easily. An inability to retract the prepuce is called *phimosis*; an inability to replace it is called *paraphimosis*. Untreated, these conditions can impair local circulation and lead to edema and even gangrene.

Inquire whether the patient has noticed sores, lumps, or ulcers on their penis. These can signal a sexually transmitted infection (STI). Ask about scrotal swelling. This can indicate an inguinal hernia, a hematocele, epididymitis, or a testicular tumor. Also ask whether the patient has penile discharge or bleeding.

Drug connection

Ask what medications the patient regularly takes, including over-the-counter, prescription, herbal, and illicit or recreational drugs. Some drugs can affect the appearance of urine or alter GU function.

Asking about sexual health and practices

Finally, ask the patient about their sexual partners and practices so that you can assess risk-taking behaviors. How many sexual partners does the patient currently have? How many has the patient had in the past? Ask about history of STIs and whether treatment was received for them. Inquire about precautions the patient takes to prevent contracting STIs. Find out about human immunodeficiency virus status. Also ask about birth control measures and whether the patient has had a vasectomy. (See *Don't forget to ask older patients*, page 372.)

Assessing urine appearance

How your patient's urine looks can provide clues about their general health and the source of their genitourinary problem. During the health history, ask the patient whether they have noticed any change in urine color. If they have, use this list to help interpret the changes:

- Pale and diluted—diabetes insipidus, diuretic therapy, excessive fluid intake
- Dark yellow or amber and concentrated—acute febrile disease, dehydration, gallbladder disease
- Blue-green—methylene blue ingestion
- Green-brown—bile duct obstruction
- Dark brown or black—acute glomerulonephritis, intake of such drugs as chlorpromazine
- Orange-red or orange-brown—obstructive jaundice, urobilinuria, intake of such drugs as rifampin or phenazopyridine
- Red or red-brown—hemorrhage, porphyria, intake of such drugs as phenazopyridine.

Handle with care

Don't forget to ask older patients

Most people erroneously believe that sexual performance normally declines with age. Some also believe—also erroneously—that older people are incapable of having sex, that they aren't interested in sex, or that they can't find partners of similar ages who are also interested in sex.

Harboring these beliefs could prevent you from asking your older male patients about their sexual health. The truth is, patients may be experiencing sexual problems that they're too embarrassed to bring up on their own. Therefore, be sure to ask older patients about their sexual health and provide support as needed. If the patient is dissatisfied with their sexual performance, bring this to the attention of the doctor. The doctor can then investigate the cause of the problem and initiate treatment as needed. Be aware that organic disease must be ruled out before counseling to improve sexual performance can start.

Taking precautions

Also ask the patient about sexual health. Have they ever had trauma to their penis or scrotum? Were they ever diagnosed with an undescended testicle? Have they ever had surgery involving their penis or reproductive system? Have they ever been diagnosed with a low sperm count? If so, caution them that hot baths, frequent bicycle or motorcycle riding, and tight underwear or athletic supporters can elevate scrotal temperature and temporarily decrease sperm count. If the patient participates in sports, ask how they protect from possible genital injuries. This is also a good time to ask them whether they know how to examine their testicles for signs of testicular cancer. (See *Testicular self-examination*.)

Assessing the male GU system

To perform a physical assessment of the male GU system, use the techniques of inspection, percussion, palpation, and auscultation. Assessment of the urinary system may be done with assessment of the GU system or as part of the GI assessment.

Examining the urinary system

In many ways, assessing the male urinary system is similar to assessing the female urinary system. Before examining specific structures, check the patient's blood pressure and weight.

Testicular self-examination

During the patient history, ask your patient whether they perform monthly testicular self-examinations (TSE). If not, explain that testicular cancer, the most common cancer in male adults ages 20 to 35, can be treated successfully when it's detected early.

Teaching the technique
Advise the patient to perform TSE after a shower or bath, when the scrotum is warm and most relaxed. To do this examination, the patient should grasp the testes with both hands and palpate gently between the thumb and fingers. The testes should feel smooth and egg-shaped and be firm to the touch. Both testicles should be the same size, although the left one is usually lower than the right because the left spermatic cord is longer. The epididymis, found behind the testes, should feel like a soft tube.

If the patient finds any abnormalities, they should notify their primary care provider immediately.

Scan the skin

Also, observe the patient's skin. A person with decreased renal function may be pale because of a low hemoglobin level or may even have uremic frost—snowlike crystals on the skin from metabolic wastes. Also look for signs of fluid imbalance, such as dry mucous membranes, sunken eyeballs, edema, or ascites.

Before performing an assessment, ask the patient to urinate; then help them into the supine position with their arms at their sides. As you proceed, expose only the areas being examined.

Inspection

First, inspect the patient's abdomen. When the patient is supine, their abdomen should be symmetrical and smooth, flat, or concave. The skin should be free from lesions, bruises, discolorations, and prominent veins.

Silvery streaks of striae

Watch for abdominal distention with tight, glistening skin and striae (silvery streaks caused by rapidly developing skin tension). These are signs of ascites, which may accompany nephrotic syndrome. This syndrome is characterized by edema, increased urine protein levels, and decreased serum albumin levels.

Percussion and palpation

First, tell the patient what you're going to do; otherwise, they may be startled and you could mistake the reaction for a feeling of acute tenderness. Percuss the kidneys, checking for pain or tenderness, which suggests a kidney infection. Remember to percuss both sides of the body to assess both kidneys. Then percuss the bladder to elicit tympany or dullness. (See *Performing fist percussion*.)

Dullness = retention

A dull sound instead of the normal tympany may indicate retained urine in the bladder caused by bladder dysfunction or infection. You can also palpate the bladder to check for distention. Because the kidneys aren't usually palpable, detecting an enlarged kidney may prove important. Kidney enlargement may accompany hydronephrosis, a cyst, or a tumor.

Auscultation

Auscultate the renal arteries to rule out bruits, which signal renal artery stenosis. You can do this during assessment of the GU system or as part of an abdominal assessment.

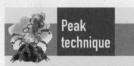

Peak technique

Performing fist percussion

To assess the kidneys by indirect fist percussion, ask the patient to sit up with their back to you. Warn them that you'll be gently striking their back. Then place one hand at the costovertebral angle and strike it with the ulnar surface of your other hand, as shown below.

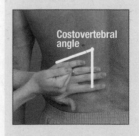

Costovertebral angle

Examining the reproductive system

Before examining the reproductive system, put on gloves. Make the patient as comfortable as possible, and explain what you're doing every step of the way. Make sure that the privacy curtain is fully drawn or that the door is closed to help the patient feel less embarrassed.

Inspection

Inspect the penis, scrotum, and testicles as well as the inguinal and femoral areas.

Penis

Start by examining the penis. Penis size depends on the patient's age and overall development. The penile skin should be slightly wrinkled and pink to light brown in patients with light skin and light brown to dark brown in patients with dark skin. Check the penile shaft and glans for lesions, nodules, inflammations, and swelling. Inspect the glans of an uncircumcised penis by retracting the prepuce. Also check the glans for smegma, a cheesy secretion commonly found beneath the prepuce.

Pressing the point

Then gently compress the tip of the glans to open the urethral meatus. It should be located in the center of the glans and be pink and smooth. Inspect it for swelling, discharge, lesions, inflammation, and, especially, genital warts. If you note discharge, obtain a culture specimen. (See *Examining the urethral meatus*.)

Scrotum and testicles

Have the patient hold the penis away from the scrotum so you can observe the scrotum's general size and appearance. The skin here is darker than on the rest of the body. Spread the surface of the scrotum, and examine the skin for swelling, nodules, redness, ulceration, and distended veins.

It's perfectly normal!

Sebaceous cysts—firm, white to yellow, nontender cutaneous lesions—are a normal finding. Also check for pitting edema, a sign of cardiovascular disease. Spread the pubic hair and check the skin for lesions and parasites. If the patient is a child, check especially for penile enlargement. (See *Assessing pediatric patients*.)

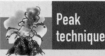

Peak technique

Examining the urethral meatus

To inspect the urethral meatus, compress the tip of the glans, as shown below.

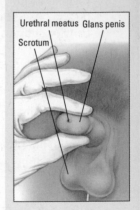

Urethral meatus Glans penis
Scrotum

Assessing pediatric patients

Before palpating a child's scrotum for a testicular examination, explain what you'll be doing and why. A younger child may want a parent or caregiver present for comfort; however, an older child will probably want privacy. Make sure the patient is comfortably warm and as relaxed as possible. Cold and anxiety may cause the testicles to retract so that you can't palpate them.

If the child has an exaggerated or inappropriate response to the examination, consider the possibility that they may have been sexually abused.

Hernia and hydroceles

If you see an enlarged scrotum in a child younger than age 2, suspect a scrotal extension of an inguinal hernia, a hydrocele, or both. Hydroceles, usually associated with inguinal hernias, are common in children of this age group. To differentiate between the two, remember that hydroceles transilluminate and aren't tender or reducible.

Obesity

An adolescent who's obese may appear to have an atypically small penis. You may have to retract the fat pad over the symphysis pubis to properly assess penis size.

Palpating the testicles

Gently palpate both testes between your thumb and first two fingers of your gloved hand, as shown below. Assess their size, shape, and response to pressure. A normal response is a deep visceral pain.

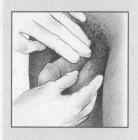

Inguinal and femoral areas

Have the patient stand. Then ask them to hold their breath and bear down while you inspect the inguinal and femoral areas for bulges or hernias. A hernia is a loop of bowel that comes through a muscle wall.

Palpation

Palpate the penis, testicles, epididymides, spermatic cords, inguinal and femoral areas, and prostate gland.

Penis

Use your thumb and forefinger to palpate the entire penile shaft. It should be somewhat firm, and the skin should be smooth and movable. Note swelling, nodules, or indurations.

Testicles

You'll also need to palpate the testicles. Make sure they're equal in size, move freely in the scrotal sac, and feel firm, smooth, and rubbery. (See *Palpating the testicles*.)

The shadow knows

If you note hard, irregular areas or lumps, transilluminate them by darkening the room and pressing the head of a flashlight against the scrotum, behind the lump. The testicle and any lumps, masses, warts, or blood-filled areas will appear as opaque shadows.

Transilluminate the other testicle to compare your findings. This is also a good time to reinforce the methods for and importance of doing a monthly testicular self-examination.

Epididymides

Next, palpate the epididymides, which are usually located in the posterolateral area of the testicles. They should be smooth, discrete, nontender, and free from swelling and induration.

Spermatic cords

Palpate both spermatic cords, which are located above each testicle. Palpate from the base of the epididymis to the inguinal canal. The vas deferens is a smooth, movable cord inside the spermatic cord.

It's a "no glow"

If you feel swelling, irregularity, or nodules, transilluminate the problem area, as described above. If serous fluid is present, you won't see a glow.

Inguinal area

To assess the patient for a direct inguinal hernia, place two fingers over each external inguinal ring and ask the patient to bear down. If there is a hernia, you'll feel a bulge. Two types of groin hernias include inguinal and femoral hernias. These may be direct or indirect. Approximately 96% of groin hernias are inguinal, and 4% are femoral.

A direct inguinal hernia emerges from behind the external inguinal ring and protrudes through it. This type of hernia seldom descends into the scrotum and usually affects male patients older than age 40.

An indirect inguinal hernia is the most common type of hernia; it occurs in males of all ages. It can be palpated in the internal inguinal canal with its tip in or beyond the canal, or the hernia may descend into the scrotum.

Stand up, please!

To assess the patient for an indirect inguinal hernia, examine them while they are standing and then while they are in a supine position with their knee flexed on the side you're examining. (See *Palpating for an indirect inguinal hernia.*)

Place your index finger on the neck of the scrotum and gently push upward into the inguinal canal. When you've inserted your finger as far as possible, ask the patient to bear down or cough. A hernia feels like a mass of tissue that withdraws when it meets the finger.

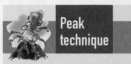

Peak technique

Palpating for an indirect inguinal hernia

To palpate for an indirect inguinal hernia, place your gloved finger on the neck of the scrotum and insert it into the inguinal canal, as shown below. Then ask the patient to bear down. If the patient has a hernia, you'll feel a soft mass at your fingertip.

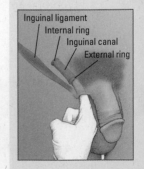

Inguinal ligament
Internal ring
Inguinal canal
External ring

Femoral area

Although you can't palpate the femoral canal, you can estimate its location to help detect a femoral hernia. Place your right index finger on the right femoral artery with your finger pointing toward the patient's head. Keep your other fingers close together. Your middle finger will rest on the femoral vein and your ring finger, on the femoral canal. Note tenderness or masses. Use your left hand to check the patient's left side. Although femoral hernias are the least common type of hernia, 40% present as emergencies with incarceration or strangulation.

Prostate gland

Tell the patient that you need to place your finger in their rectum to examine the prostate gland, and warn them that they'll feel some pressure during the examination. Have them stand and lean over the examination table. If they can't do this, have them lie on their left side, with their right knee and hip flexed or with both knees drawn toward their chest. Inspect the skin of the perineal, anal, and posterior scrotal areas. It should be smooth and unbroken, with no protruding masses.

Probing the issue

Then lubricate the gloved index finger of your dominant hand and insert it into the rectum. Tell the patient to relax to ease the passage of the finger through the anal sphincter. If they're having difficulty relaxing the anal sphincter, ask them to bear down as if having a bowel movement while you gently insert your finger. With your finger pad, palpate the prostate gland on the anterior rectal wall just past the anorectal ring. The gland should feel smooth, rubbery, and about the size of a walnut. (See *Palpating the prostate gland*.)

A growing problem

If the prostate gland protrudes into the rectal lumen, it's probably enlarged. An enlarged prostate gland is classified from grade 1 (protruding less than ⅜" [1 cm] into the rectal lumen) to grade 4 (protruding more than 1¼" [3.2 cm] into the rectal lumen). Also note tenderness or nodules.

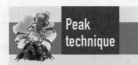

Peak technique

Palpating the prostate gland

To palpate the prostate gland, insert a lubricated, gloved index finger into the rectum. Palpate the prostate on the anterior rectal wall, just past the anorectal ring.

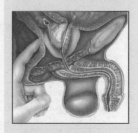

Abnormal findings

Your assessment may uncover abnormalities of the GU system. Although the urinary problems discussed below also occur in women, the causes described are unique to men. (See *Male GU abnormalities*, pages 378 and 379.)

Interpretation station

Male GU abnormalities

After you assess the patient, a group of findings may lead you to suspect a particular disorder. The chart below shows common groups of findings for the male genitourinary (GU) system, along with their signs and symptoms and probable causes.

Sign or symptom and findings	Probable cause
Penile lesions	
• Fluid-filled vesicles on the glans penis, prepuce (foreskin), or penile shaft • Painful ulcers • Tender inguinal lymph nodes • Fever • Malaise • Dysuria	Genital herpes
• Painless warts (tiny pink swellings that grow and become pedunculated) near the urethral meatus • Lesions that spread to the perineum and the perianal area • Cauliflower appearance of multiple swellings	Genital warts
• Sharply defined, slightly raised, scaling patches on the inner thigh or groin (bilaterally) or on the scrotum or penis • Severe pruritus	Tinea cruris (jock itch)
Scrotal swelling	
• Swollen scrotum that's soft or unusually firm • Bowel sounds that may be auscultated in the scrotum	Hernia
• Gradual scrotal swelling • Scrotum that's soft and cystic or firm and tense • Painless • Round, nontender scrotal mass on palpation • Glowing when transilluminated	Hydrocele

Sign or symptom and findings	Probable cause
• Scrotal swelling with sudden and severe pain • Unilateral elevation of the affected testicle • Nausea and vomiting	Testicular torsion
Penile discharge	
• Purulent or milky urethral discharge • Sudden fever and chills • Lower back pain • Perineal fullness • Myalgia • Arthralgia • Urinary frequency and urgency • Cloudy urine • Dysuria • Tense, boggy, very tender, warm prostate palpated on digital rectal examination	Prostatitis
• Opaque, gray, yellowish, or blood-tinged discharge that's painless • Dysuria • Eventual anuria	Urethral neoplasm
• Scant or profuse urethral discharge that's thin and clear, mucoid, or thick and purulent • Urinary hesitancy, frequency, and urgency • Dysuria • Itching and burning around the meatus	Urethritis

(Continued)

Male GU abnormalities *(continued)*

Sign or symptom and findings	Probable cause
Urinary hesitancy	
• Reduced caliber and force of urinary stream • Perineal pain • Feeling of incomplete voiding • Inability to stop urine stream • Urinary frequency • Urinary incontinence • Bladder distention	Benign prostatic hyperplasia
• Urinary frequency and dribbling • Nocturia • Dysuria • Bladder distention • Perineal pain • Constipation • Hard, nodular prostate palpated on digital rectal examination	Prostate cancer

Sign or symptom and findings	Probable cause
• Dysuria • Urinary frequency and urgency • Hematuria • Cloudy urine • Bladder spasms • Costovertebral angle tenderness • Suprapubic, low back, pelvic, or flank pain • Urethral discharge	Urinary tract infection

Urinary problems

Possible urinary problems include hematuria; urinary frequency, urgency, and hesitancy; nocturia; and urinary incontinence.

Hematuria

Hematuria (presence of blood in the urine) may indicate urinary tract infection (UTI), renal calculi, or trauma to the urinary mucosa. It may be a temporary condition after urinary tract or prostate surgery or after urethral catheterization. It can be classified as gross hematuria or microscopic hematuria. Gross hematuria is suspected because of the presence of red or brown urine. Microscopic hematuria refers to blood detectable only on examination of the urine sample by microscopy.

A red flag

A patient with hematuria may have brown or bright red urine. Bleeding at the end of urination signals a disorder of the bladder neck, urethra, or prostate gland.

Urinary frequency, urgency, and hesitancy

Urinary frequency (abnormally frequent urination) and urgency (intense and immediate desire to urinate) are classic symptoms of a

UTI. Urinary frequency also occurs with benign prostatic hyperplasia, urethral stricture, and a prostate tumor, which can put pressure on the bladder.

Incomplete passage

Urinary hesitancy (hesitancy in beginning the urine stream) is most common in the older patient who has an enlarged prostate gland, which can cause partial obstruction of the urethra.

Nocturia

Excessive urination at night, or nocturia, is a common sign of renal or lower urinary tract disorders. It can result from benign prostatic hyperplasia, when significant urethral obstruction develops, or from prostate cancer. It may also result from increased fluid intake or diuretic medications.

Urinary incontinence

Urinary incontinence (involuntary release of urine) may be caused by benign prostatic hyperplasia, prostate infection, prostate cancer, or radical prostatectomy.

Reproductive system problems

A number of reproductive system problems may occur, many of which are discussed below.

Penile lesions

Lesions on the penis can vary in appearance. A hard, nontender nodule, especially in the glans or inner lip of the prepuce, may indicate penile cancer. Lesions may also indicate genital herpes, genital warts, or syphilis. (See *Male genital lesions*.)

Penile discharge

A profuse, yellow discharge from the penis suggests gonococcal urethritis. Other symptoms may include urinary frequency, burning, and urgency. Without treatment, the prostate gland, epididymis, and periurethral glands become inflamed. A copious, watery, purulent urethral discharge may indicate chlamydial infection; a bloody discharge may indicate infection or cancer in the urinary or reproductive tract.

Paraphimosis

In paraphimosis, the prepuce is so tight that, when retracted, it gets caught behind the glans and can't be replaced. Edema can result and there can be painful swelling at the end of the penis.

Male genital lesions

Several types of lesions may affect the male genitalia. Some of the more common types are described here.

Penile cancer

Penile cancer causes a painless, ulcerative lesion on the glans or prepuce (foreskin), possibly accompanied by discharge.

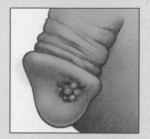

Genital warts

Genital warts are flesh-colored, soft, moist papillary growths that occur singly or in cauliflower-like clusters. They may be barely visible or several inches in diameter.

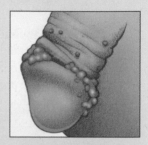

Genital herpes

Genital herpes causes a painful, reddened group of small vesicles or blisters on the prepuce, shaft, or glans. Lesions eventually disappear but tend to recur.

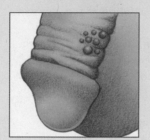

Syphilis

Syphilis causes a hard, round papule on the penis. When palpated, this syphilitic chancre may feel like a button. Eventually, the papule erodes into an ulcer. You may also note swollen lymph nodes in the inguinal area.

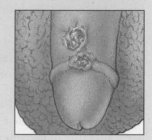

Cleaning up

Instruct uncircumcised patients to retract the prepuce each time they clean the glans and then to replace it afterward. Frequent retraction and cleaning of the prepuce prevents excessive tightness, which in turn prevents the prepuce from closing off the urinary meatus and constricting the glans.

Displacement of the urethral meatus

When the urethral meatus is located on the underside of the penis, the condition is called hypospadias. When the urethral meatus is located on the top of the penis, the condition is called epispadias. Both conditions are congenital and may contribute to infertility.

Testicular tumor

A painless scrotal nodule that can't be transilluminated may be a testicular tumor. This disorder occurs most commonly in patients ages 20 to 35. The tumor can grow, enlarging the testicle.

Scrotal swelling

Scrotal swelling occurs when a condition affecting the testicles, epididymis, or scrotal skin produces edema or a mass. It commonly results from a hydrocele or hernia.

Checking the fluid level

A hydrocele is a fluid-filled sac along the spermatic cord within the scrotum. It may occur on one or both sides. It's associated with conditions that cause poor fluid reabsorption, such as cirrhosis, heart failure, and testicular tumor. A hydrocele can be transilluminated during assessment.

Butting in

A hernia is a protrusion of an organ through an abnormal opening in the muscle wall. It may be direct or indirect, inguinal or femoral.

A direct inguinal hernia emerges from behind the external inguinal ring and protrudes through it. This type of hernia seldom descends into the scrotum and usually affects patients older than age 40.

The indirect approach

An indirect inguinal hernia is the most common type of hernia; it occurs in patients of all ages. It can be palpated in the internal inguinal canal with its tip in or beyond the canal, or the hernia may descend into the scrotum.

A femoral hernia feels like a soft tumor below the inguinal ligament in the femoral area. It may be difficult to distinguish from a lymph node and is uncommon in males.

Prostate gland enlargement

A smooth, firm, symmetrical enlargement of the prostate gland indicates benign prostatic hyperplasia, which typically starts after age 50. It is extremely common, with prevalence reaching 60% at age 60, and 80% at age 80. Although it can be asymptomatic, many patients can experience symptoms which include nocturia, urinary hesitancy and frequency, and recurring urinary tract infections.

In acute prostatitis, the prostate gland is firm, warm, and extremely tender and swollen. Because bacterial infection causes the condition, the patient usually has a fever and is acutely ill. The most common symptoms include fever, chills, dysuria, pelvic and perineal pain, and cloudy urine.

Prostate gland lesions

Hard, irregular, fixed lesions that make the prostate feel asymmetrical suggest prostate cancer. Palpation may be painful. This condition also causes urinary dysfunction. Back and leg pain may occur with bone metastases in advanced stages.

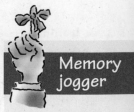

Memory jogger

To remember which findings suggest prostate cancer, think of the mnemonic **PAINS**:

Prostate cancer

Asymmetric

Irregular

Nodules

Stony (hard) and fixed.

Erectile dysfunction

Erectile dysfunction is the inability to achieve and maintain penile erection sufficient to complete satisfactory sexual intercourse; ejaculation may or may not be affected. Erectile dysfunction varies from occasional and minimal to permanent and complete. It may result from psychological, vascular, neurologic, or hormonal disorders or malfunctions. Fatigue, poor health, age, and drugs can also disrupt normal sexual function.

Priapism

A urologic emergency, priapism is a persistent, painful erection that's unrelated to sexual excitation. It may last for several hours or days and is usually accompanied by a severe, constant, dull aching in the penis. Unfortunately, the patient may be too embarrassed to seek medical help right away. Lack of prompt treatment can cause penile ischemia and thrombosis. Priapism may result from a blood disorder (such as sickle cell anemia), a neoplasm, trauma, or the use of certain drugs.

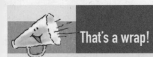

That's a wrap!

Male GU system review

Anatomy and physiology
• Urinary structures: similar to those in the female GU system, including kidneys, ureters, bladder, and urethra; extra 8″ (20 cm) in male urethra to pass through the penis
• Penis: consists of the shaft, glans, urethral meatus, corona, and prepuce (foreskin); discharges urine as well as sperm
• Scrotum: loose, wrinkled sac that contains the testicles, epididymides, and portions of the spermatic cords
• Testicles: oval, rubbery structures that produce testosterone and sperm
• Epididymis: a reservoir for mature sperm located on the posterolateral surface of each testicle
• Vas deferens: storage site and pathway for sperm
• Seminal vesicles: saclike glands found on the lower posterior surface of the bladder whose secretions help form seminal fluid
• Prostate gland: produces a thin, milky fluid that mixes with seminal fluid to enhance sperm activity

The health history
• Determine the patient's presenting problem.
  – Common urinary problems include pain on urination and changes in voiding pattern or urine color or output.
  – Common reproductive problems include penile discharge, erectile dysfunction, infertility, scrotal or inguinal masses, and pain or tenderness.
• Ask about past health and family health, especially about the presence or history of diabetes or hypertension.

(Continued)

Male GU system review *(continued)*

• Ask about current health, such as circumcision status; penile sores, lumps, ulcers, or discharge; and scrotal swelling.
• Ask about sexual health and practices, including any history of sexually transmitted infections and performance of testicular self-examination.

Assessment of the urinary system
• Follow same technique as for female urinary assessment.
• Inspect the patient's skin and abdomen.
• Percuss and palpate the kidneys and bladder.
• Auscultate over the renal arteries to check for bruits.

Assessment of the reproductive system
• Inspect the penis for size, skin color, and abnormalities; compress the tip of the glans to inspect the urethral meatus.
• Inspect the scrotum, testicles, and pubic hair.
• Inspect the inguinal and femoral areas for bulges or hernias.
• Palpate the entire penile shaft.
• Gently palpate both testicles, assessing their size, shape, and response to pressure; transilluminate hard, irregular areas or lumps.
• Palpate the epididymides and both spermatic cords.

• Palpate the prostate gland by performing a rectal examination.

Abnormal urinary findings
• Hematuria: presence of blood in urine
• Urinary frequency: abnormally frequent urination
• Urinary urgency: intense and immediate desire to urinate
• Urinary hesitancy: delay in starting urine stream
• Nocturia: excessive urination at night

Abnormal reproductive system findings
• Paraphimosis—tight prepuce that, when retracted, gets caught behind the glans and can't be replaced
• Hypospadias—urethral meatus located on the underside of the penis
• Epispadias—urethral meatus located on top of the penis
• Hydrocele—collection of fluid in the testicle
• Hernia—protrusion of an organ through a muscle wall
• Erectile dysfunction—inability to achieve and maintain penile erection sufficient to complete satisfactory sexual intercourse
• Priapism—persistent, painful erection unrelated to sexual excitation

Quick quiz

1. Stress to the patient the importance of performing testicular self-examination every:
   A. day.
   B. week.
   C. month.
   D. 6 months.

Answer: C. A monthly testicular self-examination can help detect testicular cancer early.

2. An inguinal hernia is best palpated with the patient:
   A. sitting.
   B. in a supine position.
   C. standing.
   D. lying on their right side.

Answer: C. To check for an inguinal hernia, have the patient stand and then hold their breath and bear down while you palpate the area.

3. Signs of benign prostatic hyperplasia include:
   A. an irregular, pea-shaped gland.
   B. an enlarged, hard gland with asymmetric swelling.
   C. smooth, firm symmetrical prostate enlargement.
   D. a firm, warm, tender prostate gland accompanied by a fever.

Answer: C. In male adults older than age 50, a smooth, firm, symmetrical enlargement of the prostate gland may be a normal finding.

4. Although the male and female urinary systems function in the same way, there's a difference in the length of the:
   A. bladder neck.
   B. ureter.
   C. epididymis.
   D. urethra.

Answer: D. Because the male urethra passes through the erectile tissue of the penis, it's about 6″ (15 cm) longer than the female urethra.

Scoring

☆☆☆   If you answered all four questions correctly, incredible! You've shown that you're a hands-down master of the material in this chapter.

☆☆   If you answered three questions correctly, congratulations! You're making history as an awesome assessor.

☆   If you answered fewer than three questions correctly, hang in there! Why not take a break and then try the quiz again?

Just for fun

Learn more about your patient's urinary health by asking about any noticeable urine changes. Match the urine color change in column 1 with the possible cause in column 2.

Urine color change

1. Pale and diluted

2. Orange-red or orange-brown
   _____

3. Blue-green _____

4. Dark yellow or amber and concentrated
   _____

5. Green-brown _____

6. Dark brown or black _____

7. Red or red-brown _____

Possible cause

A. Methylene blue ingestion

B. Acute glomerulonephritis, intake of chlorpromazine

C. Diabetes insipidus, diuretic therapy, excessive fluid intake

D. Bile duct obstruction

E. Hemorrhage, porphyria, intake of phenazopyridine

F. Obstructive jaundice, urobilinuria, intake of rifampin or phenazopyridine

G. Acute febrile disease, inadequate fluid intake, severe diarrhea or vomiting

Answer: 1. C, 2. F, 3. A, 4. G, 5. D, 6. B, 7. E

Identify the structures of the male reproductive system indicated on this illustration.

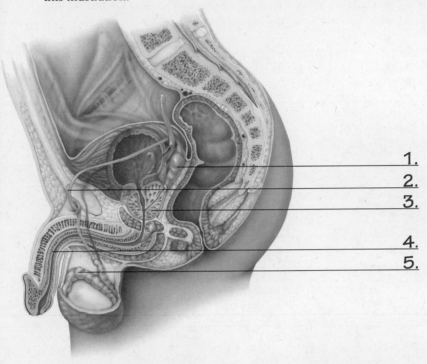

1.
2.
3.
4.
5.

Answer: 1. Seminal vesicles, 2. Vas deferens, 3. Prostate gland, 4. Urethra, 5. Epididymis.

Sound out each group of pictures and symbols to reveal information about the urinary system.

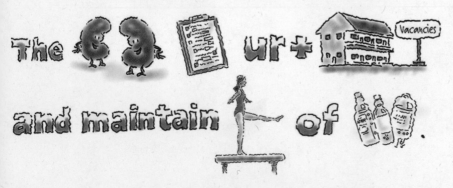

Answer: The kidneys form urine and maintain balance of fluids.

Chapter 15

Musculoskeletal system

Just the facts

In this chapter, you'll learn:

♦ structures of the musculoskeletal system

♦ questions to ask during a health history of the musculoskeletal system

♦ techniques to assess the musculoskeletal system

♦ causes and characteristics of abnormal findings of the musculoskeletal system.

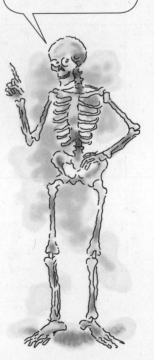

Besides giving the body its shape, my 206 bones serve as storage sites for minerals and my bone marrow produces blood cells.

A look at the musculoskeletal system

During a musculoskeletal assessment, you'll use sight, hearing, and touch to determine the health of the patient's muscles, bones, joints, tendons, and ligaments. These structures give the human body its shape and ability to move. Your sharp assessment skills will help uncover musculoskeletal abnormalities and evaluate the patient's ability to perform activities of daily living (ADLs).

Anatomy and physiology

The three main parts of the musculoskeletal system are the bones, joints, and muscles.

Bones

The 206 bones of the skeleton form the body's framework, supporting and protecting organs and tissues. The bones also serve as storage sites for minerals and contain bone marrow, the primary site for blood cell production. (See *A close look at the skeletal system*, page 390.)

A close look at the skeletal system

Of the 206 bones in the human skeletal system, 80 form the axial skeleton (skull, facial bones, vertebrae, ribs, sternum, and hyoid bone) and 126 form the appendicular skeleton (arms, legs, shoulders, and pelvis). Shown below are the body's major bones.

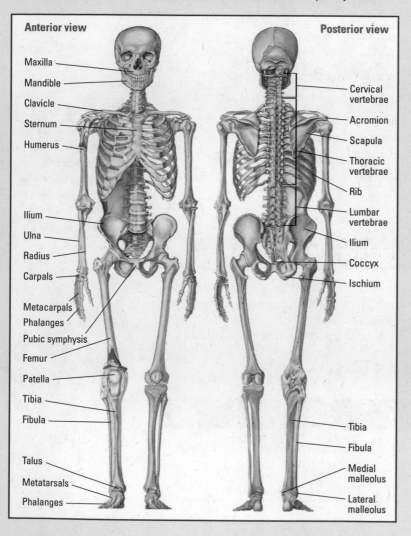

Anterior view

Posterior view

Maxilla
Mandible
Clavicle
Sternum
Humerus

Ilium
Ulna
Radius
Carpals

Metacarpals
Phalanges
Pubic symphysis
Femur
Patella
Tibia
Fibula

Talus
Metatarsals
Phalanges

Cervical vertebrae
Acromion
Scapula
Thoracic vertebrae
Rib
Lumbar vertebrae
Ilium
Coccyx
Ischium

Tibia
Fibula
Medial malleolus
Lateral malleolus

Joints

The junction of two or more bones is called a *joint*. Joints stabilize the bones and allow a specific type of movement. The two types of joints are nonsynovial and synovial.

Nonsynovial

In nonsynovial joints, the bones are connected by fibrous tissue, or cartilage. The bones may be immovable, like the sutures in the skull, or slightly movable, like the vertebrae.

Synovial

Synovial joints move freely; the bones are separate from each other and meet in a cavity filled with synovial fluid, a lubricant. (See *A close look at a synovial joint*.) In synovial joints, a layer of resilient cartilage covers the surfaces of opposing bones. This cartilage cushions the bones and allows full joint movement by making the surfaces of the bones smooth. (See *Types of joint motion*, page 392.) These joints are surrounded by a fibrous capsule that stabilizes the joint structures. The capsule also surrounds the joint's ligaments—the tough, fibrous bands that join one bone to another.

The joint's a-jumpin'!

Synovial joints come in several types, including ball-and-socket joints and hinge joints. Ball-and-socket joints—the shoulders and hips being the only examples of this type—allow for flexion, extension, adduction, and abduction. These joints also rotate in their sockets and are assessed by their degree of internal and external rotation. Hinge joints, such as the knee and elbow, typically move in flexion and extension only. (See *Popular joints*.)

A close look at a synovial joint

Normally, bones fit together. Cartilage—a smooth, fibrous tissue—cushions the end of each bone, and synovial fluid fills the joint space. This fluid lubricates the joint and eases movement, much as the brake fluid functions in a car.

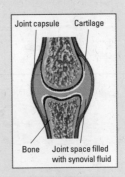

Joint capsule   Cartilage

Bone   Joint space filled with synovial fluid

Popular joints

Ball-and-socket joints	Hinge joints
• Located in the shoulders and hips • Allow flexion, extension, adduction, and abduction • Rotate in their sockets • Are assessed by their degree of internal and external rotation	• Include the knee and elbow • Move in flexion and extension

Types of joint motion

The illustrations below show various areas of the body and what types of movements their joints allow.

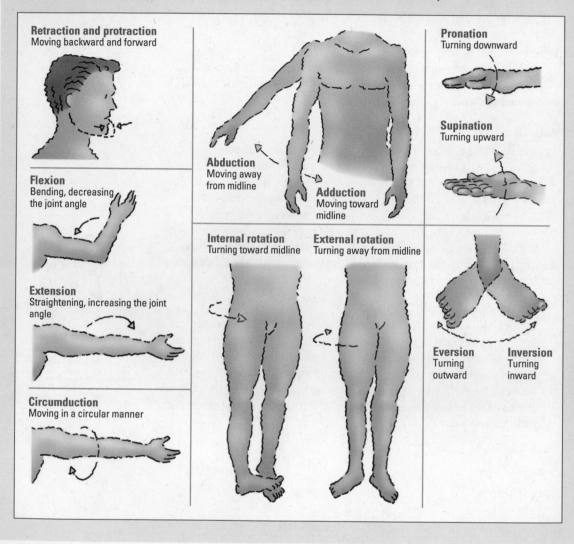

Retraction and protraction
Moving backward and forward

Flexion
Bending, decreasing the joint angle

Extension
Straightening, increasing the joint angle

Circumduction
Moving in a circular manner

Abduction
Moving away from midline

Adduction
Moving toward midline

Internal rotation
Turning toward midline

External rotation
Turning away from midline

Pronation
Turning downward

Supination
Turning upward

Eversion
Turning outward

Inversion
Turning inward

A close look at muscles

These illustrations show the major muscles of the body.

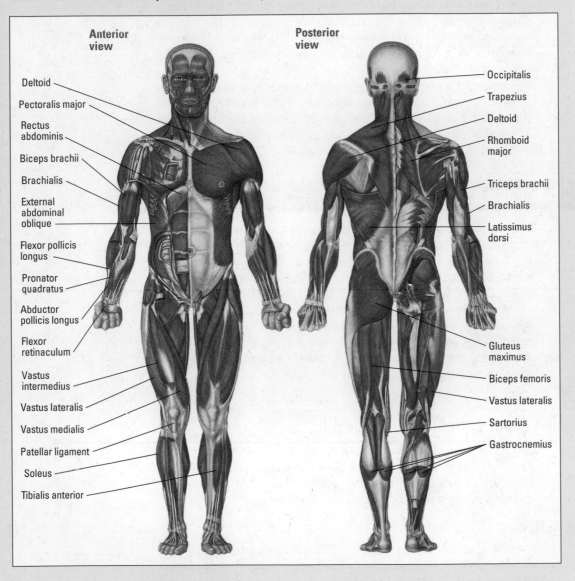

Anterior view

- Deltoid
- Pectoralis major
- Rectus abdominis
- Biceps brachii
- Brachialis
- External abdominal oblique
- Flexor pollicis longus
- Pronator quadratus
- Abductor pollicis longus
- Flexor retinaculum
- Vastus intermedius
- Vastus lateralis
- Vastus medialis
- Patellar ligament
- Soleus
- Tibialis anterior

Posterior view

- Occipitalis
- Trapezius
- Deltoid
- Rhomboid major
- Triceps brachii
- Brachialis
- Latissimus dorsi
- Gluteus maximus
- Biceps femoris
- Vastus lateralis
- Sartorius
- Gastrocnemius

Muscles

Muscles are groups of contractile cells or fibers that affect movement of an organ or a part of the body. Skeletal muscles, the focus of this chapter, contract and produce skeletal movement when they receive a stimulus from the central nervous system (CNS). The CNS is responsible for both involuntary and voluntary muscle function. (See *A close look at muscles*, page 393.)

Tendons are tough fibrous portions of muscle that attach the muscles to bone. Bursae are sacs filled with friction-reducing synovial fluid; they're located in areas of high friction such as the knee. Bursae allow adjacent muscles or muscles and tendons to glide smoothly over each other during movement.

Obtaining a health history

The patient's reason for seeking care is important because it can determine the focus of your examination. Patients with joint injuries usually report pain, swelling, or stiffness, and they may have noticeable deformities. Deformity can also occur with a bone fracture, which causes sharp pain when the patient moves the affected area.

Muscle injuries are commonly accompanied by pain, swelling, stiffness, and weakness. Because many musculoskeletal injuries are emergencies, you might not have time for a thorough assessment. In these cases, the PQRSTU device explained in Chapter 1 can help you remember which key areas to focus on.

Asking about current and past health

Ask about the patient's past and current health status. Are the patient's ADLs affected by their condition? Ask whether they have noticed grating sounds when they move certain parts of their body. Do they use ice, heat, or other remedies to treat the problem?

Ancient history

Inquire whether the patient has ever had gout, arthritis, tuberculosis, or cancer, which may cause bony metastases. Has the patient been diagnosed with osteoporosis?

Ask whether they have had a recent blunt or penetrating trauma or any surgery on their muscles, joints, or bones. If so, when was the trauma or surgery? What was the reason for any surgery? For example, did they suffer knee and hip injuries after being hit by a car, or did they ever have surgery for a broken bone? This information can help guide your assessment and predict hidden trauma.

Also ask the patient whether they use an assistive device, such as a cane, walker, or brace. If they do, watch them use the device to assess how they move.

Asking about medications

Question the patient about the medications they take regularly. Many drugs can affect the musculoskeletal system. Corticosteroids, for example, can cause muscle weakness, myopathy, osteoporosis, pathologic fractures, and avascular necrosis of the heads of the femur and humerus. Potassium-depleting diuretics can cause muscle cramping and weakness. Cholesterol-lowering agents can cause generalized muscle soreness.

Asking about lifestyle

Ask the patient about their job, hobbies, and personal habits. Knitting, playing football or tennis, working at a computer, or doing construction work can all cause repetitive stress injuries or injure the musculoskeletal system in other ways. Even carrying a heavy knapsack or purse can cause injury or increase muscle size.

Assessing the musculoskeletal system

Because the CNS and the musculoskeletal system are interrelated, you should assess them together. To assess the musculoskeletal system, use the techniques of inspection and palpation to test all the major bones, joints, and muscles. Perform a complete examination if the patient has generalized symptoms such as aching in several joints. Perform an abbreviated examination if they have pain in only one body area.

Go head to toe

Before starting your assessment, have the patient undress down to their underwear and have them put on an examination gown. If possible, make sure the room is warm. Explain each procedure as you perform it. The only special equipment you'll need is a tape measure and possibly a reflex hammer.

Begin your examination with a general observation of the patient. Then systematically assess the whole body, working from head to toe and from proximal to distal structures. Because muscles and joints are interdependent, interpret these findings together. As you work your way down the body, follow these general rules:

- Note the size and shape of joints, limbs, and body regions.
- Inspect and palpate the skin and tissues around the joints, limbs, and body regions.

Muscular dystrophy

Muscular dystrophy is a group of congenital disorders characterized by progressive symmetrical wasting of skeletal muscles without neural or sensory defects. The most common form is Duchenne (pseudohypertrophic) muscular dystrophy. Duchenne occurs during early childhood; onset is insidious and occurs between ages 3 and 5. The disorder initially affects the legs, pelvis, and shoulders. Findings include the following:

- enlarged, firm calf muscles
- waddling gait, toe-walking, lumbar lordosis, and positive Gower sign
- difficulty climbing stairs
- history of frequent falls.

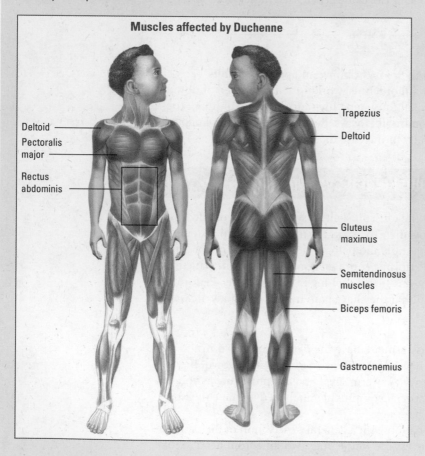

Muscles affected by Duchenne

Deltoid
Pectoralis major
Rectus abdominis

Trapezius
Deltoid
Gluteus maximus
Semitendinosus muscles
Biceps femoris
Gastrocnemius

(Continued)

Muscular dystrophy *(continued)*

Gower sign
A positive Gower sign—an inability to lift the trunk without using the hands and arms to brace and push—indicates pelvic muscle weakness, as occurs in muscular dystrophy and spinal muscle atrophy. To check for Gower sign, place the patient in the supine position and ask the patient to rise.

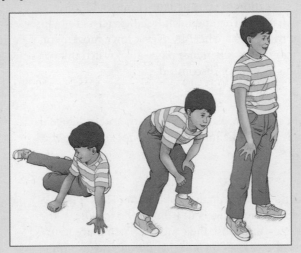

- Have the patient perform active range-of-motion (ROM) exercises of a joint, if possible. Active ROM exercises are joint movements the patient can do without assistance.
- If the patient can't perform active ROM exercises, perform passive ROM exercises. Passive ROM exercises don't require the patient to exert any effort.
- During passive ROM exercises, support the joint firmly on either side and move it gently to avoid causing pain or spasm. Never force movement.

Walk the walk

Whenever possible, observe how the patient stands and moves. Watch them walk into the room or, if they're already in, ask them to walk to the door, turn around, and walk back toward you. Their torso should sway only slightly, their arms should swing naturally at their sides, their gait should be even, and their posture should be erect.

As they walk, each foot should flatten and bear their weight completely, and their toes should flex as they push off with their foot. In midswing, their foot should clear the floor and pass the other leg. If you note a child with a waddling, ducklike gait (an important sign of muscular dystrophy), check for a positive Gower's sign, which indicates pelvic muscle weakness. (See *Muscular dystrophy*.)

Assessing the bones and joints

Perform a head-to-toe evaluation of your patient's bones and joints using inspection and palpation. Then perform ROM exercises to help you determine whether the joints are healthy. Never force movement. Ask the patient to tell you if they experience pain. Also, watch their facial expression for signs of pain or discomfort.

Head, jaw, and neck

First, inspect the patient's face for swelling, symmetry, and evidence of trauma. The mandible should be in the midline, not shifted to the right or left.

Is the TMJ A-OK?

Next, evaluate ROM in the temporomandibular joint (TMJ). Place the tips of your first two or three fingers in front of the middle of the ear. Ask the patient to open and close their mouth. Then place your fingers into the depressed area over the joint, and note the motion of the mandible. The patient should be able to open and close their jaw and protract and retract their mandible easily, without pain or tenderness.

If you hear or palpate a click as the patient's mouth opens, suspect an improperly aligned jaw. TMJ dysfunction may also lead to swelling of the area, crepitus, or pain. (See *Evaluating the temporomandibular joint.*)

Peak technique

Evaluating the temporomandibular joint

- Place the tips of your index fingers in front of the middle of each ear, as shown at right.
- Ask the patient to open and close the mouth. The patient should be able to open and close the jaw and protract and retract the mandible easily, without pain or tenderness. Your fingertips should drop into the depressed areas over the joints as the patient's mouth opens.
- If you hear or palpate a click as the patient's mouth opens, suspect an improperly aligned jaw. Swelling of the area, crepitus, or pain may occur.

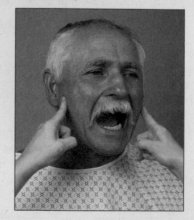

Check the neck

Inspect the front, back, and sides of the patient's neck, noting muscle asymmetry or masses. Palpate the spinous processes of the cervical vertebrae and the areas above each clavicle (supraclavicular fossae) for tenderness, swelling, or nodules.

To palpate the neck area, stand facing the patient with your hands placed lightly on the sides of the neck. Ask them to turn their head from side to side, flex their neck forward, and then extend it backward. Feel for any lumps or tender areas.

As the patient moves their neck, listen and palpate for crepitus. Crepitus is an abnormal grating sound. Note that this sound is different than the occasional crack that can be heard from joints.

Head circles and chin-ups

Now, check ROM in the neck. Ask the patient to try touching their right ear to their right shoulder and their left ear to their left shoulder without lifting their shoulders. The usual ROM is 40° on each side. Next, ask them to touch their chin to their chest and then to point their chin toward the ceiling. The neck should flex forward 45° and extend backward 55°.

To assess rotation, ask the patient to turn their head to each side without moving their trunk. Their chin should be parallel to their shoulders. Finally, ask them to move their head in a circle—normal rotation is 70°. (See *Assessing neck range of motion.*)

Spine

Open the patient's examination gown in the back so you can observe their spine. First check their spinal curvature as they stand in profile. In this position, the spine has a reverse "S" shape.

Next, observe the spine posteriorly. It should be in midline position, without deviation to either side. Lateral deviation suggests scoliosis. You may also notice that one shoulder is lower than the other. To assess for scoliosis, have the patient bend at the waist. This position makes deformities more apparent. Normally, the spine remains at midline. (See *Testing for scoliosis.*)

Spinal tape

Next, assess the range of spinal movement. Ask the patient to straighten up, and use a measuring tape to measure the distance from the nape of their neck to their waist. Then ask them to bend forward at the waist. Continue to hold the tape at their neck, letting it slip through your fingers slightly to accommodate the increased distance as the spine flexes.

The length of the spine from neck to waist usually increases by at least 2″ (5 cm) when the patient bends forward. If it doesn't, the patient's mobility may be impaired, and you'll need to assess them further. (See *Assessing the range of spinal movement.*)

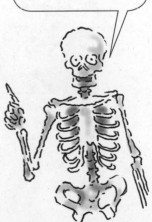

The length of the spine from neck to waist increases when I bend over. I'm a pretty flexible guy!

Assessing neck range of motion

- Ask the patient to try touching right ear to right shoulder and left ear to left shoulder. The usual range of motion is 40° on each side.

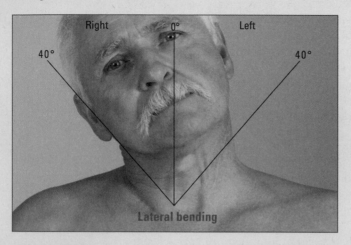

- Ask the patient to touch chin to chest and then to point the chin up toward the ceiling. While doing this, the patient's neck should flex forward 45° and extend backward 55°.

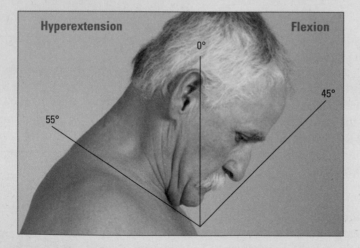

- To assess rotation, watch while the patient moves the head side to side without moving the trunk of the body. During this movement, the chin should remain parallel to the shoulders.
- Finally, ask the patient to move the head in a circle—normal rotation is 70°.

Spine-tingling procedure

Finally, palpate the spinal processes and the areas lateral to the spine. Have the patient bend at the waist and let their arms hang loosely at their sides. Palpate the spine with your fingertips. Then repeat the palpation using the side of your hand, lightly striking the areas lateral to the spine. Note tenderness, swelling, or spasm.

Shoulders and elbows

Start by observing the patient's shoulders, noting asymmetry, muscle atrophy, or deformity. Swelling or loss of the normal rounded shape could mean that one or more bones are dislocated or out of alignment. Remember, if the patient's reason for seeking care is shoulder pain, the problem may not have originated in the shoulder. Shoulder pain may be referred from other sources and may be due to a heart attack or ruptured ectopic pregnancy.

Palpate the shoulders with the palmar surfaces of your fingers to locate bony landmarks; note crepitus or tenderness. Using your entire hand, palpate the shoulder muscles for firmness and symmetry. Also palpate the elbow and the ulna for subcutaneous nodules that occur with rheumatoid arthritis.

Lift and rotate

If the patient's shoulders don't appear to be dislocated, assess rotation. Start with the patient's arm straight at their side—the neutral position. Ask them to lift their arm straight up from their side to shoulder level and then to bend their elbow horizontally until their forearm is at a 90° angle to their upper arm. Their arm should be parallel to the floor, and their fingers should be extended with palms down.

To assess external rotation, have them bring their forearm up until their fingers point toward the ceiling. To assess internal rotation, have them lower their forearm until their fingers point toward the floor. Normal ROM is 90° in each direction.

Flex and extend

To assess flexion and extension, start with the patient's arm in the neutral position (at their side). To assess flexion, ask them to move their arm anteriorly over their head, as if reaching for the sky. Full flexion is 180°. To assess extension, have them move their arm from the neutral position posteriorly as far as possible. Normal extension ranges from 30° to 50°.

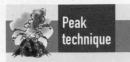

Peak technique

Testing for scoliosis

When testing for scoliosis, have the patient remove their shirt and stand as straight as possible with their back to you. Look for:
• uneven shoulder height and shoulder blade prominence
• unequal distance between the arms and the body
• asymmetrical waistline
• uneven hip height
• sideways lean.

Bend over

Then have the patient bend forward, keeping their head down and palms together. Look for:
• asymmetrical thoracic spine or prominent rib cage (rib hump) on either side
• asymmetrical waistline.

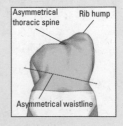

Swing into position

To assess abduction, ask the patient to move their arm from the neutral position laterally as far as possible. Normal ROM is 180°. To assess adduction, have the patient move their arm from the neutral position across the front of their body as far as possible. Normal ROM is 50°.

Up to the elbows

Next, assess the elbows for flexion and extension. Have the patient rest their arm at their side. Ask them to flex their elbow from this position and then extend it. Normal ROM is 90° for both flexion and extension.

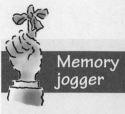

Memory jogger

Here's an easy way to keep adduction and abduction straight:

Adduction is moving a limb toward the body's midline; think of it as adding two things together.

Abduction is moving a limb away from the body's midline; think of it as taking something away, like abducting, or kidnapping.

Peak technique

Assessing the range of spinal movement

• Ask the patient to straighten up.
• Use a measuring tape to measure the distance from the nape of the neck to the waist.
• Ask the patient to bend forward at the waist.
• Continue to hold the tape at the patient's neck, letting it slip through your fingers slightly to accommodate the increased distance as the spine flexes.
• The length of the spine from neck to waist usually increases by at least 2″ (5 cm) when the patient bends forward. If it doesn't, the patient's mobility may be impaired, and you'll need to assess this further.

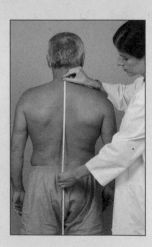
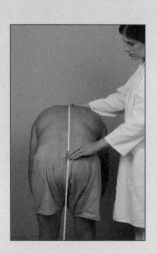

(Continued)

Assessing the range of spinal movement *(continued)*

Normal position of spine

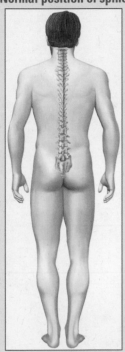

Normal curvature of spine

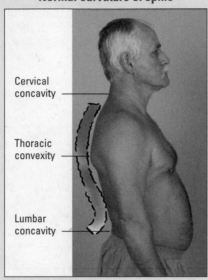

Cervical concavity

Thoracic convexity

Lumbar concavity

To assess supination and pronation of the elbow, have the patient place the side of their hand on a flat surface with the thumb on top. Ask them to rotate their palm down toward the table for pronation and upward for supination. The normal angle of elbow rotation is 90° in each direction.

Wrists and hands

Inspect the wrists and hands for contour, and compare them for symmetry. Also check for nodules, redness, swelling, deformities, and webbing between fingers.

Use your thumb and index finger to palpate both wrists and each finger joint. Note any tenderness, nodules, or sponginess. To avoid causing pain, be especially gentle with older patients and those with arthritis.

Wristy business

Assess ROM in the wrists. Ask the patient to rotate each wrist by moving their entire hand—first laterally then medially—as if waxing a car. Normal ROM is 55° laterally and 20° medially.

Observe the wrist while the patient extends their fingers up toward the ceiling and down toward the floor, as if flapping their hand. They should be able to extend their wrist 70° and flex it 90°. If these movements cause pain or numbness, they may have carpal tunnel syndrome. (See *Testing for carpal tunnel syndrome*.)

Peak technique

Testing for carpal tunnel syndrome

Two simple tests—Tinel sign and Phalen maneuver—can confirm carpal tunnel syndrome.

Tinel sign

Lightly percuss the transverse carpal ligament over the median nerve where the patient's palm and wrist meet. If this action produces discomfort, such as numbness and tingling shooting into the palm and finger, the patient has Tinel sign and may have carpal tunnel syndrome.

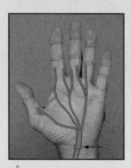

Phalen maneuver

If flexing the patient's wrist for about 30 seconds causes pain or numbness in their hand or fingers, they have a positive Phalen maneuver. The more severe the carpal tunnel syndrome, the more rapidly the symptoms develop.

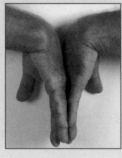

Lift a finger; make a fist

To assess extension and flexion of the metacarpophalangeal joints, ask the patient to keep their wrist still and move only their fingers—first up toward the ceiling and then down toward the floor. Normal extension is 30°; normal flexion, 90°.

Next, ask the patient to touch their thumb to the little finger of the same hand. They should be able to fold or flex their thumb across the palm of their hand so that it touches or points toward the base of their little finger.

To assess flexion of all of the fingers, ask the patient to form a fist. Then have them spread their fingers apart to demonstrate abduction and draw them back together to demonstrate adduction.

At arm's length

If you suspect that one arm is longer than the other, take measurements. Put one end of the measuring tape at the acromial process of the shoulder and the other on the tip of the middle finger. Drape the tape over the outer elbow. The difference between the left and right extremities should be no more than ⅜″ (1 cm).

Hips and knees

Inspect the hip area for contour and symmetry. Inspect the position of the knees, noting whether the patient is bowlegged, with knees that point out, or knock-kneed, with knees that turn in. Then watch the patient walk.

Palpate each hip over the iliac crest and trochanteric area for tenderness or instability. Palpate both knees. They should feel smooth, and the tissues should feel solid. (See *Bulge sign*.)

Hip, hip, hooray!

Assess ROM in the hip. These exercises are typically done with the patient in a supine position.

To assess hip flexion, place your hand under the patient's lower back and have the patient bend one knee and pull it toward their abdomen and chest as far as possible. You'll feel the patient's back touch your hand as the normal lumbar lordosis of the spine flattens. As the patient flexes their knee, the opposite hip and thigh should remain flat on the bed. Repeat on the opposite side.

To assess hip abduction, stand alongside the patient and press down on the superior iliac spine of the opposite hip with one hand to stabilize the pelvis. With your other hand, hold the patient's leg by the ankle and gently abduct the hip until you feel the iliac spine move. That movement indicates the limit of hip abduction. Then, while still stabilizing the pelvis, move the ankle medially across the patient's

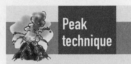

Peak technique

Bulge sign

The bulge sign indicates excess fluid in the joint. To assess the patient for this sign, ask them to lie down so that you can palpate their knee. Then give the medial side of their knee two to four firm strokes, as shown here, to displace excess fluid.

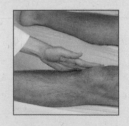

body to assess hip adduction. Repeat on the other side. Normal ROM is about 45° for abduction and 30° for adduction.

To assess hip extension, have the patient lie prone (face down), and gently extend the thigh upward. Repeat on the other thigh. (See *Assessing hip ROM.*)

Peak technique

Assessing hip ROM

These illustrations show you how to assess range of motion (ROM) in a patient's hips.

Flexion
To assess flexion, have the patient lie on their back. Then have them bend one knee and pull it toward their abdomen and chest as far as possible. As they flex their knee, the opposite hip and thigh should remain flat. Repeat the test on the opposite side.

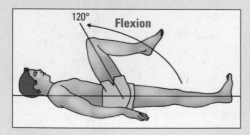

Extension
To assess extension, have the patient lie in a prone position (face down) and gently extend the thigh upward. Repeat the test on the other thigh.

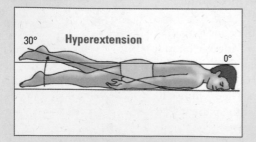

Internal and external rotation
To assess internal and external rotation, ask the patient to bend their knee and turn their leg inward. Then ask them to turn their leg outward. Normal ROM for internal rotation is 40°; for external rotation, 45°.

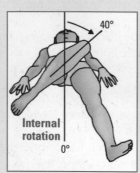

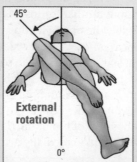

Abduction and adduction
To test abduction and adduction, stand alongside the patient and press down on the superior iliac spine of the opposite hip with one hand to stabilize the pelvis.

With your other hand, hold the patient's leg by the ankle and gently abduct the hip until you feel the iliac spine move. That movement indicates the limit of hip abduction. Next, while still stabilizing the patient's pelvis, move the ankle medially across the patient's body to assess hip adduction. Repeat on the other side. Normal ROM is about 45° for abduction and 30° for adduction.

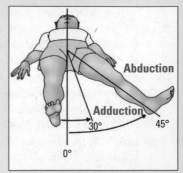

As the hip turns

To assess internal and external rotation of the hip, ask the patient to lift one leg up and, keeping their knee straight, turn their leg and foot medially and laterally. Normal ROM for internal rotation is 40°; for external rotation, 45°.

On bended knees

Assess ROM in the knee. If the patient is standing, ask them to bend their knee as if trying to touch their heel to their buttocks. Normal ROM for flexion is 120 to 130°. If the patient is lying down, have them draw their knee up to their chest. Their calf should touch their thigh.

Knee extension returns the knee to a neutral position of 0°; however, some knees may normally be hyperextended 15°. If the patient can't extend their leg fully or if their knee pops audibly and painfully, consider the response abnormal.

Other abnormalities include pronounced crepitus, which may signal a degenerative disease of the knee, and sudden buckling, which may indicate a ligament injury. (See *Assessing knee ROM*, page 407.)

Peak technique

Assessing knee ROM

To assess knee range of motion (ROM) in a patient who's standing, ask them to bend their knee as if trying to touch their heel to their buttocks, as shown. Normal range of motion for flexion is 120° to 130°. If the patient is lying down, you can assess ROM by having them draw their knee up to their chest. Their calf should touch their thigh.

Knee extension returns the knee to a neutral position of 0°; however, some knees may normally be hyperextended 15°. If the patient can't extend their leg fully or if their knee pops audibly and painfully, consider the response abnormal. Pronounced crepitus may signal a degenerative disease of the knee. Sudden buckling may indicate a ligament injury.

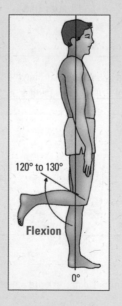

120° to 130°

Flexion

0°

Ankles and feet

Inspect the ankles and feet for swelling, redness, nodules, and other deformities. Check the arch of the foot and look for toe deformities. Also note edema, calluses, bunions, corns, ingrown toenails, plantar warts, trophic ulcers, hair loss, or unusual pigmentation.

Peak technique

Assessing ankle and foot range of motion

- Have the patient sit in a chair or on the side of a bed.
- Test plantar flexion of the ankle by asking the patient to point the toes toward the floor.
- Test dorsiflexion by having the patient point toes toward the ceiling.
- Normal range of motion (ROM) for plantar flexion is about 45°; for dorsiflexion, 20°.

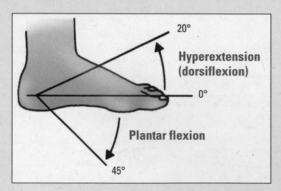

- Ask the patient to demonstrate inversion by turning the feet inward, and eversion by turning the feet outward. Normal ROM for inversion is 30°; for eversion, 20°.

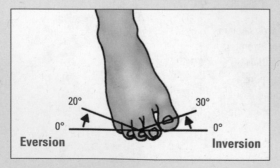

- To assess the metatarsophalangeal joints, ask the patient to first flex the toes and then straighten them.

Use your fingertips to palpate the bony and muscular structures of the ankles and feet. Palpate each toe joint by compressing it with your thumb and fingers.

The ankle angle

To examine the ankle, have the patient sit in a chair or on the side of a bed. To test plantar flexion, ask them to point their toes toward the floor. Test dorsiflexion by asking them to point their toes toward the ceiling. Normal ROM for plantar flexion is about 45°; for dorsiflexion, 20°.

Next, assess ROM in the ankle. Ask the patient to demonstrate inversion by turning their feet inward, and eversion by turning their feet outward. Normal ROM for inversion is 45°; for eversion, 30°.

To assess the metatarsophalangeal joints, ask the patient to flex their toes and then straighten them. (See *Assessing ankle and foot range of motion.*)

The long and short of it

If you suspect that one leg is longer than the other, take measurements. Put one end of the tape at the medial malleolus at the ankle and the other end at the anterior iliac spine. Cross the tape over the medial side of the knee. A difference of more than ⅜″ (1 cm) is abnormal.

Assessing the muscles

Start assessing the muscles by inspecting all major muscle groups for tone, strength, and symmetry. If a muscle appears atrophied or hypertrophied, measure it by wrapping a tape measure around the largest circumference of the muscle on each side of the body and comparing the two numbers.

Other muscle abnormalities include contracture and abnormal movements, such as spasms, tics, tremors, and fasciculations (twitches).

Tuning in to muscle tone

Muscle tone describes muscular resistance to passive stretching. To test the patient's arm muscle tone, move their shoulder through passive ROM exercises. You should feel a slight resistance. Then let their arm drop. It should fall easily to their side.

Test leg muscle tone by putting the patient's hip through passive ROM exercises and then letting the leg fall to the examination table or bed. Like the arm, the leg should fall easily.

Abnormal findings include muscle rigidity and flaccidity. Rigidity indicates increased muscle tone, possibly caused by an upper motor neuron lesion such as from a stroke. Flaccidity may result from a lower motor neuron lesion.

Wrestling with muscle strength

Observe the patient's gait and movements to form an idea of their general muscle strength. Grade muscle strength on a scale of 0 to 5, with 0 representing no strength and 5 representing normal strength. Document the results as a fraction, with the score as the numerator and maximum strength as the denominator. (See *Grading muscle strength* and *Documenting muscle strength*.)

To test specific muscle groups, ask the patient to move the muscles while you apply resistance; then compare the contralateral muscle groups. (See *Testing muscle strength*.)

Documenting muscle strength

See below for an example of proper documentation of patient muscle strength.

3/14/24	1730	Pt. alert and oriented to person, place,
		and time. Finished 80% of dinner tray.
		No difficulty swallowing. Feeds self
		with minimal effort. Full ROM upper
		extremities. Strong bilateral hand-
		grip. Weakness in left leg unchanged,
		muscle strength 3/5 left leg and 5/5
		right leg. Son visiting with patient.
		Mary Petty, RN

Grading muscle strength

Grade muscle strength on a scale of 0 to 5, as follows:
- 5/5—Normal: Patient moves joint through full range of motion (ROM) and against gravity with full resistance.
- 4/5—Good: Patient completes ROM against gravity with moderate resistance.
- 3/5—Fair: Patient completes ROM against gravity only.
- 2/5—Poor: Patient completes full ROM with gravity eliminated (passive motion).
- 1/5—Trace: Patient's attempt at muscle contraction is palpable but without joint movement.
- 0/5—Zero: No evidence of muscle contraction.

Peak technique

Testing muscle strength

To test specific muscle groups, ask the patient to move the muscles while you apply resistance; then compare the contralateral muscle groups. Use the techniques shown here to test the muscle strength of your patient's arm and ankle muscles.

Biceps strength

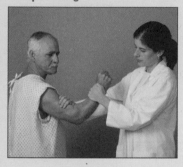

Triceps strength

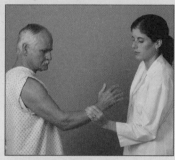

Ankle strength: Plantar flexion

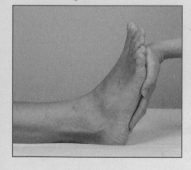

Ankle strength: Dorsiflexion

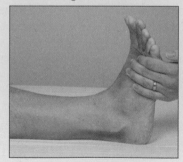

Shoulder, arm, wrist, and hand strength

Test the strength of the patient's shoulder girdle by asking them to extend their arms with the palms up and hold this position for 30 seconds. If they can't lift both arms equally and keep their palms up, or if one arm drifts down, they probably have shoulder girdle weakness on that side.

If they pass the first part of the test, gauge their strength by placing your hands on their arms and applying downward pressure as they resist you.

Testing the bi's and tri's

Next, have the patient hold their arm in front of them with the elbow bent. To test biceps strength, pull down on the flexor surface of their forearm as they resist. To test triceps strength, have them try to straighten their arm as you push upward against the extensor surface of their forearm.

Forcing their hand

Assess the strength of the patient's flexed wrist by pushing against it. Test the strength of the extended wrist by pushing down on it. Test the strength of finger abduction, thumb opposition, and handgrip the same way. (See *Testing handgrip strength*.)

Leg strength

Ask the patient to lie supine or in a sitting position on the examination table or bed and lift both legs at the same time. Note whether they lift both legs at the same time and to the same distance. To test quadriceps strength, have them lower their legs and raise them again while you press down on their anterior thighs.

Then ask the patient to flex their knees and put their feet flat on the bed. Assess lower leg strength by pulling their lower leg forward as they resist and then by pushing it backward as they extend their knee.

If the patient is sitting, ask them to extend both legs simultaneously while you press in on the anterior surface of the lower legs. Then have the patient pull back (flexion) both lower legs against your hands as you provide resistance.

Finally, assess ankle strength by having the patient push their foot down against your resistance and then pull their foot up as you try to hold it down.

Peak technique

Testing handgrip strength

- Face the patient.
- Extend the first and second fingers of each hand, and ask the patient to grasp your fingers and squeeze.
- Don't extend fingers with rings on them; a strong handgrip on those fingers can be painful.

Abnormal findings

Abnormalities in the musculoskeletal system occur for many reasons. Some general abnormalities have already been discussed; more specific abnormalities are described below.

A call to arms

Arm pain (pain anywhere from the hand to the shoulder) usually results from musculoskeletal disorders, but it can also stem from neurovascular or cardiovascular disorders. In some cases, it may be referred pain from another area, such as the chest, neck, or abdomen.

Crunching crepitus

Crepitus is an abnormal crunching or grating you can hear and feel when a joint with roughened articular surfaces moves. It occurs in patients with rheumatoid arthritis or osteoarthritis or when broken pieces of bone rub together. (See *Rheumatoid arthritis*.)

Rheumatoid arthritis

A chronic, systemic inflammatory immune disorder, rheumatoid arthritis commonly affects bilateral joints of the fingers, wrists, elbows, knees, or ankles as well as surrounding muscles, tendons, ligaments, and blood vessels. Spontaneous remissions and unpredictable exacerbations mark the course of this potentially crippling disease. Swollen, painful, and stiff joints, especially of the hands, are typical in acute rheumatoid arthritis.

As the disease progresses, bone atrophy and misalignment cause visible deformities, restriction of movement, and muscle atrophy. In chronic rheumatoid arthritis, deformities of the interphalangeal joints develop. Swan-neck deformity—hyperextension of the proximal interphalangeal joints with flexion of the distal interphalangeal joints—may occur. A less common deformity is the boutonnière deformity—flexion of the proximal interphalangeal joint with hyperextension of the distal interphalangeal joint.

Acute rheumatoid arthritis

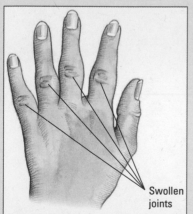

Swollen joints

Chronic rheumatoid arthritis

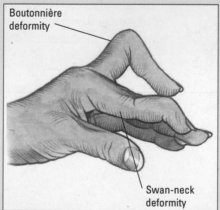

Boutonnière deformity

Swan-neck deformity

Unsure footing

Footdrop—plantar flexion of the foot with the toes bent toward the instep—results from weakness or paralysis of the dorsiflexor muscles of the foot and ankle. A characteristic and important sign of certain peripheral nerve or motor neuron disorders, footdrop may also stem from prolonged immobility when inadequate support, improper positioning, or infrequent passive exercise produces shortening of the Achilles tendon.

What kind of joint is this?

Heberden and Bouchard nodes are hard nodes that develop on the distal and proximal joints of the fingers in patients with osteoarthritis. (See *Heberden and Bouchard nodes*, page 414.) Patients with osteoarthritis may also experience joint swelling, pain, crepitus, limited movement, and contracture. Gait may be affected if knees and hips are involved. Joint mobility can also be impacted by a ganglion. (See *Ganglion*.) Patients with gout may experience pain and swelling in their joints. (See *Gout*.)

Heberden and Bouchard nodes

Heberden and Bouchard nodes are typically seen in patients with osteoarthritis.

Heberden nodes

Heberden nodes appear on the distal interphalangeal joints. Usually hard and painless, these bony and cartilaginous enlargements typically occur in middle-aged and older patients with osteoarthritis.

Bouchard nodes

Bouchard nodes are similar but less common and appear on the proximal interphalangeal joints.

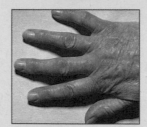

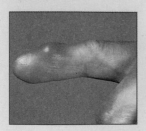

Ganglion

A ganglion is a round, enlarged, fluid-filled cyst commonly found on the dorsal side of the wrist. A ganglion may be nontender, but when it develops near a tender sheath, it may be painful and may limit joint mobility.

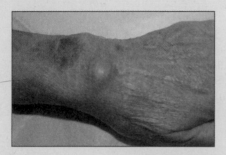

Gout

Gout is a metabolic disorder in which uric acid deposits in the joints cause the joints to become painful, arthritic, red, and swollen. Skin temperature may be elevated due to the irritation and inflammation.

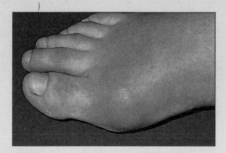

Not a leg to stand on

Although leg pain commonly indicates a musculoskeletal disorder, it can also result from more serious vascular or neurologic disorders. The pain may occur suddenly or gradually and may be localized or affect the entire leg. Constant or intermittent, it may feel dull, burning, sharp, shooting, or tingling.

Wasting away

Muscle atrophy, or muscle wasting, results from denervation or prolonged muscle disuse. When deprived of regular exercise, muscle fibers lose both bulk and length, which produces a visible loss of muscle size and contour and apparent emaciation or deformity in the affected area. It usually results from neuromuscular disease or injury but may also stem from metabolic and endocrine disorders and prolonged immobility. Some muscle atrophy also occurs with aging.

Muscle spasms

Muscle spasms, or cramps, are strong, painful contractions. They can occur in virtually any muscle but are most common in the calf and foot. Muscle spasms typically occur from simple muscle fatigue, after exercise, and during pregnancy. However, they may also develop in electrolyte imbalances and neuromuscular disorders or as the result of taking certain drugs.

Feeble finding

Muscle weakness may be reported to you by the patient, or you may detect it by observing and measuring the strength of an individual muscle or muscle group. It can result from a malfunction in the cerebral hemispheres, brain stem, spinal cord, nerve roots, peripheral nerves, or myoneural junctions and within the muscle itself.

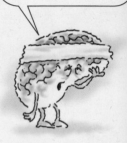

Muscle weakness can result from several causes, including a malfunction in the brain stem or spinal cord. I'm not feeling so well...

Feeling wounded

Most musculoskeletal emergencies result from trauma. Specific traumatic injuries include fractures, dislocations, amputations, crush injuries, and serious lacerations. The patient is usually alert and able to describe how the injury occurred.

If their level of consciousness deteriorates, suspect shock or drug or alcohol ingestion, and assess them further. Remember, even if the patient has ingested drugs or alcohol, they can still go into shock. (See *The 5 Ps of musculoskeletal injury.*)

The 5 Ps of musculoskeletal injury

Pain—Does the patient feel pain? If so, assess its location, severity, and quality.

Paresthesia—Assess for loss of sensation by touching the injured area with the tip of an open safety pin. Abnormal sensation or loss of sensation indicates neurovascular involvement.

Paralysis—Can the patient move the affected area? If not, the patient may have nerve or tendon damage.

Pallor—Paleness, discoloration, and coolness on the injured side may indicate neurovascular compromise.

Pulse—Check all pulses distal to the injury site. If a pulse is decreased or absent, blood supply to the area is reduced.

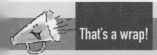 That's a wrap!

Musculoskeletal system review

Anatomy and physiology
Bones
- Support and protect organs and tissues
- Serve as storage sites for minerals
- Produce red blood cells in bone marrow

Joints
- Defined as the junction of two or more bones
- Consist of two types
  - Nonsynovial: immovable or slightly movable bones connected by fibrous tissue or cartilage (such as sutures in the skull and vertebrae)
  - Synovial: freely movable bones that meet in a cavity filled with synovial fluid (a lubricant); include ball-and-socket and hinge joints
- Perform different types of motion:
  - Circumduction: moving in a circular manner
  - Flexion: bending, decreasing the joint angle
  - Extension: straightening, increasing the joint angle
  - Abduction: moving away from midline
  - Adduction: moving toward midline
  - Retraction and protraction: moving backward and forward
  - Pronation: turning downward
  - Supination: turning upward
  - Internal rotation: turning toward midline
  - External rotation: turning away from midline
  - Eversion: turning outward
  - Inversion: turning inward

Muscles
- Consist of groups of contractile cells or fibers
- Attach to bone by tendons (tough fibrous portions of muscle)

The health history
- Determine the patient's reason for seeking care, such as pain, swelling, stiffness, and obvious deformities.
- Ask about current health, such as effects on ADLs and the use of ice, heat, or other remedies to treat the problem.
- Ask about past health, including arthritis, cancer, osteoporosis, and trauma, and inquire about the patient's use of assistive devices, such as a walker or cane.
- Ask about medications, especially those that may affect the musculoskeletal system (such as corticosteroids and potassium-depleting diuretics).
- Ask about lifestyle, including the patient's job, hobbies, and personal habits.

Assessing the musculoskeletal system
- Work from head to toe and from proximal to distal.
- Note the size and shape of joints, limbs, and body regions.
- Inspect and palpate around joints, limbs, and body regions.
- Have the patient perform active ROM exercises; if they can't, perform passive ROM exercises. Never force any movement!
- Observe the patient's posture and gait whenever possible.

Assessing bones and joints
Head, jaw, and neck
- Inspect the patient's face.
- Evaluate ROM in the TMJ.
- Inspect the front, back, and sides of the patient's neck.
- Palpate the cervical vertebrae and the neck area. Listen for crepitus as the patient moves their neck.
- Assess ROM in the neck.

Spine
- Inspect the patient's spine posteriorly and as they stand in profile.
- Assess for scoliosis by having the patient bend at the waist.

(Continued)

Musculoskeletal system review *(continued)*

- Assess the range of spinal movement.
- Palpate the spinal processes and areas lateral to the spine as the patient bends at the waist.

Shoulders and elbows

- Inspect and palpate the shoulders.
- Assess internal and external rotation, flexion and extension, and abduction and adduction of the shoulders.
- Assess flexion and extension as well as supination and pronation of the elbows.

Wrists and hands

- Inspect and palpate the wrists and hands. Also palpate each finger joint.
- Assess ROM in the wrist: rotation, flexion, and extension. Assess for carpal tunnel syndrome if these movements cause pain or numbness.
- Assess extension and flexion of the metacarpophalangeal joints.
- Assess flexion, extension, abduction, and adduction of all the fingers.
- Measure both arms if you suspect one is longer than the other.

Hips and knees

- Inspect the hip area and knees.
- Palpate the hips and knees.
- Perform the bulge sign to assess for excess fluid in the knee joint.
- Assess hip flexion, extension, abduction, and adduction as well as internal and external hip rotation.
- Assess flexion and extension in the knee.

Ankles and feet

- Inspect and palpate the ankles and feet.
- Assess dorsiflexion, plantar flexion, inversion, and eversion of the ankles.

- Assess the metatarsophalangeal joints by having the patient flex and extend their toes.
- Measure both legs if you suspect one is longer than the other.

Assessment of the muscles

- Assess muscle tone as you move each limb through passive ROM exercises.
- Assess shoulder, arm, wrist, and hand strength.
- Assess leg strength.

Abnormal musculoskeletal findings

- Crepitus: abnormal crunching or grating that may be heard or felt when a joint with roughened articular surfaces moves
- Footdrop: plantar flexion of the foot with the toes bent toward the instep
- Heberden nodes: hard nodes on the distal interphalangeal joints in patients with osteoarthritis
- Bouchard nodes: hard nodes on the proximal interphalangeal joints in patients with osteoarthritis
- Muscle atrophy: muscle wasting
- Muscle spasms: muscle cramps; strong, painful muscle contractions

The 5 Ps of musculoskeletal injury

- Pain
- Paresthesia
- Paralysis
- Pallor
- Pulse

Quick quiz

1. If you hear crepitus while moving a patient's joint, the joint must be:
    A. synovial.
    B. nonsynovial.
    C. fixed.
    D. slightly movable.

Answer: A. Crepitus occurs when roughened articular surfaces of bone or bone fragments rub together. Thus it can only occur in joints that are freely movable such as the synovial joints.

2. If your patient's arm drifts down after they extend it for 10 seconds, they probably have:
    A. carpal tunnel syndrome.
    B. broken metatarsal bones.
    C. weakness of shoulder girdle muscles.
    D. a fractured rib.

Answer: C. Inability to lift and extend an arm for 30 seconds indicates weakness of the shoulder girdle muscles on that side.

3. Your patient can't move their right arm away from their side, so you document this as impaired:
    A. supination.
    B. abduction.
    C. adduction.
    D. eversion.

Answer: B. Abduction is the ability to move a limb away from the midline. In adduction, the limb is moved toward the midline.

4. To assess a swollen knee, perform the:
    A. bulge sign test.
    B. straight leg raise test.
    C. Ortolani sign test.
    D. Phalen maneuver test.

Answer: A. A swollen knee suggests excess fluid in the joint. The bulge sign occurs when you apply pressure to the knee and a bulge of fluid appears on the opposite side.

Scoring

⭐⭐⭐ If you answered all four questions correctly, hooray! No bones about it, you're a master of musculoskeletal assessments.

⭐⭐ If you answered three questions correctly, yeah! You're really beginning to flex your assessment muscles.

⭐ If you answered fewer than three questions correctly, that's okay! Building knowledge, just like building muscles, takes persistence.

Just for fun

Can you pass the muscle strength test? Match the grade level in column 1 with the muscle strength response in column 2.

Grade

1. 5/5 _____
2. 4/5 _____
3. 3/5 _____
4. 2/5 _____
5. 1/5 _____
6. 0/5 _____

Muscle strength response

A. Poor: Completes ROM with gravity eliminated (passive motion)
B. Normal: Moves joint through full ROM and against gravity with full resistance
C. Trace: Attempt at muscle contraction is palpable but without joint movement
D. Good: Completes ROM against gravity with moderate resistance
E. Zero: No evidence of muscle contraction
F. Fair: Completes ROM against gravity only

Answer: 1. B, 2. D, 3. F, 4. A, 5. C, 6. E

Appendices and index

Practice makes perfect 422

Glossary 445

Selected references 448

Index 451

Questions

1. A 3-year-old client is admitted for an elective procedure. Which of the following actions should be the nurse's first priority when performing this client's admission assessment?
1. Having the client's legal guardian sign the admission forms
2. Establishing rapport with the client and legal guardian
3. Obtaining the necessary equipment
4. Taking the client's vital signs

2. A 56-year-old client is admitted with a diagnosis of heart failure. He tells the nurse, "I have trouble breathing when I try to lie flat." The nurse replies, "You have difficulty breathing while lying flat?" What communication strategy is this nurse using?
1. Reflection
2. Facilitation
3. Confirmation
4. Summarization

3. An occupational health nurse is performing a physical assessment on a prospective company employee. Which assessment should the nurse perform first?
1. Vital signs
2. Presence of skin lesions
3. Anthropometric measurements
4. General survey

4. A 52-year-old client is admitted with unstable angina. The nurse assigned to the client notes an irregular rhythm when assessing pulse. To further assess the irregular pulse, the nurse knows it is necessary to determine the client's pulse deficit. Which pulses help identify pulse deficit?
1. Carotid and apical
2. Apical and radial
3. Radial and brachial
4. Carotid and radial

5. An 85-year-old client is admitted with severe abdominal pain, nausea, and vomiting for 3 days. The nurse performs an abdominal assessment. Which sound should the nurse hear when percussing over dense tissue?
1. Tympany
2. Dullness
3. Flatness
4. Resonance

6.   A nurse is assessing the blood pressure of a client with diabetic ketoacidosis. What instructions should the nurse follow when inflating the blood pressure cuff before releasing the valve and listening for the blood pressure?
   1.   Inflate the cuff until the radial pulse disappears, and then inflate it an additional 30 mm Hg.
   2.   Inflate the cuff to 200 mm Hg; if the sound can be heard immediately, inflate to 220 mm Hg.
   3.   Inflate the cuff until the needle on the manometer stops bouncing.
   4.   Inflate the cuff until the client reports feeling a tingling sensation in the hand.

7.   A 73-year-old female client with Alzheimer disease is admitted to the hospital with dehydration. Her daughter, who has been caring for the client at home, verbalizes frustration that the client refuses to eat or drink. The nurse performs anthropometric arm measurements on the client, and the result is 85% of the standard. What does this result suggest?
   1.   Caloric deprivation
   2.   Normalcy
   3.   Protein malnutrition
   4.   Caloric excess

8.   A 76-year-old client is diagnosed with liver disease. Which finding should the nurse expect when assessing this client's nails?
   1.   Dark, yellowish color
   2.   Transverse bands of white
   3.   White patches
   4.   Spoon shape

9.   A 23-year-old client is admitted to an inpatient psychiatric unit with severe depression. To develop rapport with the client, the nurse initiates a contract. What should the contract include?
   1.   Expectations and responsibilities for the nurse and the client
   2.   A description of the therapies the client will undergo
   3.   A prediction of the length of the hospitalization
   4.   The client's insurance and financial information

10.   During an assessment, an 18-year-old client reports using an addictive substance. Which response by the nurse is most appropriate?
   1.   "How do you obtain the substance?"
   2.   "What substance do you use?"
   3.   "Does your employer know about this?"
   4.   "You really shouldn't do that."

11. A nurse is assessing a child's visual acuity using the Snellen chart. The result is 20/40 in both eyes. Which explanation should the nurse give to the child's parent?
  1. "What normal eyes see at a distance of 40 feet, your child's eyes see at a distance of 20 feet."
  2. "What normal eyes see at a distance of 20 feet, your child's eyes see at a distance of 40 feet."
  3. "To see what the normal eye sees at a distance of 20 feet, your child's eyes need a 40% magnification increase."
  4. "Your child's eyes see 20% of what children with normal vision see at 40 feet."

12. During an interview, a client has episodes in which they repeat the interviewer's words. Which term identifies this type of speech?
  1. Neologisms
  2. Echolalia
  3. Confabulation
  4. Flight of ideas

13. A 25-year-old client was brought to the emergency room by their mother. The mother states that the client has been acting "strange" the last week and thinks they have superpowers. The client's behavior and unrealistic statement are most consistent with which diagnosis?
  1. Schizophrenia
  2. Personality disorder
  3. Anxiety disorder
  4. Obsessive-compulsive disorder

14. A 40-year-old client is admitted with excessive vomiting. To assess the client's skin turgor for signs of dehydration, the nurse should:
  1. squeeze the skin on their forearm or sternum.
  2. palpate the skin on the dorsum of their hand.
  3. press on their nail beds to cause blanching.
  4. transilluminate the skin over the forearm.

15. A nurse notes a number of small, firm, inflamed, blisterlike lesions on a client's abdomen and back. The nurse should chart these findings as:
  1. macules.
  2. pustules.
  3. papules.
  4. plaques.

16. A 49-year-old client with a history of alcohol misuse is admitted with bleeding esophageal varices. The nurse assessing the client notes several small, weblike, vascular lesions on their cheeks. The nurse should chart these findings as:
  1. purpura.
  2. telangiectases.
  3. angiomas.
  4. petechiae.

17. A 65-year-old client comes to the plastic surgeon's office for a follow-up appointment after having a basal cell lesion removed from their face. When teaching the client how to inspect their skin for signs of melanoma, the nurse should tell the client to look for:
1. pale patches on the skin.
2. skin flaking that won't go away.
3. black or purple irregularly shaped nodules.
4. flat areas of discoloration.

18. A 9-year-old child tells his school nurse that his eye itches and tears much more than usual. When the nurse examines his eye, his sclera is reddened. Which eye abnormality do these signs and symptoms most suggest?
1. Cataracts
2. Ptosis
3. Glaucoma
4. Conjunctivitis

19. A nurse is inspecting a 10-year-old child's pupils as part of a routine eye examination. When the nurse shines indirect light into the child's right eye, the normal response would be:
1. both eyes dilate.
2. both eyes constrict.
3. the right eye constricts, and the left eye dilates.
4. no response.

20. A nurse is performing a mental health assessment of a client seeking help to control her overwhelming depression. During the mental health assessment, what should be the nurse's focus?
1. To state goals for care of the client
2. To determine outcomes for the client
3. To distinguish medical problems from mental health problems
4. To gather information from the client

21. An 11-year-old child reports to the school nurse with an earache and a sore throat. The nurse inspects the tympanic membrane using an otoscope. Which color suggests an ear infection?
1. Clear
2. Yellow
3. Gray
4. Red

22. A nurse is performing an otoscopic examination on a 3-year-old child who has an earache and a fever. In which direction should the nurse pull the child's auricle to straighten the ear canal?
1. Down and forward
2. Up and forward
3. Up and back
4. Down and back

23. A mother states that her daughter has been complaining for 3 days of a sore throat, which has increased in severity. The nurse palpates the girl's neck and identifies a swollen lymph node directly under the mandible. Which lymph node is this?

1. Preauricular
2. Submandibular
3. Submental
4. Supraclavicular

24. A 19-year-old college student is brought to the emergency department with dyspnea and asymmetrical breathing patterns after falling down a flight of steps at a party. His admission chest x-ray shows right-sided pneumothorax. During inspection, what other characteristic of pneumothorax might the nurse observe?

1. Funnel chest
2. Barrel chest
3. Finger clubbing
4. Tracheal deviation

25. After a fall from a scaffold, a 32-year-old construction worker reports shortness of breath and has labored breathing. His admission chest x-ray reveals a large, right-sided pneumothorax. What sound should the nurse expect when percussing over the right lung?

1. Tympany
2. Dullness
3. Hyperresonance
4. Flatness

26. A nurse is performing an admission assessment of a 63-year-old client with pneumonia. While auscultating his lungs, the nurse asks him to repeatedly say "ninety-nine." For what sound is the nurse checking?

1. Bronchophony
2. Egophony
3. Pectoriloquy
4. Crepitus

27. A client develops pneumothorax after an attempted central line insertion. What breath sounds should the nurse expect to hear over the affected lung?

1. Crackles
2. Rhonchi
3. Diminished sounds
4. Wheezes

28. A nurse is evaluating a 46-year-old client with left lower lobe pneumonia who reports shortness of breath. Identify the area where the nurse may hear fine crackles associated with this condition.

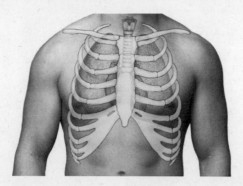

29. A 63-year-old client is hospitalized in the coronary care unit after experiencing an anterior myocardial infarction (MI). While performing the initial assessment, the nurse palpates the pulses on the inner wrist. What are these pulses?
1. Radial pulses
2. Dorsalis pedis pulses
3. Posterior tibial pulses
4. Anterior tibial pulses

30. A 57-year-old client comes to the emergency department with reports of chest pain that developed while he was climbing the stairs. The nurse asks the client to describe his chest pain. Which type of chest pain is most commonly associated with MI?
1. Sore and aching
2. Dull and stabbing
3. Sharp and burning
4. Tightness and pressure

31. A 19-year-old client is admitted to the coronary care unit after experiencing a syncopal episode while playing basketball. When auscultating his heart sounds, the nurse hears a "lub-dub" sound. What mechanical event in the heart is associated with the "dub" sound?
1. Closure of the mitral and aortic valves
2. Closure of the tricuspid and aortic valves
3. Closure of the aortic and pulmonic valves
4. Closure of the mitral and tricuspid valves

32. A nurse is inspecting a 58-year-old client's chest wall to locate the apical impulse. Where should the nurse look?
1. At the fifth intercostal space medial to the left midclavicular line
2. Over the base of the heart
3. Over the aortic area
4. At the third intercostal space to the left of the sternum

33. A nurse is assessing a 53-year-old client who's beginning to undergo menopause. Which finding is **not** a change associated with menopause?
1. Breast enlargement
2. Flattened nipples
3. Irregular periods
4. Weight gain

34. Identify on the illustration below where a nurse should place the diaphragm of a stethoscope to auscultate the pulmonic valve.

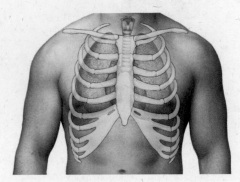

35. During examination of a 36-year-old client's right breast, the nurse palpates a lump. Which characteristic most suggests that the lump may be malignant?
1. Softness
2. Mobility
3. Irregular shape
4. Nontender

36. A 28-year-old client asks, "When should I perform breast self-examination (BSE)?" The best response by the nurse would be:
1. "On the first day of your menstrual cycle each month."
2. "On the last day of your menstrual cycle each month."
3. "On the first day of every month."
4. "2 to 3 days after your menstrual cycle ends each month."

37. When palpating a client's breast, the nurse should use:
1. the whole palm of the palpating hand.
2. one index finger.
3. three middle finger pads.
4. the pad of the thumb.

38. A 47-year-old client reports burning abdominal pain after eating at a restaurant. Burning abdominal pain is most commonly associated with:
1. cholecystitis.
2. appendicitis.
3. peptic ulcer disease.
4. pancreatitis.

39. A client comes to the emergency department reporting right upper quadrant pain and nausea. His temperature is 100.7° F (38.2° C). The nurse plans to assess the client's abdomen. Place the steps below in the order in which the nurse should perform them for an abdominal assessment.

1. Palpation
2. Percussion
3. Inspection
4. Auscultation

40. A physician orders daily measurement of abdominal girth for a 35-year-old client with upper GI bleeding. At which point on the abdomen should the nurse take the measurement?
  1. Just below the rib cage
  2. Just above the pelvis
  3. Across the umbilicus
  4. At the fullest point

41. A 27-year-old client comes to the emergency department reporting abdominal pain. Deep palpation of the abdomen shouldn't be performed if the client:
  1. has ascites.
  2. reports constipation.
  3. is ticklish.
  4. has abdominal rigidity.

42. A nurse is assisting a physician with a routine pelvic examination. Which lubricant should the nurse use on the speculum?
  1. Water-soluble jelly
  2. Petroleum jelly
  3. Warm water
  4. Mineral oil

43. A nurse is teaching a group of fifth-grade girls about menstruation. She tells them that menses occurs every 21 to 38 days and that the duration is normally:
    1. 2 to 4 days.
    2. 2 to 8 days.
    3. 3 to 5 days.
    4. 4 to 7 days.

44. A client with a urinary tract infection reports pain when the nurse percusses her back at the costovertebral angle. This finding suggests:
    1. a ureteral stone.
    2. an ovarian cyst.
    3. kidney inflammation.
    4. bladder cancer.

45. A school nurse is performing an annual screening on a 12-year-old student. To assess for scoliosis, the nurse should:
    1. palpate for crepitus.
    2. measure the length of the spine from neck to waist.
    3. ask the client to bend forward at the waist.
    4. palpate the spinous processes.

46. A 28-year-old client tells a nurse that he discovered a lump in his scrotum. Before palpating his testicles, the nurse should know that an abnormal testicle is:
    1. smooth.
    2. oval.
    3. rubbery.
    4. nodular.

47. A nurse is assessing a client with an abdominal aortic aneurysm. Identify in the illustration below the area of the abdomen where the nurse should auscultate for a bruit over the aorta.

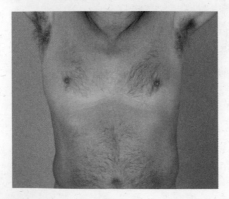

48. A 46-year-old client comes to the clinic for his annual physical examination. During the assessment, the nurse palpates his inguinal area for what reason?
1. To check for herniation
2. To locate a pulse
3. To check for a nondescended testicle
4. To assess the prostate gland

49. A 62-year-old client reports urinary hesitancy. During the assessment, the nurse palpates his prostate gland. The nurse should know that a normal prostate gland is about the size of a:
1. marble.
2. grape.
3. walnut.
4. peach.

50. After slipping in her bathroom, an 80-year-old client is brought to the emergency department with a deformed right hip and hip pain that she rates as an 8 on a scale of 1 to 10. The nurse examining her notices gross internal rotation of the right hip. Which of the following findings is indicative of internal rotation?
1. A misshapen pelvis
2. Inward pointing of the foot
3. Dorsiflexion of the right foot
4. Unequal leg lengths

51. A 34-year-old client reports pain and tingling in her right wrist. During the assessment, the client reports pain when the nurse flexes the wrist for 30 seconds. The nurse knows that this finding indicates:
1. a fractured wrist.
2. carpal tunnel syndrome.
3. a stroke.
4. paralysis.

52. A 58-year-old client comes to the clinic for his annual physical examination. The nurse notices that the client's urine specimen has a cloudy appearance. What does this finding suggest?
1. Hypervolemia
2. Benign prostatic hyperplasia
3. Urinary tract infection
4. Hematuria

53. A nurse is assessing the leg of a client who has come to the emergency department with a suspected fractured femur. To perform a quick and accurate assessment, the nurse should evaluate the affected leg for which of the following signs and symptoms? Select all that apply.
    1. Pain
    2. Pliability
    3. Paresthesia
    4. Paralysis
    5. Pallor
    6. Pulses

54. A 30-year-old client is brought to the emergency department with head injuries from a motorcycle accident. During the neurologic assessment, the client displays Babinski reflex. The nurse knows that this finding is:
    1. an abnormal response.
    2. a normal response.
    3. a hyperactive response.
    4. a diminished response.

55. During a routine physical examination, a 68-year-old client can't take a deep breath and hold it while stopping or starting to walk. The nurse knows that this abnormal finding indicates:
    1. apraxia.
    2. aphasia.
    3. graphesthesia.
    4. impaired stereognosis.

56. A client comes to the emergency department with a rash that appears to be in a confluent pattern. Which graphic shows a reticular pattern?

    1.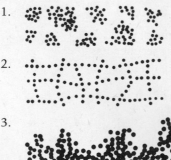

    2.

    3.

    4.

57. A client's sense of balance is assessed by performing:
1. deep tendon reflex (DTR) testing.
2. passive range-of-motion (ROM) exercises.
3. Romberg test.
4. constructional ability testing.

58. An 84-year-old client reports leg pain. A nurse assesses his legs and discovers an ulcerated area close to the ankle on his left leg. The nurse knows that this finding indicates:
1. arterial insufficiency.
2. chronic venous insufficiency.
3. skin infection.
4. skin allergy.

59. A nurse records a client's weight as 180 lb and his height as 70″. What's this client's body mass index (BMI)? Round your answer to one decimal place.

60. A nurse is assessing a client using the Glasgow Coma Scale. The client reports pain in his lower abdomen, is confused about place and time, and anxiously watches the nurse perform the assessment. Using the scale (shown below), what score should the nurse assign to this client?
1. 9
2. 11
3. 13
4. 15

Assessment

Glasgow Coma Scale

Test	Client's reaction	Score
Eye opening response	Opens spontaneously	4
	Opens to verbal command	3
	Opens to pain	2
	No response	1
Best motor response	Obeys verbal command	6
	Localizes painful stimuli	5
	Flexion-withdrawal	4
	Flexion-abnormal (decorticate rigidity)	3
	Extension (decerebrate rigidity)	2
	No response	1
Best verbal response	Oriented and converses	5
	Disoriented and converses	4
	Inappropriate words	3
	Incomprehensible sounds	2
	No response	1

Answers

1. 2. The first priority of a successful physical assessment is establishing rapport with the client and the legal guardian. Having the legal guardian sign the admission forms, taking vital signs, and obtaining equipment are also important but aren't the nurse's first priority in most cases.

> Client needs category: Psychosocial integrity
> Client needs subcategory: None
> Cognitive level: Application

2. 1. Reflection is a technique that involves repeating something a client has just said. It can help the nurse obtain more specific information. Facilitation involves using phrases that encourage the client to continue with his story. Confirmation helps clear misconceptions. Summarization restates the information that the client has given.

> Client needs category: Psychosocial integrity
> Client needs subcategory: None
> Cognitive level: Application

3. 4. After assembling the necessary equipment, the nurse should perform the first part of the assessment—forming an initial impression of the client by performing a general survey. Vital signs should follow this initial observation. Assessment for skin lesions and anthropometric measurements should occur later in the assessment process.

> Client needs category: Health promotion and maintenance
> Client needs subcategory: None
> Cognitive level: Application

4. 2. When determining a pulse deficit, the nurse should palpate the radial pulse while auscultating the apical pulse. The apical pulse rate minus the radial pulse rate equals the pulse deficit. Pulse deficit isn't identified using the carotid or brachial pulses.

> Client needs category: Health promotion and maintenance
> Client needs subcategory: None
> Cognitive level: Analysis

5. 3. When percussing over dense tissue, such as muscle, the nurse should expect to hear flatness. Tympany is heard over an area of air collection, dullness is heard over organs, and resonance is a low-pitched sound heard over normal lung tissue.

> Client needs category: Health promotion and maintenance
> Client needs subcategory: None
> Cognitive level: Application

6. 1. The nurse should neither underinflate nor overinflate the cuff. The ideal method is to palpate the radial pulse while inflating the cuff. When the radial pulse disappears, the nurse should inflate the cuff an additional 30 mm Hg and then close the valve. The other methods of obtaining blood pressure are incorrect.

> Client needs category: Physiological integrity
> Client needs subcategory: Reduction of risk potential
> Cognitive level: Comprehension

7. 1. Anthropometric arm measurements help assess nutritional status. Less than 90% of the standard indicates caloric deprivation. This result doesn't indicate a normal measurement and doesn't show caloric excess. Protein malnutrition is determined by albumin levels.

> Client needs category: Physiological integrity
> Client needs subcategory: Reduction of risk potential
> Cognitive level: Analysis

8. 1. Clients with liver disease typically have dark, yellowish nails. Spoon-shaped nails are associated with iron deficiency anemia. White, transverse bands are associated with hypoalbuminemia. White patches on the nails may be associated with fungal infection.

> Client needs category: Physiological integrity
> Client needs subcategory: Reduction of risk potential
> Cognitive level: Analysis

9. 1. A contract with a psychiatric client should include the nurse's expectations and responsibilities as well as the client's. A description of the client's therapies, the length of hospitalization, and insurance and financial information wouldn't be included in a contract.

> Client needs category: Psychosocial integrity
> Client needs subcategory: None
> Cognitive level: Application

10. 2. When a client identifies a history of substance misuse, the nurse should assess the risk of withdrawal, which includes determining the substance being used. Determining how the substance was obtained and asking if the client's employer knows about her behavior aren't relevant. Telling the client she really shouldn't use an addictive substance is judgmental and inappropriate.

> Client needs category: Physiological integrity
> Client needs subcategory: Pharmacological and parenteral
>   therapies
> Cognitive level: Analysis

11. 1. The Snellen chart measures visual acuity and provides readings such as 20/40. A person with 20/40 vision can view from 20′ that which a person with normal vision can view from 40′. The other explanations are incorrect.

> Client needs category: Health promotion and maintenance
> Client needs subcategory: None
> Cognitive level: Comprehension

12. 2. A repetition of the interviewer's words is called *echolalia*. Flight of ideas is the continuous flow of speech in which the client jumps abruptly from topic to topic. Neologism is the distortion or invention of words. Confabulation is the fabrication of events to fill in for memory loss.

> Client needs category: Psychosocial integrity
> Client needs subcategory: None
> Cognitive level: Comprehension

13. 1. Impaired perception of reality such as having superpowers suggests schizophrenia. Pervasive maladaptive patterns of behavior suggest a personality disorder. An anxiety disorder is characterized by anxiety and avoidant behavior. Obsessive-compulsive disorder involves recurrent obsessions and compulsions.

> Client needs category: Psychosocial integrity
> Client needs subcategory: None
> Cognitive level: Analysis

14. 1. To evaluate skin turgor, the nurse should gently squeeze the skin on the forearm or sternum. If the skin quickly returns to its original shape, the client's skin turgor is normal. If it returns to its original shape slowly over 30 seconds or maintains a tented position, the skin has poor turgor, which is a sign of dehydration. Palpating or transilluminating the skin doesn't detect dehydration. Pressing on the nail beds helps evaluate circulation.

> Client needs category: Physiological integrity
> Client needs subcategory: Reduction of risk potential
> Cognitive level: Analysis

15. 2. Pustules are small, inflamed, blisterlike lesions. Papules are small, raised, circumscribed, solid lesions. Macules are flat lesions. Plaques are broad, raised areas on the skin.

> Client needs category: Physiological integrity
> Client needs subcategory: Reduction of risk potential
> Cognitive level: Analysis

16. 2. Telangiectases are small, dilated vessels that form a weblike pattern. They're commonly seen on the face, especially in clients with a history of alcohol misuse. Purpura is red or purple discoloration of the skin. Angiomas are benign tumors near the surface of the skin. Petechiae are pinpoint hemorrhages in the skin or mucous membranes.

> Client needs category: Physiological integrity
> Client needs subcategory: Reduction of risk potential
> Cognitive level: Analysis

17. 3. Typically, melanomas are black or purple nodules that are irregularly shaped. Pale patches on the skin, skin flaking, and flat areas of discoloration aren't signs of melanoma.

> Client needs category: Health promotion and maintenance
> Client needs subcategory: None
> Cognitive level: Application

18. 4. Conjunctivitis causes redness of the eye as well as itching and increased tearing. A child would be unlikely to develop a cataract or glaucoma. Ptosis refers to a drooping eyelid.
> Client needs category: Physiological integrity
> Client needs subcategory: Reduction of risk potential
> Cognitive level: Analysis

19. 2. Shining a light in the right eye should cause right eye constriction (direct) and left eye constriction (consensual). The other papillary responses aren't normal and may indicate a neurologic problem.
> Client needs category: Health promotion and maintenance
> Client needs subcategory: None
> Cognitive level: Application

20. 4. The focus of the mental health assessment should be to gather information from the client so the nurse can develop a care plan. Goals for care and client outcomes shouldn't be determined until after the assessment is complete. The mental health assessment primarily focuses on the client's mental health, not medical problems.
> Client needs category: Physiological integrity
> Client needs subcategory: Reduction of risk potential
> Cognitive level: Analysis

21. 4. A red eardrum (tympanic membrane) can indicate an ear infection. A gray or clear eardrum indicates a normal eardrum. Yellow findings may indicate wax buildup.
> Client needs category: Physiological integrity
> Client needs subcategory: Reduction of risk potential
> Cognitive level: Analysis

22. 3. To perform an otoscopic examination on a client age 3 or older, the nurse should pull the auricle up and back to straighten the ear canal. Pulling the auricle in the other manners described may cause injury to the child's eardrum.
> Client needs category: Physiological integrity
> Client needs subcategory: Reduction of risk potential
> Cognitive level: Application

23. 2. The submandibular lymph nodes are under the mandible. The submental lymph node is located directly under the chin. The preauricular lymph node is located in front of the ear, and the supraclavicular nodes are above the clavicle.
> Client needs category: Physiological integrity
> Client needs subcategory: Reduction of risk potential
> Cognitive level: Comprehension

24. 4. With right-sided pneumothorax, the nurse may observe tracheal deviation to the left. Funnel chest is a chest deformity. Barrel chest and finger clubbing occur with chronic obstructive pulmonary disease.
> Client needs category: Physiological integrity
> Client needs subcategory: Physiological adaptation
> Cognitive level: Comprehension

25. 1. For a client with a large pneumothorax, the pleural space on the affected side is increased resulting in tympanic sounds due to trapped air. A patient with a small pneumothorax produces a hyperresonant sound on percussion. Dullness is heard over a solid area, such as in pneumonia, and flatness occurs with consolidation.
    Client needs category: Physiological integrity
    Client needs subcategory: Physiological adaptation
    Cognitive level: Comprehension

26. 1. When testing for bronchophony, the client is asked to say "ninety-nine" or "blue moon" while the nurse auscultates his lungs. Over normal tissue, the words sound muffled; over consolidated areas, such as those that occur with pneumothorax, the words sound unusually loud. To test for egophony, the nurse would ask the client to say "E." To test for pectoriloquy, the nurse would ask the client to whisper "1, 2, 3." Crepitus is air under the skin that is felt on palpation.
    Client needs category: Physiological integrity
    Client needs subcategory: Reduction of risk potential
    Cognitive level: Comprehension

27. 3. With pneumothorax, air movement is diminished or absent in the affected lung, so breath sounds are diminished in that area. Crackles are related to collapsed or fluid-filled alveoli. Rhonchi result from fluid in the large airways. Wheezes are caused by blocked airflow.
    Client needs category: Physiological integrity
    Client needs subcategory: Physiological adaptation
    Cognitive level: Comprehension

28.

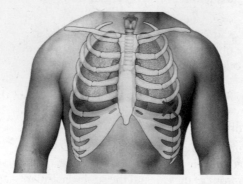

To auscultate the left lower lobe from the anterior chest, the nurse should use the landmarks of the left anterior axillary line, between the fifth and sixth intercostal spaces.
    Client needs category: Physiological integrity
    Client needs subcategory: Physiological adaptation
    Cognitive level: Comprehension

29. 1. The radial pulses are located above the wrist joint near the base of the thumb. The dorsalis pedis pulses are located on the tops of the feet. The posterior tibial pulse is found posterior to the medial malleolus. The anterior tibial pulse is located anterior to the ankle.

> Client needs category: Physiological integrity
> Client needs subcategory: Reduction of risk potential
> Cognitive level: Analysis

30. 4. The pain typically associated with an MI is characterized by tightness and pressure. The other types of pain described could be associated with an MI but are less common.

> Client needs category: Physiological integrity
> Client needs subcategory: Physiological adaptation
> Cognitive level: Comprehension

31. 3. The second heart sound, S_2, or the "dub" sound, is a result of closure of the aortic and pulmonic valves. The first heart sound, S_1, which produces the "lub" sound, is associated with closure of the mitral and tricuspid valves. The other choices are incorrect.

> Client needs category: Physiological integrity
> Client needs subcategory: Reduction of risk potential
> Cognitive level: Comprehension

32. 1. The apical impulse, also usually the point of maximum impulse, can be found at the fifth intercostal space medial to the left midclavicular line. The other areas are incorrect.

> Client needs category: Physiological integrity
> Client needs subcategory: Reduction of risk potential
> Cognitive level: Application

33. 1. Breast enlargement is most common during puberty and pregnancy. After menopause, glandular tissues atrophy and are replaced with fatty deposits. The breasts become flabbier and smaller, and the nipples flatten and become less erectile. Irregular periods and weight gain are common symptoms associated with menopause

> Client needs category: Physiological integrity
> Client needs subcategory: Reduction of risk potential
> Cognitive level: Comprehension

34.

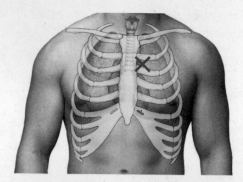

The pulmonic valve is best heard at the second intercostal space, just left of the sternum.
> Client needs category: Physiological integrity
> Client needs subcategory: Reduction of risk potential
> Cognitive level: Application

35. 3. An irregularly shaped lump in the breast suggests malignancy. A malignant mass may also be firm and not easily moved.
> Client needs category: Physiological integrity
> Client needs subcategory: Physiological adaptation
> Cognitive level: Comprehension

36. 4. Because certain changes take place in the breasts during the menstrual cycle, a BSE should be performed 2 to 3 days after the menstrual cycle ends. The other choices aren't optimal times.
> Client needs category: Health promotion and maintenance
> Client needs subcategory: None
> Cognitive level: Comprehension

37. 3. The preferred method for palpating a client's breast is to use three middle finger pads and to gently rotate them around the breast, moving in concentric circles. Using the whole palm, one index finger, or the pad of the thumb doesn't allow the nurse to adequately feel the breast tissue and identify abnormalities.
> Client needs category: Health promotion and maintenance
> Client needs subcategory: None
> Cognitive level: Application

38. 3. Burning abdominal pain is most commonly associated with peptic ulcer disease. Cholecystitis and pancreatitis cause stabbing abdominal pain. Appendicitis causes severe abdominal cramping.
> Client needs category: Physiological integrity
> Client needs subcategory: Physiological adaptation
> Cognitive level: Comprehension

39.

3.	Inspection

4.	Auscultation

2.	Percussion

1.	Palpation

The proper order for abdominal assessment is inspection, auscultation, percussion, and palpation. Palpating or percussing the abdomen before auscultation can change the character of the client's bowel sounds and lead to an inaccurate assessment.
> Client needs category: Physiological integrity
> Client needs subcategory: Reduction of risk potential
> Cognitive level: Application

40. 4. When measuring abdominal girth, the nurse should measure the abdomen at its fullest point. Measuring at the other points may not accurately evaluate an increase in abdominal size.
> Client needs category: Physiological integrity
> Client needs subcategory: Reduction of risk potential
> Cognitive level: Application

41. 4. Because abdominal rigidity may indicate peritoneal inflammation, the nurse should avoid palpation because it may lead to pain or organ rupture. Performing deep palpation on a client who has ascites, is constipated, or is ticklish may be difficult, but it isn't contraindicated.
> Client needs category: Physiological integrity
> Client needs subcategory: Physiological adaptation
> Cognitive level: Comprehension

42. 3. Water should be used to lubricate the speculum before an internal vaginal examination. Other lubricants are discouraged because they can alter the results of a Papanicolaou test.
> Client needs category: Physiological integrity
> Client needs subcategory: Reduction of risk potential
> Cognitive level: Application

43. 2. Although menses duration may vary, the duration in a normal menstrual cycle is 2 to 8 days.
> Client needs category: Health promotion and maintenance
> Client needs subcategory: None
> Cognitive level: Comprehension

44. 3. Pain during percussion over the costovertebral angle suggests kidney inflammation. Clients with ureteral stones, ovarian cysts, or bladder cancer more commonly report abdominal pain.

    Client needs category: Physiological integrity
    Client needs subcategory: Physiological adaptation
    Cognitive level: Comprehension

45. 3. To assess for scoliosis, the nurse should inspect the spine for abnormalities while the client is bending forward at the waist. This position can make spinal deformities more apparent. The other actions don't assist with the diagnosis of scoliosis.

    Client needs category: Health promotion and maintenance
    Client needs subcategory: None
    Cognitive level: Application

46. 4. A nodular testicle may indicate malignancy. A normal testicle is smooth, oval, and rubbery.

    Client needs category: Physiological integrity
    Client needs subcategory: Physiological adaptation
    Cognitive level: Analysis

47.

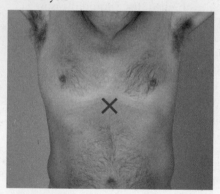

An aortic bruit is best heard with the stethoscope bell placed at the midline of the abdomen, slightly below the xiphoid process.

    Client needs category: Physiological integrity
    Client needs subcategory: Physiological adaptation
    Cognitive level: Application

48. 1. The purpose of palpating a client's inguinal area during assessment is to check for herniation. The nurse wouldn't find a pulse, testicle, or prostate gland in this area.

    Client needs category: Health promotion and maintenance
    Client needs subcategory: None
    Cognitive level: Application

49. 3. A normal prostate gland is about the size of a walnut. The other choices are incorrect.

    Client needs category: Physiological integrity
    Client needs subcategory: Reduction of risk potential
    Cognitive level: Comprehension

50. 2. With internal rotation of the hip, inward turning and pointing of the foot to a pigeon-toed position occurs. A misshapen pelvis, dorsiflexion of the foot, and unequal leg length don't indicate rotation.

Client needs category: Physiological integrity
Client needs subcategory: Physiological adaptation
Cognitive level: Comprehension

51. 2. Pain or numbness in the hand or fingers that occurs when the client's wrist is flexed is called *Phalen maneuver*. This finding is indicative of carpal tunnel syndrome. A fractured wrist would cause pain with any movement. Stroke and paralysis aren't indicated by pain with wrist flexion.

Client needs category: Physiological integrity
Client needs subcategory: Reduction of risk potential
Cognitive level: Analysis

52. 3. A client with cloudy urine may be a sign of an infection or urinary tract infection. Hematuria may have brown or bright red urine. With hypervolemia, urine would be pale in appearance. Benign prostatic hyperplasia usually don't affect urine color.

Client needs category: Physiological integrity
Client needs subcategory: Reduction of risk potential
Cognitive level: Analysis

53. 1, 3, 4, 5, 6. To perform a swift assessment of a musculoskeletal injury, the nurse should remember the 5 P's: pain, paresthesia, paralysis, pallor, and pulses. The nurse wouldn't assess pliability with a suspected fracture.

Client needs category: Physiological integrity
Client needs subcategory: Reduction of risk potential
Cognitive level: Application

54. 1. Although Babinski reflex is a normal finding in infants and children younger than age 2, it's always an abnormal finding in adults. It wouldn't be classified as hyperactive or diminished.

Client needs category: Physiological integrity
Client needs subcategory: Physiological adaptation
Cognitive level: Comprehension

55. 1. Apraxia is the inability to perform coordinated movements. Aphasia is a language deficit. The ability to identify a common object by touching and manipulating it is called stereognosis. Graphesthesia is the ability to recognize writing on the skin.

Client needs category: Physiological integrity
Client needs subcategory: Physiological adaptation
Cognitive level: Analysis

56. 3. In a confluent configuration in which lesions merge so that individual lesions aren't visible or palpable. Option 1 shows a grouped configuration in which lesions are clustered together. Option 2 shows a reticular pattern, the lesions form a meshlike network. Option 4 shows a discrete configuration in which the individual lesions are separate and distinct.

   Client needs category: Physiological integrity
   Client needs subcategory: Physiological adaptation
   Cognitive level: Analysis

57. 3. The Romberg test evaluates balance. DTRs reflect neurological function. ROM tests muscle tone, which represents muscular resistance to passive stretching, is assessed by performing passive range of motion. Constructional ability testing assesses the client's ability to perform simple tasks and use various objects.

   Client needs category: Health promotion and maintenance
   Client needs subcategory: None
   Cognitive level: Comprehension

58. 2. A client with chronic venous insufficiency is likely to have ulceration around the ankle. Arterial insufficiency is more likely to cause ulceration around the toes. A skin infection or allergy would be characterized by multiple areas of skin disruption, not an ulceration.

   Client needs category: Health promotion and maintenance
   Client needs subcategory: None
   Cognitive level: Analysis

59. 25.8

BMI is a measure of body fat based on height and weight. To determine a client's BMI, the nurse should use the formula:

$$BMI = \frac{\text{weight in pounds}}{\text{height in inches} \times \text{height in inches}} \times 703$$

Therefore:

$$BMI = \frac{180}{70 \times 70} \times 703$$
$$BMI = 25.82 \text{ or } 25.8$$

   Client needs category: Health promotion and maintenance
   Client needs subcategory: None
   Cognitive level: Application

60. 3. The Glasgow Coma Scale is used to assess level of consciousness, based on testing and scoring the client's best eye opening, motor response, and verbal response. In this case, the client spontaneously keeps his eyes open as he watches the nurse's actions (eye opening score of 4), can express and localize the area of pain (motor response score of 5), and is disoriented about place and time (verbal response score of 4). Therefore, his total score is 13.

   Client needs category: Physiological integrity
   Client needs subcategory: Physiological adaptation
   Cognitive level: Application

Glossary

accommodation: a change in the shape of the lens that allows the eye to focus on a nearby object; accompanied by constriction of the pupils and convergence of the eyes

adnexa: appendages of the uterus, including the ovaries, fallopian tubes, and supporting tissues

alert: term used to describe a patient who can follow commands, comprehend verbal and written language, and express ideas freely and is oriented to time, place, and person

alopecia: hair loss

amplitude: strength of a pulse or other force; recorded as bounding, normal, weak, or absent

anisocoria: inequality of the diameter of the pupils

ankylosis: fixation of a joint due to fibrous or bony union; results from a disease process

anorexia: loss of appetite

anthropometric measurements: measurements of the human body taken as part of a comprehensive nutritional assessment; include midarm circumference, skin-fold thickness, and midarm muscle circumference

aphasia: language disorder characterized by difficulty expressing or comprehending speech

apraxia: inability to perform coordinated movements, even though no motor deficit is present

ascites: accumulation of fluid in the abdominal cavity

ataxia: uncoordinated actions when voluntary muscle movements are attempted

auscultation: physical assessment technique by which the examiner listens (usually with a stethoscope) for sounds coming from the heart, lungs, abdomen, or other organs

bimanual palpation: method of palpation involving the use of two hands to locate body structures and assess their texture, size, consistency, mobility, and tenderness

borborygmus: loud, gurgling, splashing sounds produced by hyperactive intestinal peristalsis

bruit: abnormal sound heard on auscultation over an artery, organ, or gland that indicates turbulent blood flow through a narrow or partially occluded vessel

cardiac cycle: the period from the beginning of one heartbeat to the beginning of the next; includes two phases, systole and diastole

cataract: opacity of the lens of the eye

cerumen: waxlike secretion in the external ear

choreiform: involuntary jerking movement associated with certain neurologic conditions

closed questions: questions that elicit yes-or-no answers

coma: unconscious state in which the patient appears to be asleep, doesn't speak, and responds to neither body nor environmental stimuli

consensual light reflex: reflex constriction of both pupils when one eye is exposed to bright light

crackles: intermittent, nonmusical, crackling breath sounds that are caused by collapsed or fluid-filled alveoli popping open at the end of inspiration

cremasteric reflex: superficial reflex of the testicles elicited by stroking the upper inner thigh, which causes brisk retraction of the testicle on the side of the stimulus

crepitus: noise or vibration produced by irregular cartilage surfaces or broken ends of a bone rubbing together; also the sound heard when air in subcutaneous tissue is palpated

diastolic blood pressure: the minimum pressure exerted on the arterial wall during left ventricular relaxation

dimpling: puckering or depression of the surface of the body or an organ; also called retraction

diplopia: double vision

dorsal lithotomy position: position commonly used for female pelvic examinations in which the patient lies on their back with hips and knees flexed and thighs abducted and rotated externally

dysarthria: speech defect commonly related to a motor deficit of the tongue or speech muscles

dysphagia: difficulty swallowing

Erb point: auscultatory point on the precordium at the third intercostal space to the left of the sternum

exophthalmos: abnormal protrusion of the eyeball

expressive aphasia: inability to express words or thoughts

flaccidity: decreased muscle tone, which causes muscle to become weak or flabby

fluid wave: rippling across the abdomen during percussion; indicative of the presence of ascites

fremitus: palpable vibration that results from air passing through the bronchopulmonary system and transmitting vibrations to the chest wall

gynecomastia: enlargement of breast tissue in the male breast

hematuria: presence of blood in the urine

hernia: abnormal protrusion of a structure through an opening; for example, the protrusion of a loop of bowel through a muscle wall

hirsutism: excessive hair growth; may be hereditary, a sign of an endocrine disorder, or an effect of certain drugs

hordeolum: inflammation of the sebaceous gland of the eyelid; also called stye

hydrocele: accumulation of serous fluid in a saclike structure such as the testicle

hyperopia: defect in vision that allows a person to see objects clearly at a distance but not at close range; also called farsightedness

hyperresonance: increased resonance produced by percussion

inspection: critical observation of the patient during which the examiner may use sight, hearing, or smell to make informed observations

intensity: degree of strength; for example, the loudness of a heart murmur recorded as soft, medium, or loud

introitus: entrance to a canal or cavity, such as the vagina

jaundice: yellowish discoloration of the skin caused by the accumulation of bilirubin

kwashiorkor: protein-deficiency malnutrition that occurs in young children and involves a loss of visceral protein

lethargy: slowed responses, sluggish speech, and slowed mental and motor processes in a person oriented to time, place, and person

lichenification: thickening and hardening of the skin often resulting from the irritation caused by repeated scratching of a pruritic lesion

mammogram: x-ray of the breast used to detect tumors and other abnormalities

marasmus: protein and calorie malnutrition that primarily affects children ages 6–18 months; results from a chronic lack of nutrients

meatus: opening or passageway in the body

menarche: first menstrual period

menopause: cessation of the menstrual period

murmur: abnormal sound heard on auscultation of the heart; caused by abnormal blood flow through a valve

mydriasis: dilation of the pupil due to paralysis of the oculomotor muscles or the effects of drugs

myopia: defect in vision that allows a person to see objects clearly at close range but not at a distance; also called nearsightedness

nipple inversion: inward turning or depression of the central portion of the nipple

nystagmus: involuntary, rhythmic movement of the eyes

objective data: information verifiable through direct observation, laboratory tests, screening procedures, or physical examination

occult blood: blood hidden in stool or urine that can be detected with a guaiac test

open-ended question: question that requires an answer in a sentence form rather than a yes-or-no form

palpation: physical assessment technique by which the examiner uses the sense of touch to feel pulsations and vibrations or to locate body structures and assess their texture, size, consistency, mobility, and tenderness

peau d'orange: orange-peel appearance of breast skin associated with breast cancer

percussion: physical assessment technique by which the examiner taps on the skin surface with their fingers to assess the size, border, and consistency of internal organs and to detect and evaluate fluid in a body cavity

peristalsis: sequence of muscle contractions that propels food through the GI tract

pitch: frequency of a sound, measured in the number of sound waves generated per second

point of maximum impulse (PMI): point at which the upward thrust of the heart against the chest wall is greatest, usually over the apex of the heart

precordium: area of the chest over the heart

protein-calorie malnutrition (PCM): spectrum of disorders resulting from either prolonged or chronic inadequate protein or calorie intake or from high metabolic requirements for protein and energy

pruritus: severe itching

ptosis: drooping of the eyelid

rebound tenderness: sharp, stabbing pain that occurs when the abdomen is pushed in deeply and then suddenly released; usually associated with peritoneal inflammation

receptive aphasia: inability to understand spoken word

resonance: clear, hollow, low-pitched sound produced by percussion; typically heard over normal lungs

rhonchi: low-pitched, snoring, rumbling breath sounds that may be heard on inhalation but are more pronounced on exhalation

strabismus: lack of coordination of eye muscles

striae: stripes or lines of tissue differing in color and texture from the surrounding tissue

stridor: loud, high-pitched crowing sound usually heard during inspiration without the need for a stethoscope

stupor: state in which a patient lies quietly with minimal spontaneous movement and is unresponsive except to vigorous and repeated stimuli

subjective data: information that the patient, their family, or their friends give about the patient's current health care status during the health history; reflects the personal perspective of the patient, family, and friends

synovial joint: type of freely movable joint lined with a synovial membrane that secretes synovial fluid for lubrication

systolic blood pressure: the maximum pressure exerted on the arterial wall at the peak of left ventricular contraction

tail of Spence: extension of breast tissue that projects from the upper outer quadrant of the breast toward the axilla

telangiectasis: permanently dilated small blood vessels that form a web-like pattern; may be the result of

scleroderma, lupus erythematosus, or cirrhosis or may be normal in healthy, older adults

thrill: palpable vibration felt over the heart or vessel that results from turbulent blood flow

tinnitus: ringing sound in one or both ears

tone: normal degree of vigor and tension; in muscle, the normal degree of tension

tympany: musical, drumlike sound heard during percussion over a hollow organ such as the stomach; a normal sound

vertigo: sensation that one's body is moving in space or that an object is moving around the body

vitiligo: a benign acquired skin condition of unknown cause consisting of complete absence of melanin pigment leading to patchy areas of white or light skin

wheezes: high-pitched, musical breath sounds heard continuously during inspiration and expiration but are louder during exhalation

Selected references

American Heart Association (Ed.). (2022, December 2). *Monitoring your blood pressure at home.* https://www.heart.org/en/health-topics/high-blood-pressure/understanding-blood-pressure-readings/monitoring-your-blood-pressure-at-home

American Psychiatric Association. (2022). *Diagnostic and statistical manual of mental disorders* (7th ed.). American Psychiatric Association.

The American Cancer Society medical and editorial content team. (2022, January 14). *ACS breast cancer screening guidelines.* American Cancer Society. https://www.cancer.org/cancer/breast-cancer/screening-tests-and-early-detection/american-cancer-society-recommendations-for-the-early-detection-of-breast-cancer.html

Bickley, L. (2020). *Bates' guide to physical examination and history taking* (13th ed.). Lippincott Williams & Wilkins.

Burns, C. E. (2021). *Burns' Pediatric Primary Care* (7th ed.). W.B. Saunders.

Centers for Disease Control and Prevention. (n.d.). https://www.cdc.gov/

Campos, M. C., Nery, T., Starke, A. C., de Bem Alves, A. C., Speck, A. E., & S Aguiar, A. (2022). Post-viral fatigue in COVID-19: A review of symptom assessment methods, mental, cognitive, and physical impairment. *Neurosci Biobehav Rev, 142,* 104902, https://doi-org.frontier.idm.oclc.org/10.1016/j.neubiorev.2022.104902

Cooper, K., & Gosnell, K. (2022). *Foundations and adult health nursing* (9th ed.). Mosby.

Estes, M. E. (2013). *Health assessment and physical examination* (5th ed.). Clifton Park.

Fenske, C., D'Amico, D., Watkins, K., Saunders, T., & Barbarito, C. (2019). *Health & physical assessment in nursing* (4th ed.). Prentice Hall.

Flugelman, M. (2021). History-taking revisited: Simple techniques to foster patient collaboration, improve data attainment, and establish trust with the patient. *GMS J Med Educ, 38*(6), Doc109–11. https://doi-org.frontier.idm.oclc.org/10.3205/zma001505

Gross, J. M., Fetto, J., & Rosen, E. (2015). *Musculoskeletal examination* (4th ed.). Wiley-Blackwell.

Gubrud, P., Bauldoff, G., & Carno, M. (2019). *LeMone and Burke's medical-surgical nursing: Clinical reasoning in patient care* (7th ed.). Pearson Education.

Harding, M. M. (2020). *Lewis's medical-surgical nursing assessment and management of clinical problems* (11th ed.). Mosby.

Hinkle, J. L., Cheever, K. H., & Overbaugh, K. (2021). *Brunner & Suddarth's textbook of medical-surgical nursing* (15th ed.). Lippincott Williams & Wilkins.

Hockenberry, M. J., & Wilson, D. (2018). *Wong's nursing care of infants and children* (11th ed.). Mosby.

Ingram, S. (2017). Taking a comprehensive health history: learning through practice and reflection. *Br J Nurs, 26*(18), 1033–1037. https://doi-org.frontier.idm.oclc.org/10.12968/bjon.2017.26.18.1033

Jarvis, C. (2019). *Physical examination and health assessment* (8th ed.). Saunders.

Jensen, S. (2018). *Nursing health assessment: A best practice approach* (3rd ed.). Lippincott Williams & Wilkins.

Lapum, J., Hughes, M., St-Amant, O., Garcia, W., Verkuyl, M., Petrie, P., Dimaranan, F., Pemasani, M., & Savicevic, N. (2021, January 1). *Palpation.* Physical Examination Techniques A Nurses Guide. https://pressbooks.library.torontomu.ca/ippa/chapter/palpation/

Merck Manuals: Professional Version. (n.d.). Merck & Co. https://www.merckmanuals.com/professional

Nettina, S. M. (2018). *Lippincott manual of nursing practice* (11th ed.) Wolters Kluwer.

Perpetua, E.M. & Keegan, P. (2020). *Cardiac Nursing* (7th ed.). Wolters Kluwer.

Potter, P.A., et al. (2021). *Fundamentals of nursing* (11th ed.). Mosby.

O'Rae, A., Ferreira, C., Hnatyshyn, T., & Krut, B. (2021). Family nursing telesimulation: Teaching therapeutic communication in an authentic way. *Teaching and Learning in Nursing, 16*(4), 404–409. https://doi-org.frontier.idm.oclc.org/10.1016/j.teln.2021.06.013

Swartz, M. (2020). *Textbook of physical diagnosis: History and examination* (8th ed.). W.B. Saunders.

Taylor, C.R., et al. (2018). *Fundamentals of nursing: The art and science of person-centered care* (9th ed.). Lippincott Williams & Wilkins.

Toney-Butler, T. J., & Unison-Pace, W. J. (2022). *Nursing Admission Assessment and Examination.* In: *StatPearls.* StatPearls Publishing. Available from https://www.ncbi.nlm.nih.gov/books/NBK493211

Waterhouse, C., Woodward, S., Foster, E., Lockhart, L., Richmond, A., Smith, N., Sutherill, R., Vickerman, K., & Woodhead, E. (2021). *Oxford handbook of neuroscience nursing* (2nd ed). (Waterhouse, C. & Woodward, S. (Eds.). Oxford University Press.

Weber, J. R., & Kelley, J. H. (2021). *Health assessment in nursing* (7th ed.). Lippincott Williams & Wilkins.

Willis, L. (2019). *Professional Guide to Pathophysiology* (4th ed.). Wolters Kluwer.

Wilson, S. F., & Giddens, J. F. (2021). *Health assessment for nursing practice* (7th ed.). Elsevier.

Index

Note: Page numbers followed by f indicate figures, t indicate tables, and b indicate boxes.

A

Abdomen
  assessment, 295–304
  auscultation, 297–299, 299f–300f
  distention, 305, 305f
  inspection, 296–297, 373
  palpation, 301, 302f
  percussion, 298–300, 300f
  pregnancy, 342
  structures, 296f
Abdominal pain
  origins, 310t
  rebound tenderness, 309, 311
  types, 310t
Abdominal quadrants, 296f
Abdominal sounds, abnormal, 308, 308t–309t
Abruptio placentae, 351, 352f
Abuse, 12
Acceptance, communication technique, 58
Achilles reflex, 123, 123f
Acne scars, 96
Acoustic nerve, 118
Acute myocardial infarction, chest pain, 219t
Agnosia, 130
Airways, 231, 232f–234f, 233–235
Albumin, 48
Alopecia, 91t, 97
Amenorrhea, 340
Anabolism, 42
Anatomic landmarks, 37
Angina pectoris, chest pain, 219t
Anisocoria, 153
Ankle
  assessment, 408–409, 408f
  strength, 411, 411f
Anorexia, 53
Anterior chamber, eye, 138f, 140, 146
Anthropometric measurements, 46–48, 49f
Anus, assessment, 304
Anxiety, acute, chest pain, 220t
Aortic aneurysm, 222
Aortic stenosis, 224
Aphasia, 125t, 129–130
Apical impulse assessment, 208
Apnea, 257f, 259
Apocrine glands, 77
Appearance, mental health assessment, 62, 113

Appendicitis, 309
Apraxia, 126t, 130
Aqueous humor, eye, 140
Areola pigmentation, 271
Arm
  pain, 412
  strength, 412
Arrector pili, 78
Arterial insufficiency, 221f
Arterial pulses, 203, 216f
Arteries, 202–203, 202f
Arteriolar narrowing, 153
Arterioles, 203
Asbestosis, auscultation, 263t
Ascites, 303, 304f
Assessment. *See also* Physical assessment
  male genitourinary system, 372–377
  techniques, 32–36
Asthma, auscultation, 263t
Atelectasis, 263t
Atrial gallop, 212
Atrial kick, 200
Atrial systole, 199
Atrioventricular valves, 197
Atrophy, 55
Auditory impairment, 129
Auricle, 164, 172
Auscultation, 35, 373
  asthma, 263t
  heart sounds, 208–209, 209f–211f,
    212–213, 213f
  murmurs, 212, 213f
  neck, 183–184
  pericardial friction rub, 213
  respiratory disorders, 263t–264t
  vascular system, 215, 217
Autonomic nervous system, 109. *See also*
  Neurologic system

B

Babinski reflex, 122, 124b
Bacterial vaginosis, 327, 327f, 337
Ball-and-socket joints, 391, 391t
Barrel chest, 255, 256f
Bartholin glands, 319, 328
Beau lines, 97
Beck Depression Inventory, 66
Behavior, mental status assessment, 62, 113

Biceps reflex, 123, 123f
Biceps strength, 411, 411f
Bile ducts, 292
Bimanual examination, 332f
Biographic data, 8
Biot respirations, 257f, 260
Birth marks, 85, 90
Bladder, 317, 317f, 320f
Bleeding, pregnancy, 359
Blind spot, 141
Blood pressure
  measurement, 30–31, 31f
  variations, 31
Bloody stools, 311
Blowing murmur, 226
Body mass index (BMI)
  breast cancer risk and, 277b
  formula, 47
  interpretation, 47, 48t
Body temperature measurement, 26–28, 29t
Bones
  anatomy and physiology, 389, 390f
  assessment, 398–409
Bouchard nodes, 414, 414f
Bounding pulse, 223f
Bowel sounds
  abnormal, 308, 308t–309t
  examination, 298
Brachial pulse, 216f
Brachioradialis reflex, 123, 123f
Bradypnea, 257f, 259
Brain, 104f, 105–106
Brain stem, 106
Breast cancer
  body mass index and, 277b
  males, 274
Breast examinations
  men, 274
  recommended schedule, 276t
Breasts and axillae, 17
  abnormal findings, 281, 281t–282t,
    283–284
  age-related changes, 271–274, 273f
  anatomy and physiology, 270–274, 270f,
    272f–273f
  assessment, 277–284, 278f, 280f
  dimpling, 281t, 283
  health history, 274–277, 275t–276t

Breasts and axillae *(continued)*
  inspection, 277
    lesions, location identification, 280f
    lump evaluation, 275t
    lymph nodes, 271, 272f
    male concerns and, 274b
    nodule, 281t–282t, 283
    pain, 282t, 284
    postpartum assessment, 349
    younger and older male patients, 274
Breathing
  mechanics, 237f
  types, 242
Breath sounds
  abnormal, 260–262, 262f–263f
  auscultation, 249–250
  discontinuous and continuous
        adventitious, 262f–263f
  normal, 251f, 251t
Broca aphasia, 129
Bronchi, 233
Bronchiectasis, auscultation findings, 263t
Bruits, 226, 309
Bulbar conjunctiva, 138f, 139
Bulge sign, 405f

C

Café-au-lait spots, 90
Candidiasis, 337
Capillaries, 202f, 203
Cardiac circulation, 195–196, 196f
Cardiac cycle, 199–201, 200f, 210f–211f
Cardinal positions of gaze, 150, 150f
Cardiovascular disease risk, 205
Cardiovascular landmarks, 207f
Cardiovascular system
  abnormal findings, 217–218, 217t–220t,
        220–222, 223t, 224, 225t, 226
  age-related changes, 201b
  anatomy, 193–198, 194f–196f, 198f
  assessment, 45, 205–209, 207f, 209f–211f,
        212–215, 213f, 216f, 217
  health history and, 203–205
  physiology, 198–201, 199f
Carotid pulse, 216f
Carpal tunnel syndrome, 404, 404f
Catabolism, 42
Central nervous system, 104–107, 104f, 105f,
        107f. *See also* Neurologic system
Cephalopelvic disproportion (CPD), 352, 353f
Cerebellum, 106, 121
Cerebrum, 105, 105f
Cerumen variations, 175
Cervical cyanosis, 338
Cervical effacement and dilation, 348, 348f
Cervical lesions and polyps, 338, 338f

Cherry angiomas, 90
Chest
  auscultation, 249–251, 250f–251f, 251t
  deformities, 253, 255–257, 256f
  inspection, 241–242
  pain, 217–218, 219t–220t, 240
  palpation, 243–246, 244f–245f
  percussion, 246–247, 246f, 247t,
        248f–249f
Chest-wall abnormalities, 253, 255–257, 256f
Chest-wall syndrome, 220t
Cheyne-Stokes respirations, 257f, 259
Chlamydia, 338
Cholecystitis, chest pain, 220t
Cholesterol, 51
Chordae tendineae, 197
Choroid, 139
Chronic obstructive pulmonary disease
        (COPD), auscultation, 263t
Chronic venous insufficiency, 221f
Ciliary body, 138f, 140
Circulatory study, 19
Circumcision, 369
Circumstantiality, 69
Clanging, 69
Clarification, communication technique,
        7, 58
Clitoris, 319
Clubbing, 91t, 98, 98f
Coarse crackles, 261, 262f
Cochlea, 165
Cognitive Assessment Scale, 66
Cognitive Capacity Screening Examination,
        66
Cognitive function, mental status
        assessment, 63, 113, 115
Collaboration, communication technique, 58
Communication barriers, cultural, 5, 59
Communication strategies
  nonverbal, 5–6
  therapeutic, 58
  transcultural, 59
  verbal, 6–8
Complete abortion, 359
Compulsions, 69
Conceptual apraxia, 130
Conclusion, communication technique, 8
Confabulation, 69
Confirmation, communication technique, 7
Confrontation, vision assessment, 116, 149,
        149f
Congenital dermal melanocytosis, 83
Conjunctiva, 138f, 139, 145
Constipation, 307–308
Constructional apraxia, 130
Constructional impairment, 130

Contact dermatitis, 94, 94f
Contracture scar, 96
Cooper ligaments, 271
Coping mechanisms, 63–64
Cornea, 138f, 139, 146, 146f, 151
Corneal arcus, 153
Corneal light reflex, 149
Corneal sensitivity, 146, 146f
Cough, 239, 254t
Cover-uncover test, 150–151
COVID-19 pandemic
    mental health assessment, 62
    neuropsychological changes, 111
Crackles, 260–261
Cranial nerve, 108, 109f
    function assessment, 116–118
    impairment, 126–130, 127t–128t
Crepitus, 413
Crescendo, 224
Cullen sign, 307
Cultural and religious belief, mental health,
        61
Cultural background, food choice, 43
Cultural barriers, patient interview, 5, 59
Cyanosis, 83
Cystocele, 338

D

Decrescendo murmur, 224
Deep palpation, 33f
Deep tendon reflexes, 122, 123f
Delusions, 69
Demographic data, mental health
        assessment, 61
Depersonalization, 69
Depressed fibrotic scars, 96
Depressing disorders, 126
Derailment, 68
Dermis, 76
*Diagnostic and Statistical Manual of Mental
        Disorders, Fifth Edition, Text
        Revision (DSM-5-TR)*, 66–67
Diaphragmatic movement measurement,
        249, 249f
Diarrhea, 306t, 308
Diastole, 199–200
Diencephalon, 106
Digestion, 290f
Dimpling, breast, 281t, 283
Diplopia, 155
Direct percussion, 34, 34f
Dissecting aortic aneurysm, chest pain, 219t
Distention, 308
Dorsalis pedis pulse, 216f
Dressing apraxia, 130
Drooping upper eyelid, 157

Dry cerumen, 175
Duodenal ulcer, 309
Dysmenorrhea, 335t, 339–340
Dysphagia, 130, 185t, 188, 307
Dyspnea, 254t
Dysuria, 335t, 337

E

Earache, 184, 185t
Ears
 abnormal findings, 184, 185t, 186–187,
  186t–187t
 anatomy and physiology, 164–166, 164f
 assessment, 172–173, 174f, 175–176
 health history, 169–170, 170f
Ecchymoses, 93
Eccrine glands, 77
Echolalia, 69
Ectopic pregnancy, 353, 353f
Ectropion, 145, 155, 155f
Edema, 83
Elbow assessment, 401–403
Elderly patient. See also Older adults
 eye assessment, 144b
 mental health assessment, 66
 sexual health, 372b
Endocrine inquiry, 19
Entropion, 145, 155, 155f
Epidermis, 76
Epididymis, 368f, 369, 376
Epiglottis, 231
Epispadias, 381
Epistaxis, 185t, 188
Erectile dysfunction, 383
Erythema, 83
Esophagus, 288f, 289
 dysphagia, 130
 spasm, chest pain, 219t
Exophthalmos, 145
Exploration technique, 58
Expressive aphasia, 129
External ear, 164, 164f
External genitalia, female, 318–319
 inspection, 326–328
 palpation, 328
Extraocular structures, eyes, 138–139
Eyelid assessment, 145
Eyes
 abnormal findings, 153, 154t, 155–159,
  155f, 157f
 anatomy and physiology, 138–142, 138f
 assessment, 45, 144–153
 discharge, 154t, 155
 health history, 142–143
 muscle function, 149–151, 150f
 pain, 156

F

Facial nerve, 117
Facilitation, communication technique, 7
Fallopian tubes, 320f, 321
Family health, 12
 gastrointestinal system, 294
 male genitourinary system, 371
Fatigue, 217t–218t, 221
Female genitourinary system
 abnormal findings, 334, 335t–336t,
  336–340
 anatomy and physiology, 316–319,
  317f–318, 320f, 321
 assessment, 324–333
 health history, 321–323
 postpartum assessment, 349–351
Femoral pulse, 216f
Fetal engagement and station, 349, 349f
Fetal heart tone (FHT), pregnant patient,
  344, 344f
Fetal presentation, 344
Fine crackles, 261, 262f
Flight of ideas, 68
Floating ribs, 235
Fluid-filled lesions, 86
Focusing, communication technique, 58
Food intake, factors influencing, 43
Foot assessment, 408–409, 408f
Footdrop, 413
Fovea centralis, 142
Freckles, 85
Friction rubs, 309
Frontal sinuses
 palpation, 179–180, 180f
 transillumination, 180, 180f
Fundal assessment, postpartum, 349–350,
  350f
Fundal height, pregnant patient, 343
Funnel chest, 256f, 257

G

Gaits, abnormal, 131–132, 132f
Gallbladder, 288f, 291
Ganglion, 415, 416f
Gastrointestinal system
 abnormal findings, 305, 305f, 306t–307t,
  307–309, 310t, 311
 anatomy and physiology, 287–289, 288f,
  290f, 291–293, 292f
 assessment, 45, 294–301, 296f, 299f–300f,
  302f, 303–304
 health history and, 293–294
Gastrointestinal tract, 287–289, 288f
General health review, 8, 9f, 10–14
Genital herpes, 381f

Genital lesions, 337, 381f
Genital warts, 337, 381f
Gestational trophoblastic disease, 354, 354f
Glasgow Coma Scale, 114, 114f
Global aphasia, 130
Global Deterioration Scale, 66
Glossopharyngeal nerve, 118
Gout, 415, 416f
Gower sign, 397f
Grand gland, 168
Graves speculum, 329, 329f
Gynecomastia, 274

H

Hair
 abnormal findings, 91t
 abnormalities, 97, 221–222
 anatomy and physiology, 78–79, 79f
 assessment, 45, 88–89
 health history, 81–82
Hallucinations, 69
Hand
 assessment, 401–403, 404–405, 404f
 strength, 412
Handgrip strength, 412
Head assessment, 399
Head circumference measurement, child,
  28b
Health history
 breasts and axillae and, 274–277,
  275t–276t
 cardiovascular system, 203–205
 ear assessment, 169–170, 170f
 eye assessment, 144–153
 female genitourinary system, 321–323
 gastrointestinal system, 293–294
 general health review, 8, 9f, 10–14
 hair assessment, 81–82
 male genitourinary system, 370–372
 mental health assessment, 57–60
 mouth assessment, 171
 musculoskeletal system, 394–395
 nail assessment, 82
 neck assessment, 171
Health history (continued)
 neurologic assessment and, 110–111
 nose assessment, 176–178
 nutritional assessment, 42–43
 objective data, 3
 patient interview and, 4–8
 respiratory system, 238–240
 skin assessment, 81
 structures and systems review and, 14,
  15f, 16–19
 subjective data, 3
 throat assessment, 171

Hearing acuity tests, 175–176
Hearing loss, 184, 186, 187t
Heart, 17
    anatomy, 194–197, 194f–196f, 198f
    assessment, 206–209, 207f, 209f–211f, 212–213, 213f
    internal structures, 195f
    obesity effect, 205b
    physiology, 198–201, 199f–200f
    pregnancy, 342
Heart sounds
    abnormal, 224, 225t, 226
    auscultation, 208–209, 209f–211f, 212–213, 213f
    cycle of, 210f–211f
    sites for, 209f
Heberden nodes, 414, 414f
Height measurement, 26, 27b
    overcoming problems, 46
    pediatric patient, 28
Hemangiomas, 90
Hematochezia, 311
Hematocrit, 50
Hematoma, 93, 354, 354f
Hematuria, 334, 379
Hemoglobin, 48, 50
Hemoptysis, 254t–255t
Hepatomegaly, 299
Hernia, 375b
Herpes zoster, 94, 94f
Hiatal hernia, chest pain, 220
High-pitched, blowing murmur, 226
High-pitched murmur, 224
Hinge joints, 391, 391t
Hip assessment, 405–407, 406f
Hirsutism, 97
Hives, 92t, 94f
Hydroceles, 375b
Hyperpnea, 257f, 259
Hypertension, pregnancy, 355
Hyperthyroidism, 171
Hypertrophic scar, 96
Hypoglossal nerve, 118
Hypospadias, 381
Hypothalamus, 106
Hypothyroidism, 171

I

Ice-pick scars, 96
Ideal body weight, 46
Ideomotor apraxia, 130
Illuminating lesions, 86
Illusions, 69
Incoherence, 69
Incomplete abortion, 359
Indirect percussion, 34, 34f

Inevitable abortion, 359
Inguinal area, 376
Inguinal hernia, 376, 376f
Inner ear, 164f, 165–166
Inspection
    abdomen, 373
    breasts and axillae, 277
    chest, 241–242
    external genitalia, female, 326–328
    kidneys, 324
    neck, 181–183
    nostrils, 178f
    penis, 374
    scrotum, 374
    testicles, 374
    vascular system, 214
Internal genitalia, female, 319, 320f, 321
Intracranial pressure, increased, detecting, 127t
Intraocular structures, eyes, 139–142, 151–153, 151f–152f
Intrapartum fetal assessment
    cervical effacement and dilation, 348, 348f
    fetal engagement and station, 349, 349f
    fetal presentation, 344, 345f–347f, 347
Iris, 138f, 139, 146

J

Jaundice, 83, 156
Joints
    assessment, 398–409
    motion types, 392f
    nonsynovial, 391
    synovial, 391
Jugular vein distention, 215

K

Kayser-Fleischer rings, 156
Keloid scar, 96
Kidneys
    anatomy, 316, 317f
    enlargement, 301
    inspection, 324
    palpation, 325, 326f, 373
    percussion, 324, 325f, 373
Knee assessment, 407, 407f
Koilonychia, 98
Korotkoff sounds, 32f
Kussmaul respirations, 257f, 259

L

Labia majora and minora, 318–319
Laboratory studies, nutritional assessment, 48–51
Large intestine, 288f, 291

Larynx, 233
Legs
    pain, 415
    strength, 412
Lens, 138f, 140
Lens capsule, 140
Lesions, skin
    configurations, 88f
    distribution, 86
    identification, 88f
    illuminating, 86
    types, 87f
Level of consciousness (LOC)
    altered, 124
    assessment, 112–113
    decreased, 125t
Lid lag, 145
Light palpation, 33f
Lipids, nutrition and, 42
Listening, communication technique, 58
Liver, 288f, 291
    assessment, 299, 300f, 302f
    friction rubs, 309
    measurement, 299, 300f
    percussion, 299, 300f
Lobar bronchi, 233
Lobes and ducts, breasts, 271
Lochia, 351
Lochia alba, 351
Lochia rubra, 351
Lochia serosa, 351
Low-pitched murmur, 224
Low, rumbling murmur, 226
Lungs, 234–235, 234f, 342
Lymph nodes
    breasts and axillae, 271, 272f, 280
    clavicular area, 281
    head and neck, 182, 182f

M

Macula, 141, 153
Macule, 86
Male breast cancer, 274
Male genitourinary system
    abnormal findings
    anatomy and physiology, 367–370
    assessment, 372–377
    health history, 370–372
Mammary glands, 270
Maxillary sinuses
    palpation, 179–180, 179f, 180f
    transillumination, 180, 180f
Meatus, 167
Medical history, 10–12
    breast examination, 275–276
    mental health assessment, 61

Medium-pitched murmur, 224
Melanocyte, 76
Meninges, 105
Menopause, breast changes after, 273f, 274
Menstrual abnormalities, 339–340, 340b
Mental disorders, classification, 66–67
Mental health assessment
    abnormal findings, 67–69, 67t–68t
    COVID-19, 62
    health history, 57–60
    initial observations, 61–65
    interpreting findings, 67t–68t
    interview guidelines, 60
    mental status, 62–67
    patient interview, 60–62
    psychological and mental status testing, 66
Mental status assessment, 62–67, 110–116, 112t, 114f
Midarm circumference measurements, 49f
Midarm muscle circumference measurements, 49f
Middle ear, 164f, 165
Mini-Mental Status Examination, 66
Minnesota Multiphasic Personality Inventory, 66
Missed abortion, 359
Moisture, skin, 84–85
Mons pubis, 318
Montgomery glands, 271
Mood, mental status assessment, 63
Motor function assessment, 120–121
Mouth, 288, 288f
    abnormal findings, 188
    anatomy and physiology, 168f
    assessment, 180–181, 295
    health history, 171
Mucopurulent cervicitis, 327, 327f
Muddy sclera, 156
Muehrcke lines, 98
Multiple pregnancy, 356, 356f
Murmurs
    auscultating for, 212, 213f
    grading, 213, 224
    types, 224, 226
Muscles
    anatomy and physiology, 393f, 394
    assessment, 409–412, 411f
    atrophy, 415–416
    movements, abnormal, 130–131
    spasms, 416
    tone, 120, 409
    wasting, 55, 415–416
    weakness, 416
Muscle strength, 120–121
    documentation, 410

    grading, 410
    testing, 411, 411f
Muscular dystrophy, 396–397, 396f–397f
Musculoskeletal injury, 5 Ps, 416
Musculoskeletal system
    abnormal findings, 412–416
    anatomy and physiology, 389, 390f–393f, 391t, 394
    assessment, 46, 395, 396f–397f, 397–399, 400f, 401–412, 402f–403f, 406f–408f, 411f
    health history, 394–395
Myocardial infarction, acute, chest pain, 219t

N

Nails
    abnormal findings, 91t
    abnormalities, 97–99
    anatomy and physiology, 80, 80f
    assessment, 45, 89
    health history, 82
Nasal flaring, 188
Nasal obstruction, 185t–186t
Nasal stuffiness and discharge, 188
Nausea and vomiting, 306t–307t, 307
Near-vision chart, 148–149
Neck, 16
    anatomy and physiology, 167–168, 169f
    assessment, 181–184, 399, 400f
    auscultation, 183–184
    health history, 171
    inspection and palpation, 181–183
    measurement, 182b
Neologisms, 69
Neurologic system
    abnormal findings, 124, 125t–126t, 126–127, 127t, 128f, 129–132, 132f
    age-related changes, 110b
    assessment, 45, 111–113, 114f, 115–122, 123f, 124
    autonomic nervous system, 109
    central nervous system, 104–107, 104f, 105f, 107f
    health history, 110–111
    peripheral nervous system (PNS), 108, 109f
Nevi, 85
Nipple
    discharge, 283–284
    inversion, 283
    pigmentation, 271
    retraction, 282t, 283
Nitrogen, 50
Nocturia, 336, 380

Nonsynovial joints, 391
Normal breath sounds
    locations, 251f
    qualities, 251t
Normal weight, 46
Nose
    abnormal findings, 185t–186t, 188
    anatomy and physiology, 166–167
    assessment, 176–178
    health history, 171
Nosebleed, 166
Nostrils, inspection, 178f
Nutritional assessment
    abnormal findings, 51–55
    anthropometric measurements, 46–48
    body system, 45–46
    detecting problems, 44
    health history, 42–43
    interpreting findings, 52t
    laboratory studies, 48–51
Nutritional problems detection, 44
Nutrition, normal, 41–42

O

Obesity, 46, 375b
    breast cancer risk and, 277b
    heart, 205b
    menstrual disturbances, 340b
Obsessions, 69
Oculomotor nerve, 116
Offering self technique, 58
Older adults
    mental health assessment, 66b
    overcoming communication problems, 14b
    tongue surface checking, 181b
Olfactory impairment, 126
Onycholysis, 99
Open-ended questions, 6
Optic disk, 141
Optic nerve, 138f
Organ of Corti, 165
Oropharyngeal dysphagia, 130
Orthopnea, 239
Otitis externa, 170f
Otorrhea, 187
Otoscopic examination, 173, 174f, 175
Ovaries, 321
Overweight, 46, 53b

P

Pain, eye, 156
Pallor, 83
Palpation, 33–34, 218, 220
    axilla, 280

Palpation *(continued)*
  breast, 278–279, 278f
  heart, 206–207
  kidneys, 325, 326f, 373
  liver, 302f
  spleen, 302f
  types, 33f
  vascular system, 214–215
Palpebral conjunctiva, 139
Palpitation
  probable causes, 218t
  provokers, 220
Pancreas, 288f, 291–292
Papular rash, 90
Papule, 86
Paranasal sinuses, 167
Paraphimosis, 380
Para-phimosis, 371
Patellar reflex, 123, 123f
Patellar reflex arc, 106, 107, 107f
Patient interview
  activities of daily living, 13–14
  biographic data, 8
  closed questions, 6
  creating proper environment for, 4
  family history, 12
  medical history, 10–12
  mental health assessment, 60–62
  nonverbal communication strategies,
    5–6
  open-ended questions, 6
  overcoming cultural barriers, 5
  overcoming obstacles to, 5
  presenting problem, 10
  professional attitude maintenance, 14
  psychosocial history, 12–13
  transcultural communication, 59
  verbal communication strategies, 6–8
Patient Self-Determination Act, 10b
Peau d' orange, 283, 283f
Pederson speculum, 329, 329f
Pediatric patient
  Babinski reflex, 124b
  eye assessment, 144b
  head circumference measurement, 28
  hearing assessment, 176b
  height measurement, 28b
  overweight, 53b
  rebound tenderness, 303b
  skin turgor assessment, 84b
  strabismus, 158b
  testicular examination, 372b
  weight measurement, 28
Penis, 368f, 369
  cancer, 381f
  discharge, 378t, 380

inspection, 374
lesions, 378t, 380
palpation, 375f
Peptic ulcer, chest pain, 220
Perceptions
  abnormalities, 69
  validation, communication technique,
    58
Percussion, 34, 34f
  chest, 246–247, 246f, 247t, 248f–249f
  heart, 207–208
  kidneys, 324, 325f, 373
  types, 34f
Pericardial friction rub, auscultation, 213
Pericarditis, chest pain, 219t
Pericardium, 194
Perilymph fluid, 165
Perineum, postpartum assessment, 351
Periorbital edema, 156, 157f
Peripheral edema, 218t
Peripheral nervous system (PNS), 108,
    109f. *See also* Neurologic system
Perseveration, 69
Petechiae, 83, 93
PFTs. *See* Pulmonary function tests (PFTs)
Phalen maneuver, 404, 404f
Phimosis, 371
Photoreceptor neurons, 141
Physical assessment
  breasts and axillae, 277–284, 278f, 280f
  cardiovascular system, 205–209, 207f,
    209f–211f, 212–215, 213f, 216f, 217
  documenting findings, 37f
  ears, 172–173, 174f, 175–176
  eyes, 144–153, 146f, 148f–152f
  female genitourinary system, 324–333
  gastrointestinal system, 294–301, 296f,
    299f–300f, 302f, 303–304
  general survey and, 24–32
  hair, 88–89
  male genitourinary system, 372–377
  musculoskeletal system, 395, 396f–397f,
    397–399, 400f, 401–412, 402f–403f,
    406f–408f, 411f
  nails, 89
  neck, 181–184
  neurologic system, 111–113, 114f,
    115–122, 123f, 124
  nose and sinuses, 176–178
  nutritional assessment, 44–46
  respiratory system, 240–253, 244f–246f,
    247t, 248f–250f, 251t–253t, 252f
  skin, 83–88, 84f, 87f, 88f
  techniques used for, 32–36
  throat assessment, 180–181
  tools for, 23–24, 24f

Physical illnesses, mental health
    assessment, 61
Pigeon chest, 256, 256f
Pinguecula, 156
Pinna, 164
Placenta previa, 357, 357f
Pleurae, 234, 234f
Pleural effusion, auscultation findings, 263t
Pleural friction rub, 262
Pneumonia, auscultation findings, 264t
Pneumothorax
  auscultation findings, 264t
  chest pain, 219t
Polyuria, 334
Popliteal pulse, 216f
Port-wine stains, 90
Position sense, evaluation, 119
Positive splenic percussion sign, 300
Posterior chamber, eye, 140
Posterior tibial pulse, 216f
Postpartum hemorrhage, 357, 358f
Poverty of content, 69
PPROM. *See* Preterm premature rupture of
    membranes (PPROM)
PQRSTU mnemonic device, 11f
Pregnancy, 340
  abdomen, 342
  abnormal findings, 351–360
  anatomy and assessment, 341
  breasts and axillae, 275
  breast changes, 341, 342f
  estimated date of birth (EDB), 341
  fundal height, 343
  heart and lungs, 342
  intrapartum assessment, 344–349
  postpartum assessment, 349–351
  vein changes and, 204
Premature cervical dilation, 359
Premature rupture of membranes (PROM),
    360
Pressure ulcers, 92, 95, 95f
Presystolic gallop, 225t
Preterm labor, 360
Preterm premature rupture of membranes
    (PPROM), 360
Priapism, 383
Primitive reflexes, 122
Professional attitude maintenance, 14
Proptosis, 145
Propulsive gait, 131–132, 132f
Prostate gland, 368f, 370
  assessment, 377, 377f
  enlargement, 382
  lesions, 382
Protein, nutrition and, 42
Pruritus, 91t–92t, 92

Psoriasis, 94, 94f
Psychiatric illness, mental health assessment, 61
Psychological survey, 19
Psychosocial health, gastrointestinal system, 294
Psychosocial history, 12–13
Pterygium, 156
Ptosis, 157, 157f
Puberty, breast development and, 272–273, 273f
Pubic hair development, 326b
Pulmonary embolism, chest pain, 219t
Pulmonary function tests (PFTs), 252t
Pulmonic stenosis, 224
Pulsations, abnormal, 222
Pulse assessment, 28–30, 29f
Pulse waveforms, 223f
Pulsus alternans, 223f
Pulsus bigeminus, 223f
Pulsus bisferiens, 223f
Pulsus paradoxus, 223f
Pupillary changes, 128f
Pupils, 138f, 140, 146–147
Purpuric lesions, 93

R

Radial pulse, 216f
Range of motion (ROM)
    ankle and foot, 408f
    hip, 406, 406f
    knee, 407f
    neck, 400f
Rashes, 83
Rebound tenderness, 303b
Receptive aphasia, 130
Rectal bleeding, 306t
Rectocele, 339, 339f
Rectovaginal examination, 331, 333f
Rectum
    assessment, 304
    postpartum assessment, 351
Recurrent pregnancy loss, 359
Red lesions, 85
Reflex arc, 107, 107f
Reflexes, assessment, 121–124, 123f
Religion, food choice, 43
Rephrasing technique, 58
Reproduction review, 18
Reproductive system
    abnormal findings, 380–383
    anatomy, 368–370
    assessment, 326–333, 374–377
    female, 318–319, 318f, 320f, 321

health history, 322–323
    male, 368–370
Reproductive years, breast changes during, 274, 274f
Respirations, assessment, 30
Respiratory landmarks, 236f
Respiratory muscles, 235–237, 236f–237f
Respiratory patterns, abnormal, 257f, 258–260
Respiratory research, 17
Respiratory system
    abnormal findings, 253, 254t–255t, 255–262, 256f–257f, 258t, 262f–264f
    anatomy and physiology, 231, 232f–234f, 233–237, 236–237f
    assessment, 45, 240–253, 244f–246f, 247t, 248f–250f, 251f–253t, 252f
    health history, 238–240
Retina, 138f, 141–142
    anatomy and structure, 152, 152f
    assessment, 151–152, 152f
Retinal blood vessels, 141
Rheumatoid arthritis, 413, 413f
Rhonchi, 262, 263f
Ribs, 235, 236f
Rinne test, 176, 177f
Romberg test, 121, 121f
Rumbling murmur, 226

S

Scabies, 94, 94f
Scars, 96
Schlemm canal, 138f
Scissors gait, 131, 132f
Sclera, 138f, 139
Scoliosis, 401
Scrotal swelling, 378t, 382
Scrotum, 368f, 369, 374
Sebaceous glands, 77
Self-destructive behavior, 64
Self-harm, 64
Semilunar valves, 197
Seminal vesicles, 370
Sensory function assessment, 119–120
Septic abortion, 359
Seriously underweight, 46
Severely ill patient, assessment, 19
Shortness of breath, 238
Shoulders
    assessment, 401–403
    strength, 411
Silence, communication technique, 58
Sinuses

assessment, 179, 179f–180f
    transillumination, 180, 180f
Skene, 319
Skin
    abnormalities, 90–97, 91t–93t, 94f–95f, 221–222
    age-related changes, 78, 78t
    anatomy and physiology, 76–78, 77f
    assessment, 45, 83–88
    disorders, 94, 94f
    health history, 81
    layers, 76
Skin color variations
    detection, dark-skinned people, 83
    interpretation, 93t
Skin lesions
    color, 86
    configurations, 88f
    distribution, 86
    identification, 88f
    illumination, 86
    primary, 85
    secondary, 85
    types, 87f
Skin turgor, assessment, 84, 84f
Sleep apnea, snoring and, 259b
Small intestine, 288f, 289
Snellen chart, 147, 148f
Socioeconomic data, mental health assessment, 61
Socioeconomic status, food choice, 43
Solid lesions, 86
Sore throat, 189
Spastic gait, 131, 132f
Speculum
    insertion, 329–330, 330f
    types, 329, 329f
Speech
    impairment, 129–130
    mental status assessment, 113
Spermatic cords, 376
Sphygmomanometer, 31–32, 31f
Spinal cord, 104f, 106, 108f
Spinal movement assessment, 402f–403f
Spine assessment, 399, 401
Spine-tingling procedure, 401
Spleen
    assessment, 301, 302f
    enlargement, 301
    friction rubs, 309
Splenic dullard, 300
Spontaneous abortion, 358–359
Sputum production, 239–240
Steppage gait, 132, 132f
Stereognosis, 120

Stethoscope, 36
Stomach, 288f, 289
  symptom search, 17–18
Strabismus, 157, 158b
Stratum corneum, 76
Stretch marks, 96
Stridor, 262
Structures and systems review, 14, 15f, 16–19
Subarachnoid space, 105
Subconjunctival hemorrhage, 157, 157f
Subjective data, 3
Suggesting collaboration technique, 58
Suicide, warning signs, 65
Summarizing technique, 58
Superficial reflexes, 122
Swallowing impairment, 129–130
Sweat glands, 77
Symptom evaluation, 15f
Synovial joints, 391, 391f
Syphilis, 381f
Syphilitic chancre, 337
Systole, 199

T
Tachypnea, 257f, 258
Tactile fremitus, 245, 245f
Tail of Spence, 271
Telangiectases, 96
Temperature
  readings, comparison, 29t
  skin, 85
Temporomandibular joint (TMJ)
  assessment, 398, 398f
Terry nails, 99
Testicles, 368f, 369, 375–376
  inspection, 374
  palpation, 375–376, 375f
Testicular self-examination (TSE), 372b
Testicular tumor, 381
Thalamus, 106
Therapeutic communication techniques, 58
Thoracic kyphoscoliosis, 256f, 257
Thorax, 235, 236f
Thought content, abnormal, 69
Thought process
  abnormal, 68–69
  mental status assessment and, 63
Threatened abortion, 359
Throat
  abnormal findings, 189
  anatomy and physiology, 167–168, 168f
  assessment, 180–181
  as gastrointestinal tract component, 288f
  health history, 171
  pain, 186t, 189

Thyroid gland, 183f
Tics, 131
Tinea corporis (ringworm), 94, 94f
Tinel sign, 404, 404f
Transcultural communication, 59
Transferrin, 50
Tremors, 125t–126t
Triceps reflex, 123, 123f
Triceps skinfold thickness measurements, 49f
Triceps strength, 411, 411f
Trichomoniasis, 327, 327f, 338
Trigeminal nerve, 117
Triglycerides, 50
TSE. See Testicular self-examination (TSE)
Twin pregnancy presentations, 356, 356f
Tympanic membrane, 165
Tympanosclerosis, 187

U
Umbilical cord prolapse, 358, 358f
Umbilicus
  assessment, 297
  skin color changes, 307
Underweight, 46
Upper airway obstruction
  auscultation findings, 264t
  signs and symptoms, 261
Ureters, 316, 317f
Urethra, 317, 317f, 319f, 368f
Urethral meatus
  displacement, 381
  examination, 374, 374f
Urethral opening, 319
Urinary frequency, urgency, and hesitancy, 334, 336, 379–380, 379t
Urinary incontinence, 335t–336t, 336–337, 380
Urinary system, 316–317, 317f
  abnormal findings, 334, 336–337, 379–380
  anatomy, 368
  assessment, 45–46, 324–325, 325f–326f, 372–373
  health history, 321–322
  male, 368
Urine appearance, assessment, 371
Urticaria (hives), 92t, 94, 94f, 96
Uterine involution, postpartum assessment, 350, 350f
Uterine prolapse, 338–339
Uterus, 321

V
Vagina, 319, 320f
  bleeding, pregnancy, 359
  discharge, 327, 327f, 337–338

hematoma, 354
inflammation, 337–338
prolapse, 338–339
Vaginitis, 327, 327f
Valves, heart, 197
Vascular sounds, auscultation, 298, 299f
Vascular system, 201, 202–203, 202f. See also Cardiovascular system
  assessment, 214–215, 216f, 217
Vas deferens, 370
Veins, 202f, 203
  pregnancy and changes, 204
  visible, breast, 284
Ventricular gallop, 225t
Ventricular systole, 199
Venules, 203
Vertigo, 129
Vesicular rash, 97
Vessels, heart, 195–196
Vestibule, 319, 328
Vibratory sense, evaluation, 119
Visceral pleura, 234, 234f
Vision examination, 16
Vision loss, 158
Visual acuity
  charts, 148, 148f
  decreased, 153, 154t, 155
  testing, 147–149, 148f–149f
Visual field defects, 116–117
Visual floaters, 154t, 158
Visual halos, 159
Visual impairment, 127, 128f, 129
Vital signs and statistics
  interpretation, 26
  pediatric patient, 28
  recording, 26–32, 27f–29f, 29t, 31f
Vitreous chamber, 140
Vitreous humor, 138f
Vocal fremitus, 253, 253f
Vocal point, 233

W
Waddling gait, 132, 132f
Weak pulse, 223f
Weber test, 176, 177f
Weight gain, excessive, 51
Weight loss, excessive, 51
Weight measurement, 28b, 46, 47t
Wernicke aphasia, 130
Wet cerumen, 175
Wheezing, 240, 255t, 260–261
Whisper test, 175
Work schedule, food choice, 43
Wrist assessment, 404–405, 404f